1,001 BEST
HEALTH
HINTS AND TIPS

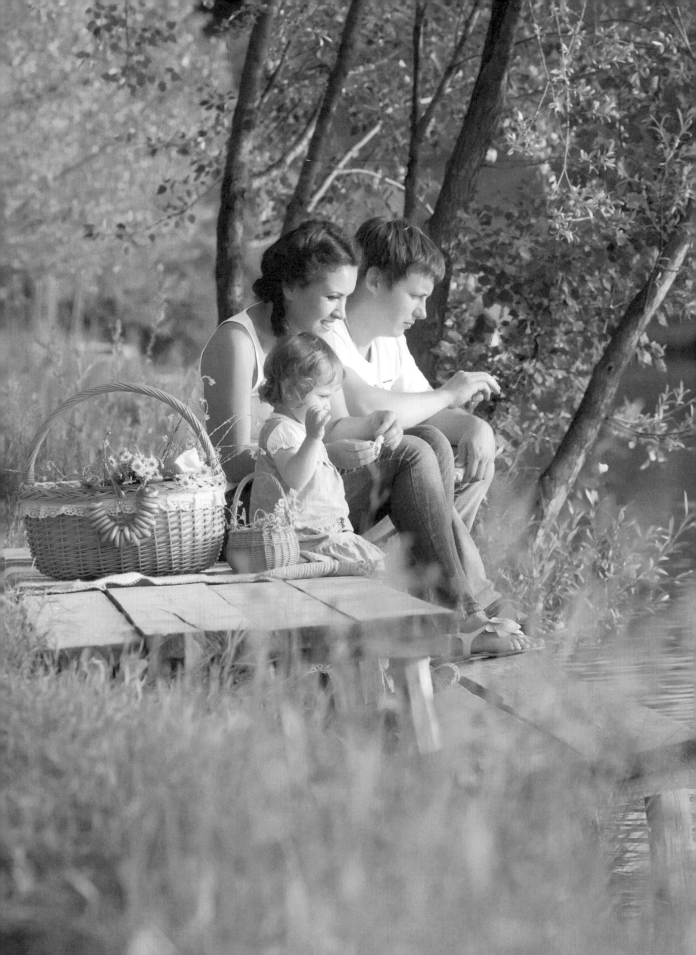

Reader's Digest

1,001 BEST HEALTH
HINTS AND TIPS

Published by
The Reader's Digest Association, Inc.
London • New York • Sydney • Montreal

Contents

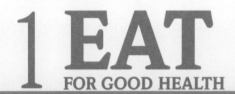
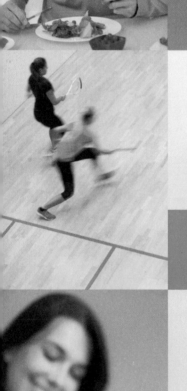

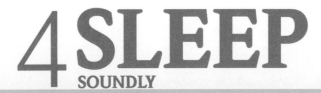

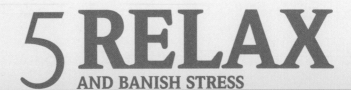

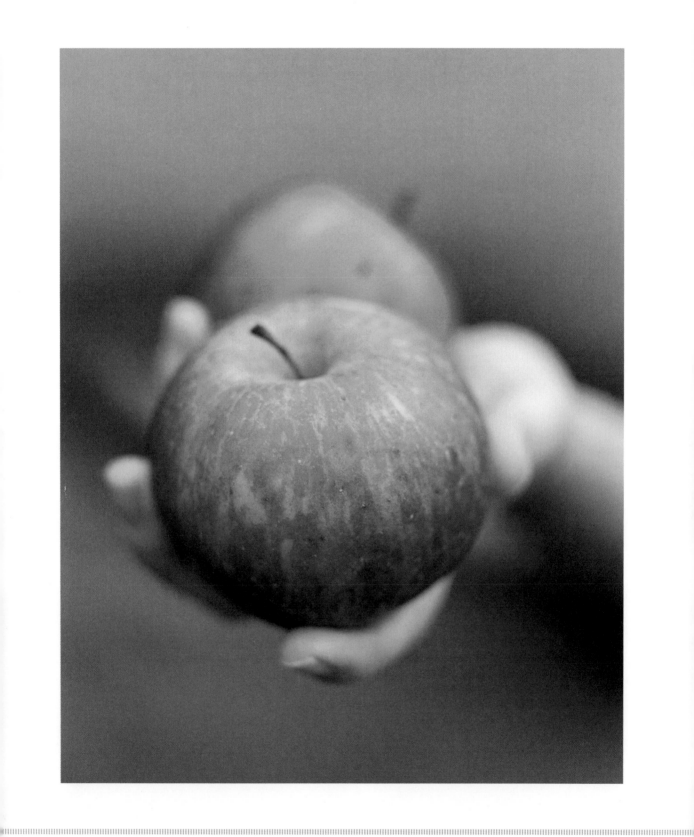

HELP YOURSELF TO
GOOD HEALTH

There are myriad diet plans or titles that advise on a single ailment such as diabetes. But few tell you precisely how to keep well, boost energy, sleep soundly and combat minor and major disorders. This new book does all these things.

1,001 Best Health Hints and Tips is packed full of clever, specific advice that you'll want to read because it addresses life's most pressing concerns – how to combat health problems and keep yourself and your loved ones as well and happy as possible. It's been compiled by digging deep into the Reader's Digest health archives to offer you the very best tips from our rich store of authoritative, doctor-approved information. None suggests a painful lifestyle overhaul. Some are as simple as sprinkling cinnamon on cereal, changing the colour of your plates or playing children's games that simultaneously strengthen your muscles. All are designed to fit easily into your everyday routine and all will cumulatively build good health.

In fact, *1,001 Best Health Hints and Tips* could best be described as a dip-in recipe book for healthy living. Its six sections address the key actions that are essential to wellbeing – Eat, Move, Sleep, Thrive, Relax, Shine. Each one outlines a wealth of diverse strategies for living well – whether it's tweaking your diet, getting active while having fun, discovering a personal formula for good sleep, conquering common ills, banishing stress, enjoying a happy sex life, or looking and feeling your best. Best-of-the-best panels, features, 'great idea!', 'try it!' and 'did you know?' boxes provide extra highlights.

Browse the colourful pages, just as you would a recipe book. There is much to learn and much to try. You can be confident that, whatever advice you choose to follow – for your own or your family's benefit – it will help to build the long, healthy life that we all aspire to lead.

Reader's Digest Health Editors

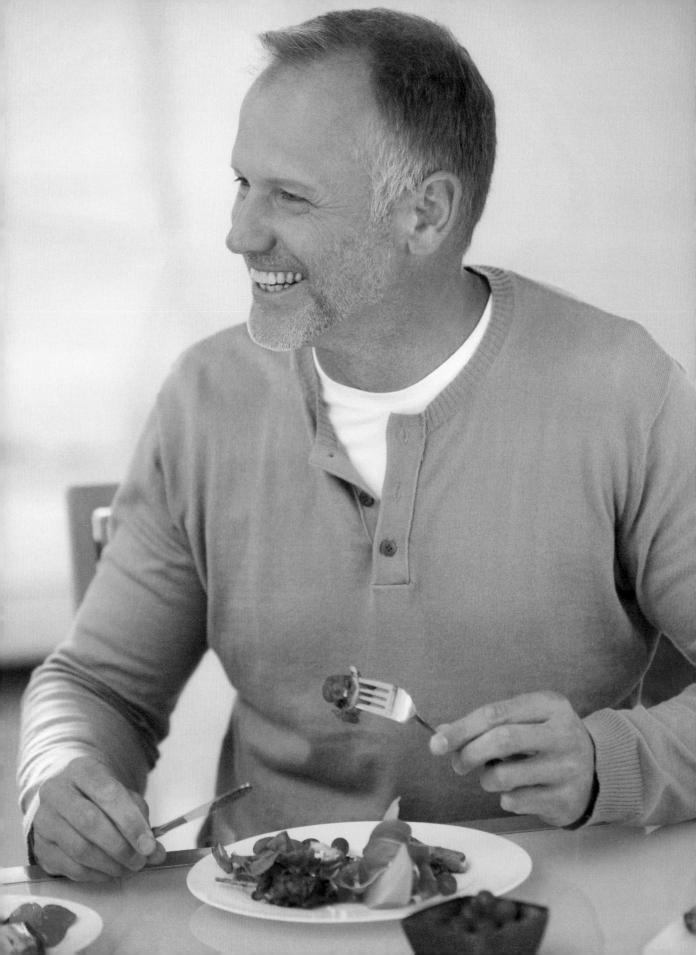

EAT
for good
health

What you put into your body largely determines its health. Poor food choices, too few essential vitamins and minerals, too much salt or sugar are all damaging, steadily eroding your immunity to disease. But eating well is not difficult and can be delicious, as this section explains with numerous examples of tasty tweaks that make all the difference.

A healthy diet makes weight control easier too, especially when combined with these effective tactics. You'll also discover new shopping and cooking tips, together with the most nutritious takeaway and restaurant foods.

FABULOUS **FIBRE**

Eating plenty of fibre – the indigestible parts of plant foods – can protect against heart disease, cancer and digestive problems. Some types of fibre can also lower cholesterol, assist weight control and regulate blood sugar. But most people eat far too little fibre, far below the recommended 24g per day. Here is a selection of easy ways to add more to your daily meals.

● **Switch to rye crackers** You mightn't think that a tiny cracker could make a difference, but two standard cream crackers contain 0.4g of fibre, while two rye crackers have 2.3g of fibre.

● **Have a yoghurt mix for breakfast** Spoon 2 tablespoons of low-fat natural yoghurt into a breakfast bowl and mix in 30g of All-Bran cereal, 1 tablespoon of ground linseeds and 5 large, halved strawberries for a whopping 12.2g of fibre – half your daily needs.

 great idea! **Every week, switch from a white food to a brown food** Replace instant white rice with instant brown rice. Instead of your usual pasta, choose wholemeal pasta. Similarly, go for wholemeal pittas and wholemeal couscous. Within two months, you should be eating only whole grains, and you should have increased your daily fibre intake by an easy 10g without radically changing your diet.

● **Spread your sandwich with hummous** Add 2 heaped tablespoons of hummous and you've got 2g of tasty fibre. Add some spinach leaves and a tomato slice for another couple of grams.

● **Use wholemeal bread for sandwiches** Even sandwich chains offer wholemeal options for lunchtime munching.

● **Make a beetroot salad** Beetroots contain virtually no fat, no cholesterol, no sodium, quite a bit of potassium and 2g of fibre. Try roasting whole, peeled beetroots for 45 minutes, chilling, then dicing into a summer salad.

● **Use wholemeal flour when baking** You can start by going half and half, eventually using only wholemeal for all your cooking needs. Adding a little baking powder helps to lighten foods made from wholemeal flour (note that you may have to add a little more liquid if using wholemeal flour).

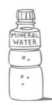 You need water to help the fibre to pass through your digestive system. So, as you're increasing the fibre in your diet, also increase your intake of water

There are a couple of rules to follow when eating more fibre

• Drink more water. You need water to help the fibre to pass through your digestive system. So, as you're increasing the fibre in your diet, also increase your intake of water or other unsweetened drinks.

• Don't increase your fibre intake all at once. Start slowly. Try one tip a week for the first couple of weeks, then two, then three. By week four or five, you should be up to the full 24g – or more.

● **Eat two apples a day** Apples are a good source of pectin, a soluble fibre that contributes to a feeling of fullness and which is also digested slowly. A 1997 study published in the *Journal of the American College of Nutrition* found that 5g of pectin was enough to leave an individual feeling satisfied for up to 4 hours.

● **Eat the skin of your baked and sweet potatoes** Eating baked potatoes with the skin on ups the fibre by at least 3g (depending on the size of the potato).

● **Choose a fibre-rich snack** Dip baby carrots into a low-fat yoghurt dip or salsa for a quick snack. You get about 5g of fibre from 150g (5½ oz) of vegetables.

● **Add kidney beans or chickpeas to salads** A 100g (3½ oz) serving of kidney beans, for example, contains 8g of fibre.

● **Add oatmeal** Use basic oatmeal instead of breadcrumbs for meatballs. Sprinkle it on top of casseroles and ice cream, bake it into biscuits and muffins, and add to homemade bread and cakes.

BEST WAYS TO EAT **BEANS**

Beans are packed with fibre (9g per 100g/3½ oz) and are readily available fresh or tinned. Rinse tinned beans before using to remove excess salt. Here are some health-boosting ideas for getting the most from your beans:

• For a tasty dip, purée a couple of handfuls of cannellini beans in a blender, adding 2 cloves of garlic and 1 tablespoon each of lemon juice and olive oil.

• Fry 2 tablespoons of mixed beans with some onion and chicken in a little oil and use to fill a soft flour tortilla.

• Mix black-eyed beans with finely chopped onion, chilli, garlic and tomatoes to make a salsa.

• Make a bean salad with black-eyed beans, fresh or frozen sweetcorn, chopped coriander, chopped onion and chopped tomato. Drizzle with olive oil and a dash of vinegar, salt and pepper.

• Make your own special chilli pizza. Top a prepared wholemeal pizza base with some kidney beans, grated cheese and minced turkey cooked with chilli.

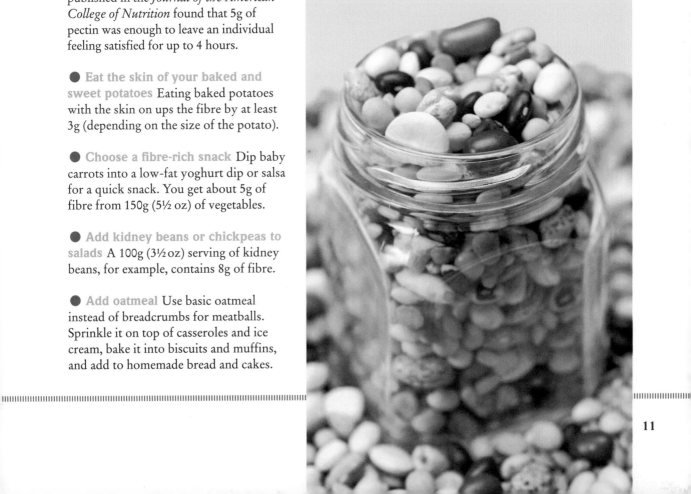

FIVE A **DAY**

If we ate more fruit and vegetables and fewer processed foods, we'd lose weight, clean out our arteries, balance our blood sugar – and slash health costs at a stroke. There is a multitude of ways to make sure you get the five or more daily servings of vegetables and fruit that health experts recommend.

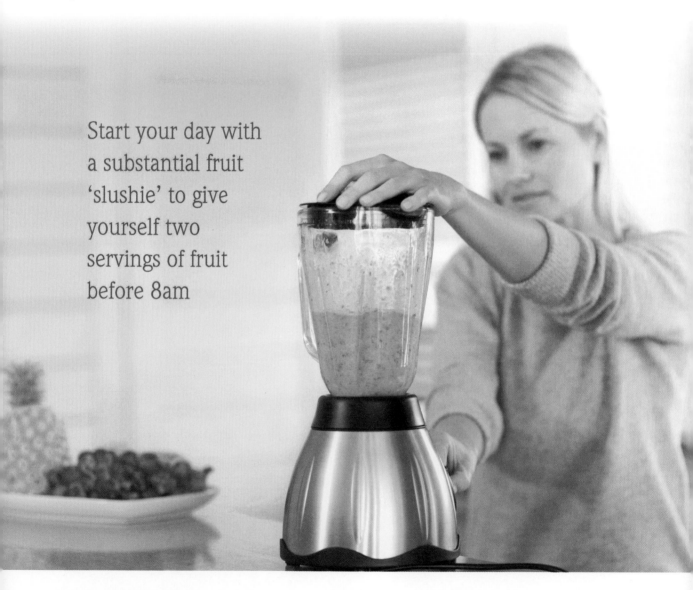

Start your day with a substantial fruit 'slushie' to give yourself two servings of fruit before 8am

● **Use vegetables as sauces** How about puréed roasted red peppers seasoned with herbs and a bit of lemon juice, then drizzled over fish? Why not purée butternut squash with carrots, grated ginger and a bit of brown sugar for a delicious topping for chicken or turkey? Cooked vegetables are easily converted into sauces. It just takes a little ingenuity and a blender.

● **Roast your vegetables** Cut hearty root vegetables such as parsnips, turnips, carrots and onions into 3cm (1in) chunks and arrange in a single layer on a baking sheet. Drizzle with olive oil and sprinkle with sea salt, freshly ground pepper and fresh or dried herbs. Roast in the oven at 230°C/450°F/gas mark 8 until soft, for about 45 minutes, turning once.

● **Purée vegetables into soup** Potatoes, carrots, cauliflower, broccoli – just about any cooked (or leftover) vegetable can be made into a creamy, comforting soup. Try this simple recipe. In a medium saucepan, sauté 160g (5½oz) of finely chopped onion in 1 tablespoon of vegetable oil until tender. Combine the onion in a blender or food processor with cooked vegetables and purée the mixture until smooth. Return the purée to the saucepan and thin it with stock or low-fat milk. Simmer and season to taste.

● **Start each dinner with a mixed green salad** Not only will it help you to eat more vegetables, but there'll be just a bit less room for the higher-calorie items that follow.

● **Serve a salad as a main course** A salade niçoise is a good example: mixed greens, steamed green beans, boiled potatoes, sliced hard-boiled egg and tuna drizzled with vinaigrette.

● **Pack your pasta sauce with vegetables** Pour a jar of low-salt prepared sauce in a pan and add green beans, peas, sweetcorn, peppers, mushrooms, tomatoes and more. Like it chunky? Cut them into big pieces. Don't want to know they're there? Grate or purée them with a bit of sauce in the blender before adding to the rest of the sauce.

● **Drink V8 or tomato juice** Although they are higher in salt, vegetable juices provide the nutrition of a vegetable serving. However, no matter how much you drink, a vegetable juice drink still counts as only one portion.

A SINGLE **SERVING**

Getting your five servings a day is less daunting than it may seem. Here are some examples of what constitutes a single serving:

• 1 medium-sized fruit (such as an apple, orange, banana or pear), half a grapefruit, 1 large slice of pineapple, 1 slice of melon or 2 slices of mango.

• 1 tablespoon of dried fruit, such as raisins, currants, sultanas or mixed fruit; 2 figs or 3 prunes.

• 2 broccoli spears, 8 cauliflower florets, 4 heaped tablespoons of kale, spring greens or green beans.

• 3 heaped tablespoons of baked, haricot, kidney, cannellini or butter beans or chickpeas. (Beans and pulses count as only 1 portion, no matter how many you eat.)

• 3 heaped tablespoons of cooked vegetables such as carrots, peas or sweetcorn (but not potatoes, which don't count).

• Salad vegetables such as 3 sticks of celery, 1 medium tomato, 7 cherry tomatoes or a 5cm piece of cucumber.

• One 150ml (¼ pint) glass of 100 per cent pure fruit or vegetable juice or smoothie (note that you can count juice as only 1 portion, no matter how much you drink).

GO **EXOTIC**

Every week, keep alive your interest in fruit by trying one exotic variety you've never had before.

- **Asian pear** Also called an Oriental, Chinese, salad or apple pear, this firm pear is meant to be eaten when hard. It's sweet, crunchy and amazingly juicy.

- **Guava** Sweet and fragrant with bright pink, white, yellow or red flesh. Buy when it is just soft enough to press, and refrigerate for up to a week in a paper bag. To use, cut in half and scoop out the flesh for salads, or peel and slice.

- **Kiwi fruit** Kiwis are ready to eat when they're slightly soft to the touch. Peel and chop, or cut in half and scoop out the flesh with a grapefruit spoon.

- **Lychee** Peel off the inedible skin and you get a white, translucent flesh similar to a grape, but sweeter, surrounding a cherry-like stone. Eat lychees like grapes, one after another.

- **Mango** Mango has a flavour that recalls peach and pineapple, but is spicier and more fragrant. Peel, then slice into wedges or cut into chunks.

- **Papaya** Soft, juicy and silky-smooth flesh with a delicate, sweet flavour. Eat like a mango, or slice in half, remove seeds and scoop out the flesh with a spoon.

- **Passion fruit** Passion fruit has golden flesh with tiny, edible black seeds and a sweet–tart taste. When ripe, it has wrinkled, dimpled, deep-purple skin. To serve, cut in half and scoop out the pulp with a spoon.

- **Persimmon** Delicate in flavour and firm in texture, it can be eaten like an apple, sliced and peeled. Great in salads.

- **Pomegranate** Each tiny, edible seed is surrounded by translucent, brilliant-red pulp that has a sparkling sweet–tart flavour. To serve, cut the fruit in half and prise out the seeds. Use them to top ice cream or sprinkle into salads.

- **Quince** Tastes like a cross between an apple and a pear, with a dry, hard, yellowish-white flesh that has a tart flavour. Better cooked than raw. Quinces are primarily used for jams, jellies and preserves.

- **Star fruit** Slice crossways for perfect five-pointed star-shaped sections as a garnish or as an ingredient in fruit salads. The star fruit's flavour combines the best of plums, pineapples and lemons.

 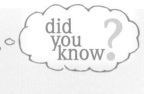

Vegetables work with every meal

If you've always thought of vegetables as no more than a side dish to your evening dinner, think again.

- Choose salad as part of your everyday lunch.

- Make scrambled egg a regular breakfast, using the egg to hold together sautéed vegetables such as peppers, mushrooms, courgettes, asparagus or onions.

- Eat leftover vegetables from last night's dinner with breakfast or lunch.

- Snack on cherry tomatoes, celery, cucumbers and carrots.

- Make vegetable sandwiches using almost any vegetable that won't roll out of the bread.

● **Go vegetarian one day a week** Simply replace your usual meat or fish portion with a vegetable serving. Or invest in a good cookbook and dabble in the world of vegetarian cooking, in which recipes are developed specifically to make a filling, robust meal out of vegetables and whole grains.

● **Grill your vegetables** Peppers, courgettes, asparagus, onions, aubergine, tomatoes – all taste wonderful when grilled. Generally, all you need to do is coat them with olive oil and put them under a hot grill. Turn every few minutes and remove when they start to soften. Or put chunks on a skewer and turn frequently.

● **Use salsa liberally** First mix a large quantity of home-made or shop-bought tomato salsa with chopped raw vegetables such as yellow peppers and courgettes. Then put salsa on everything: baked potatoes, rice, chicken breasts, sandwiches, eggs, steak. Don't save it just for tortilla chips. It's too tasty and healthy not to be used all the time.

● **Substitute fruit sorbet for ice cream** One scoop contains up to one serving of fruit.

● **Spice up shop-bought salsas with fruit** Or make your own fruit-based salsas with pineapple, mango or papaya. Mix with onions, ginger, garlic, some mint or coriander, and sprinkle on a few hot-pepper flakes for a bit of a kick.

● **Start your day with a fruit 'slushie'** Add 160g (6oz) of fresh fruit, 125ml (4fl oz) of fruit juice and a handful of ice cubes to a blender and liquidize. That will give you two servings of fruit before 8am. If you'd prefer a creamier smoothie, add 125ml (4fl oz) of plain fat-free yoghurt.

● **Have a bowl of fruit close at hand** Whether you are in an office, working at home, relaxing or doing household chores, keep a bowl of fruit near you at all times. It should contain five to eight pieces of fresh fruit, such as bananas, oranges, apples, grapes or plums. Most fruit is fine left at room temperature for three or four days.

● **Carry dried fruits with you** Dried fruits are easily portable and have a long shelf life. Take them to work, on shopping trips, or even on holiday. Raisins and prunes are classic choices. Also try dried cranberries and blueberries, which are high in phytonutrients, or dried apricots, which are full of beta carotene. Other options include dates and dried figs, peaches, pears and bananas.

● **Keep an apple in your pocket when you go for a walk** It will be your reward for getting to the midpoint of your chosen route.

● **Finish your dinner with fruit** A slice of watermelon, a peach, a bowl of blueberries – they're a delicious ending to a meal, and are so much healthier than biscuits or cake. Or try sophisticated desserts such as chocolate-covered strawberries, poached pears in red wine, or frozen fresh raspberries.

● **Take fruit with you on long car journeys** Once you're on the motorway and cruising along, an apple or a satsuma tastes great and helps to break the tedium.

● **Keep cubed or sliced melon in a container in the fridge** Use as a first course before dinner; wrap with prosciutto for a starter; mix with cottage cheese for breakfast; have a small bowl for a snack; even consider puréeing it for a quick sauce over fish.

● **Mix fruits in with your salad** A sprinkling of raisins, some chopped strawberries, a diced apple, some fresh or dried mango or some sliced kiwi all make tasty additions to the typical tossed salad.

● **Replace chocolate with raisins** Every time you want a chocolate bar, eat a small box of raisins instead. Raisins are sweet and healthy, and small boxes contain just the right amount to fulfil the need for a sweet treat.

9 key steps to a **healthier** diet

Eating healthily is all about consuming the right amount of food for your energy needs. Most adults in the UK are either overweight or obese. This means that many of us are eating more than we need, as well as eating too much of the wrong foods.

1 AIM FOR A GOOD BALANCE

When it comes to a healthy diet, balance is the key to success. This means eating a wide variety of foods in the right proportions, and consuming the right amout of food and drink to achieve and maintain a healthy body weight.

2 MIX AND MATCH FROM ALL THE FOOD GROUPS

You will get all the nutrients you need from a diet based on starchy foods such as rice and pasta; with plenty of fruit and vegetables; some protein-rich foods such as meat, fish and lentils; some dairy foods; and small quantities of fats and sugar.

3 EAT PLENTY OF PROTEIN

Meat, fish, eggs and beans are all good sources of protein – essential for growth and repair of the body. This food group should account for *slightly less than one sixth* of our total consumption. Meat is also a good source of minerals such as iron, zinc and B vitamins. Fish supplies an abundance of protein, as well as containing many vitamins and minerals. Pulses (including beans, nuts and seeds) are another good source of protein, especially for vegetarians.

4 LEARN TO LOVE YOUR FRUIT & VEG

Fruit and vegetables are a vital source of vitamins and minerals, and should make up another *one third* of all the food we consume. There is strong evidence that people who eat at least five portions of fruit and vegetables a day are at lower risk of heart disease, stroke and some cancers.

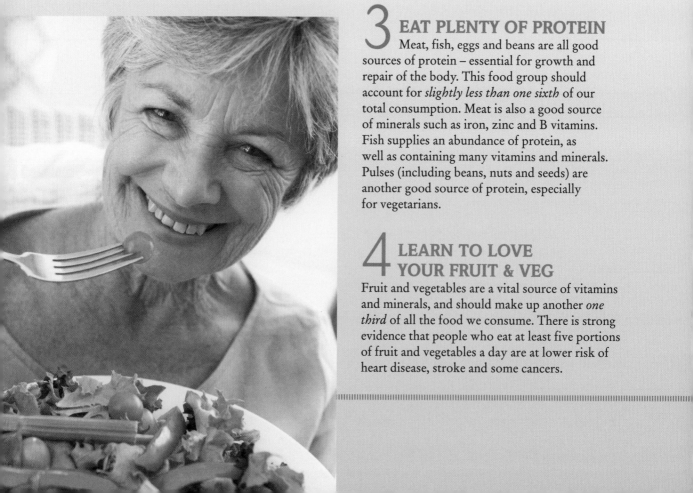

5 KNOW YOUR FATS

Take notice of the crucial difference between saturated fats and unsaturated fats. Saturated fats – found in cheese, sausages, butter, cakes, biscuits and pies – can raise your blood cholesterol level and increase the risk of heart disease. Unsaturated fats, on the other hand, can help to lower cholesterol and provide the essential fatty acids needed for good health.

6 KEEP FATS & SUGAR TO A MINIMUM

Fats and sugar both provide energy for the body, but when we eat too much of them we consume more energy than we burn, leading to weight gain and obesity, which increases the risk of diabetes, certain cancers, heart disease and stroke.

7 DON'T FORGET THE CALCIUM

Milk and dairy foods such as cheese and yoghurt are good sources of protein and they also contain calcium, which helps to keep bones healthy. They should make up *slightly less than one sixth* of our total intake. To enjoy the health benefits of dairy foods without eating too much fat, use semi-skimmed or skimmed milk, lower-fat hard cheeses or cottage cheese, and low-fat or no-fat yoghurt.

8 FUEL UP ON STARCHY FOODS

Starchy foods such as bread, cereals, potatoes, rice and pasta are a good source of energy and the main source of a range of nutrients in our diet. Starchy foods act as fuel for our bodies should make up around one third of everything we eat in the course of one day or one week.

antioxidants and free radicals

The reason why fruit and vegetables are so important to health is that they are major purveyors of disease-fighting antioxidant molecules. Antioxidants act as the body's defence system, preventing damage from molecular bombs called free radicals.

In order to breathe, move or eat, your body's cells convert food and oxygen into energy. This chemical reaction releases harmful by-products, the free radicals. Basically, a free radical is a highly reactive form of oxygen that is missing an electron. Desperate for that missing electron, it steals one from a normal cell, damaging the healthy cell and its DNA in the process. This damage eventually contributes to major health problems, including heart disease, memory loss and cancer.

Antioxidants interfere with this process by giving free radicals one of their own electrons to stabilize them, or they combine with free radicals to form different, more stable compounds. There are also antioxidant enzymes that help free radicals to react with other chemicals to produce safe substances. Antioxidants, for instance, help to prevent 'bad' LDL cholesterol from becoming stickier and forming artery-clogging plaque.

9 KNOW THE FIVE BEST FOODS TO INCLUDE IN YOUR DIET

• **Fish** supplies high-quality protein that is low in saturated fat and cholesterol. Oily fish, such as mackerel, salmon and tuna, are full of health-giving omega-3 fatty acids. Try to eat two portions of fresh fish a week, including at least one of oily fish.
• **Beans** are the richest source of vegetable protein. They're low in fat and calories, a good source of iron for vegetarians, and packed with fibre, especially soluble fibre.
• **Fruit** of all types is good for you and it's much better to eat fruits whole, rather than as processed juices. Some, including blueberries, kiwis and strawberries are particularly rich in antioxidants and fibre.
• **Oats** provides a high-fibre, high-protein source of magnesium and selenium. Studies have found that people who eat porridge oats regularly keep a stable weight and a healthy cholesterol level.
• **Sweet potatoes** contain beta carotene, which produces the antioxidant vitamin A. They're rich in vitamin C and B_6, and are also packed with fibre.

CUT DOWN ON **SUGAR**

In two decades, sugar consumption in the UK has grown by 31 per cent, to more than half a kilo per person per week. Much of the sugar is hidden in processed foods, leading to weight problems and obesity. High sugar consumption also contributes indirectly to diseases such as osteoporosis, heart disease and cancer.

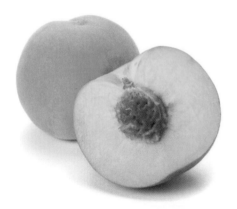

● **Reach for a peach** If you have a sweet tooth, satisfy your craving for cakes and biscuits with a piece of fruit. Next time you crave a chocolate bar, reach for a juicy peach instead. Keep a packet of dried apricots in your bag, desk or car for 'emergencies'.

● **Choose the right breakfast cereal** Many are full of sugar. You want one with less than 8g of sugar per serving or, preferably, one that is unsweetened altogether. Use diced fruit instead to sweeten your cereal.

● **Make rules about dessert** Decide to have dessert only after dinner, never after lunch, for example. Or eat dessert only on odd days of the month, or just at weekends or in restaurants.

● **Don't skip meals** When you go without breakfast, lunch or dinner, your blood-sugar levels drop, and that propels you towards high-sugar (often convenience) foods to quell your cravings.

● **Don't add sugar to foods** Many everyday recipes – including some for vegetables, soups, casseroles and sauces – call for sugar to add sweetness. In most cases, it's just not needed.

did you know?

Cracking the sugar code

Manufacturers deliberately make many products temptingly sweet. So sugar gets hidden in surprising places, including cough medicine, tinned vegetables and even meat products and some prescription medicines. The word 'sugar' may not appear on the ingredients list, but if you see one or more of the following names you can be sure that it's there: corn syrup, dextrin, dextrose, fructose, fruit juice concentrate, galactose, glucose, honey, hydrogenated starch, lactose, mannitol, maple syrup, maltose, molasses, polyols, sorghum, sucrose, sorbitol and xylitol.

● **Get your chocolate in small doses** Dip fresh strawberries into low-fat chocolate sauce, scatter chocolate sprinkles over your plain yoghurt or eat a mini-piece of dark chocolate. Think rich and decadent but in tiny portions.

● **Watch out for mixed alcoholic drinks** Have you ever thought about the sugar content of a cosmopolitan or a margarita? Drink mixers and many alcoholic beverages are thick with sugar. Stick with beer or wine, or, if you prefer spirits, mix them only with unsweetened fizzy water or drink them straight.

● **Seek out substitutes** With saccharin, aspartame, acesulfame potassium and sucralose all commercially available, you can still get the sweetness of sugar without the calories. These sweeteners can be particularly useful as part of a diabetic diet.

● **Go half and half** Mix half a standard fizzy drink with half a diet version; half a pot of sweetened yoghurt with half a pot of plain yoghurt; half a glass of juice with half a glass of fizzy water. Do this for two weeks, then cut back to a quarter sweetened to three-quarters unsweetened. Continue until you're taking only the unsweetened version.

● **Don't keep ice cream at home** A tub in the freezer is temptation writ large.

● **Cut down slowly** If you normally have two chocolate bars a day, cut down to one. Then, next week, have one every other day. The following week, have one every three days, until you're down to just one a week. If you normally take 2 teaspoons of sugar in your coffee, use the same routine, cutting down gradually to ½ teaspoon or none at all.

THE CORN-SYRUP **CONTROVERSY**

Corn syrup is a calorie-dense, nutritionally empty sweetener that may be even worse for our health than refined sugar. Often called glucose-fructose syrup in the UK, it is in many foods and drinks, including apparently healthy ones such as fruit juices, spaghetti sauces and even bread. Since its first appearance on the US market in 1966, corn syrup has been a source of controversy.

High-fructose corn syrup is generally cheaper and easier to refine than granulated sugar. So, increasingly, processed-food companies have been using it to add sweetness to their products, especially in soft drinks. That would have been the end of the story, except for recent research which suggest that the human body processes corn syrup differently from sugar.

When the body processes sugar, it triggers the production of a chemical that sends signals of 'fullness' to the brain, and also prevents the release of a chemical that indicates hunger. But, when scientists monitored how the body processes corn syrup, they noted that the fullness chemical was suppressed and the hunger chemical wasn't affected. In short, corn syrup, according to one theory, makes you hungrier. But other people believe that the issue is simply that calories consumed as liquid are less filling than calories from solid food.

Whatever the truth, corn syrup is a huge source of empty calories that interfere with the body's chemistry. So consult the label on any processed food you are thinking of buying. If corn syrup is one of the main ingredients, put the item back on the shelf.

● **Look for hidden sources of sugar** Cough syrups, chewing gum, mints, ketchup, baked beans and cold meats often contain sugar. Even some prescription medicines contain sugar. Scan every food label, and choose sugar-free and reduced-sugar alternatives when available.

CUT DOWN ON **SALT**

The average intake of salt (sodium chloride) per person in the UK is about 9g a day, most of it from processed foods. Reducing this by around 2.5g a day would greatly cut an individual's risk of stroke or heart attack. A high-salt diet can also contribute to osteoporosis, stomach cancer and obesity, as well as exacerbating asthma symptoms.

● **Prepare your own meals** Ready-meals and tinned soups usually contain a lot of salt. By preparing more food yourself, you'll cut your consumption radically. Instead of salt, use herbs, spices, a drop of lemon juice, mustard or grated horseradish, to give your meals a lift.

● **Say no to sports drinks** Endurance athletes need higher levels of salt and far more to drink than ordinary people. Sports drinks deliver both – they are rich in salt, which not only provides the necessary sodium but also stokes continued thirst. For the rest of us, the extra salt provides no benefit at all.

● **Watch out for salty nibbles** Capers, pickles and olives are packed with salt. The pickling and brining processes used to make such foods necessarily involves soaking them in a salt-dense solution.

● **Check your medicines for salt** You might not think that you'd find salt in your drugs, but you could be wrong. Particular culprits in your medicine cabinet include soluble tablets, antacids, cough medicines, pain relievers and laxatives. If you find high salt levels, talk to your doctor about alternatives.

● **Avoid salty cereals** Over a third, 35 per cent, of the salt we eat comes from cereal and cereal products (including bread). One way to reduce your intake is to choose breads with less than 1.1g of salt per 100g (3½ oz), or less than 0.4g of salt per slice. Another way is to pick breakfast cereals with no added salt, for example, porridge oats, Shredded Wheat, puffed-wheat cereals and muesli with no added salt.

● **Check salt content** You can tell if a processed food is high in salt by reading the nutritional information on the label. Look at the figure for salt or sodium per 100g (3½ oz).
• High is more than 1.5g of salt (or 0.6g of sodium) per 100g.
• Low is 0.3g of salt or less (or 0.1g of sodium) per 100g.
• If the amount of salt or sodium per 100g lies somewhere between these figures, it contains a medium level of salt.

great idea! **Make your own salt-free salad dressing** Mix 200ml (⅓ pint) olive oil, 85ml (3fl oz) balsamic vinegar, 1 pinch of sugar and 2 crushed garlic cloves in a bowl. Blend until emulsified. This tasty dressing keeps in the refrigerator for a month. Just remove it an hour before serving so it can liquefy.

THE PROBLEM WITH PROCESSED FOODS

The word sodium, rather than salt, is usually listed in the nutritional information on food labels. (It's the sodium in salt that can be bad for your health.) Other words on food labels that signal the presence of sodium include: Na, monosodium glutamate or MSG, sodium citrate, sodium bicarbonate (bicarbonate of soda) and baking powder.

Manufacturers of processed foods pile on the sodium to help to create big, attractive flavours. See the panel on the right for examples of what happens to 'real' food once manufacturers get their hands on it.

Natural food	Sodium	Processed food	Sodium
Baked potato	8mg	Potato crisps, 110g/4oz	600mg
		Large portion of chips	350mg
		Instant mashed potatoes	770mg
		Potatoes au gratin	355mg
Fresh corn-on-the-cob	15mg	Corn tortilla chips, 200g/7oz	630mg
		Cornflakes	230mg
Fresh broccoli	27mg	Frozen broccoli and cheese sauce	330mg
		Tinned cream of broccoli soup	770mg
Roast chicken breast	120mg	Chicken korma ready meal	600mg
		Chicken nuggets	765mg

● **Switch to pepper** Use freshly ground black pepper instead of salt, or look out for lemon pepper, a seasoning that adds wonderful flavour to foods.

● **Avoid meat that's been dried or cured** This includes salami, corned beef, prosciutto, ham and dried sausages. Each is laden with salt, which is used to draw out the liquid and preserve the meat.

● **Choose no-added-salt tins of vegetables and beans** When buying tinned foods such as kidney beans, chickpeas and sweetcorn, look for varieties that contain no additional salt. If you can't find beans packed in water, rinsing them thoroughly before use will help to remove some of the salt.

try it... **Put a big X on your calendar for six weeks from today** Unlike our preference for sugar, which we're born with, salt is an acquired taste, learned from habit. So it takes time to 'unlearn' your preference – about six weeks, to be exact. Slowly reduce your intake of salt between now and then, focusing on food categories where the salt will be missed the least, such as cereals, breads and dessert items. Be patient and determined; you aren't going to stop wanting salty food overnight but it comes in time. Knowing that, you won't get discouraged.

Other words on food labels that signal the presence of sodium include: Na, monosodium glutamate or MSG, sodium citrate, sodium bicarbonate and baking powder

BREAKFAST
SATISFACTION

Your choice of breakfast influences what you eat during the rest of the day, and people who eat breakfast are much less likely to be obese and have diabetes than those who don't. Indeed, breakfasting every day can make a huge, positive difference to your wellbeing. The key is to choose energy-enhancing, health-invigorating foods.

● **Have a breakfast sandwich**
Top a wholemeal roll, bread or toast with melted low-fat cheese (low-fat mozzarella is a good choice), a sliced tomato and a sliced, hard-boiled egg.

● **Choose eggs** If you're watching your weight, eggs – poached, scrambled or boiled – are a great choice for breakfast. Research has shown that on days when people ate eggs for breakfast, their overall calorie intake was lower.

● **Use omega-3-rich eggs**
They're not much more expensive than standard eggs but are much higher in all-important omega-3 fatty acids, shown to benefit everything from your mental health (reducing the risk of depression) to your heart health (reducing the risk of blocked arteries and irregular heart rhythms).

Eggs – poached, scrambled or boiled – help you to eat less later in the day

try it... **Have a bowl of sweetened brown rice**
Brown rice is full of energy-providing B vitamins, as well as being a great source of fibre. Cook the rice the night before, then, in the morning, put it in a bowl with a spoonful of honey, a handful of raisins, a cut-up apple and a sprinkle of cinnamon for a unique yet delicious treat. Don't like rice? Try other cooked grains instead, such as barley, oats, buckwheat, quinoa or millet.

● **Make your own muesli**
Many shop-bought brands are filled with sugar and fat. To make your own, mix two parts porridge oats to one part dried fruit and seeds with a little brown sugar. Store in an airtight container.

● **Sprinkle blueberries on your cereal** Studies show that these tiny purple berries are loaded with valuable antioxidants that can slow down brain ageing and protect your memory. Or try mashing them with low-fat soft cheese to spread on your toast instead of jam or marmalade.

● **Drink a glass of unsweetened orange juice** A small glass (150ml/ ¼ pint) of unsweetened fruit juice will count as one of your five-a-day. Plus, American researchers who followed almost 2,000 people for up to ten years found that the risk of developing Alzheimer's disease was 76 per cent lower in those who drank juice more than three times a week, compared to those who drank it less than once a week.

● **Add a dash of cinnamon** Several studies suggest that small amounts of cinnamon taken daily can help to keep blood sugar at a healthy level and lower cholesterol by as much as 30 per cent. Sprinkle ½ teaspoon of ground cinnamon over your daily cereal or on top of your morning coffee, or stir a generous pinch into your nutritious breakfast smoothie.

● **Enjoy a smoothie** Put a sliced banana and a sliced (but not peeled) apple, peach or pear into a blender with a handful of strawberries, blueberries or raspberries. Add some skimmed milk and a pot of low-fat yoghurt and blend them until smooth. For a dairy-free version, replace the milk and yoghurt with soya milk or blend the fruit with some fresh fruit juice.

● **Sprinkle on a teaspoon of ground linseeds** Add to cereal, yoghurt, eggs or a smoothie. After fish and omega-3-rich eggs, linseeds are one of the best sources of omega-3 fatty acids. Lightly grind the seeds in a coffee grinder or in a pestle and mortar before adding them to the food.

● **Eat half a grapefruit twice a week** Grapefruit is high in vitamin C and folic acid. According to a review of eight studies in *The Lancet*, adding folic acid to your diet may cut your stroke risk by a fifth. If you're taking regular medication, consult your doctor before eating grapefruit – the fruit can interact with medicines that have to be processed through the liver.

● **Top your cereal with soya milk** Packed with potent phyto-oestrogens, soya has been credited with everything from protecting your heart to promoting stronger bones. But make sure that it's fortified with calcium for even more of the bone-building stuff.

BEST BREAKFAST COMBINATIONS

For most people, a perfect breakfast has three components: one serving of a whole-grain carbohydrate, one serving of a dairy or high-calcium food, and one serving of fruit. Together, that would add up to roughly 300kcal. A high-protein serving (meat or an egg) is unnecessary but certainly acceptable, as long as it doesn't add too much fat or too many calories (more correctly, kilocalories – kcal – as you will see on food labels) to the mix. Here are a few winning combinations based on this formula:

• A bowl of high-fibre, multigrain cereal, with strawberries and low-fat milk on top.

• A cereal bar, an apple and a glass of cold milk.

• A pot of fat-free yoghurt with fresh blueberries mixed in, and a slice of wholemeal toast with a fruit spread.

• A mini wholemeal bagel, spread lightly with cream cheese and jam, and a peach plus a pot of yoghurt.

• A scrambled egg, a wholemeal roll, fresh-fruit salad and a cup of low-fat milk.

• A bowl of muesli or porridge with chopped banana or dried fruit.

LUNCH **MATTERS**

For many workers, the 'lunch break' is no more than an extension of an already overburdened day, with little thought given to food. Yet studies have shown that a nutritious lunch improves work performance as well as boosting energy levels. With a little forethought, there are many quick and easy ways to ensure that you eat well during the working day.

● **Graze throughout the day** One healthy option is to snack on nutritious foods whenever you get hungry, rather than having a large, formal lunch.

Spreading out your calories stabilizes blood sugar and insulin levels, provides more frequent relief from stress, tension and boredom, and avoids the fatigue that often sets in after a big meal. Plus, since you never get really hungry, you are less likely to make the regrettable food choices that you might when you feel as if you're starving.

great idea!

Create a sandwich chart and stick it on your fridge This prevents the early morning haze from overcoming your better judgment and allowing you to leave home without a packed lunch. In one category on your chart, list your bread options (wholemeal bread, pitta, tortilla wrap, and so on). In the next column, list your protein options, such as low-fat cheese, lean roast beef, hummous or tuna/chicken salad. In another column, list vegetable toppings such as spinach, lettuce, cucumber slices, tomato slices and roasted red peppers. In the last column, list your condiments, ranging from mustard to low-fat mayonnaise to Italian dressing. You can also include a list of accompaniments such as cheese sticks, apples, oranges, yoghurt, baby carrots and ready-made soup. Then, every morning (or, even better, the night before) pick one item from each column to pack.

● **Don't be tempted by meal deals** When buying lunch, especially from fast-food restaurants, don't be tempted by any 'meal deal' unless it offers healthy options as part of the deal. Otherwise you may end up eating more than you actually want.

● **Make better menu choices** If you have arranged a business lunch or lunch in a restaurant with friends or colleagues, try to be the first to order. Studies show that we're often swayed by other people's choices, so be sure you forge ahead by picking healthy options.

● **Use the office microwave** Take a low-salt, low-fat ready meal to the office and microwave it for a quick-and-easy lunch that allows plenty of time to run errands or power-walk during the rest of your lunch hour. Alternatively, pack a bean and vegetable soup, or another variety that you can put in the microwave, along with a couple of oatcakes spread with low-fat soft cheese and a carton of juice.

A nutritious lunch improves work performance

● **Enjoy teatime** Get into the routine of having a mid-afternoon cup of tea or coffee. If you have an energy dip around this time, drinking caffeine will perk you up; it will also enhance your memory and make you more productive on tasks requiring concentration. Another option is a cup of black or green tea, both of which are full of heart-healthy antioxidants that provide more than just an energy-boosting punch; as well as contributing to healthier arteries, they may also help to prevent cancer.

try it... **A superfast hot meal to have at home** Pour a tin of low-salt soup into a saucepan and add a bag of pre-cut broccoli and carrots, either fresh or frozen, heating gently. Flavour it with your preferred spices, herbs or spicy sauce. As the soup simmers, it will cook the vegetables. You have a superfast and easy lunch that's bursting with nutrition and fibre.

BEST QUICK BITES

Making your own packed lunch need not take a lot of time or creative energy. Include a source of lean protein, fruit or vegetables, and whole rather than processed grains. Leftovers from last night's dinner work wonders, as do the following quick-and-easy sandwich options:

• Chicken or tuna salad sandwich: 170g (6oz) of water-packed tuna or cooked chicken breast pieces mixed with 1 tablespoon of light mayonnaise and relish or grated carrots, served between two slices of wholemeal bread.

• A wholemeal pitta bread 'pizza': one pitta stuffed with low-fat pizza/spaghetti sauce or salsa, reduced-fat shredded mozzarella cheese, grated carrot, broccoli pieces, peppers, tomatoes, spinach, mushrooms or other vegetables of your choice, plus lean ham or fat-free vegetarian sausage. Melt in the microwave before eating if desired.

• Tortilla roll-up: 1 wholemeal tortilla spread with 1 tablespoon of low-fat soft cheese, topped with 2 slices of lean ham or wafer-thin sliced turkey and various vegetables such as chillies, lettuce or spinach, tomatoes, onion, cucumber or grated carrot.

• Cheese and salad sandwich: 2 slices of wholemeal bread spread with 1 tablespoon of light mayonnaise or mustard and filled with 1 slice of low or reduced-fat cheese, along with lettuce, sliced avocado, tomatoes and peppers.

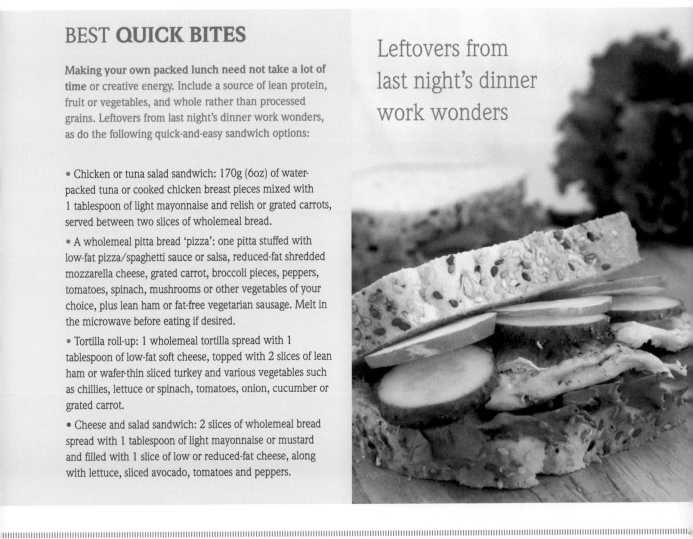

Leftovers from last night's dinner work wonders

NUTRITIOUS DINNERS

Whether we are working, caring for others, studying, volunteering or managing a home, most of us live pressurized lives. So, when it comes to dinner, we take the easy path: a pizza or frozen pie cooked in the microwave, a pre-prepared or takeaway meal. Many such dishes are filled with salt, sugar and fat, and lacking in vegetables, fibre and vitamins. With a little forethought, you can eat a lot more healthily.

● **Base a meal on good-quality stock** If you keep homemade chicken stock in the freezer or low-salt stock cubes in the store cupboard, it'll take just a few minutes to put together a vegetable soup. Use 1 litre of stock as the base. Add a variety of chopped vegetables such as spinach, carrots, sweetcorn, peas, green beans and courgettes. Be sure to include lentils, chickpeas, butter beans or other pulses; they provide excellent protein, lots of fibre, an array of micronutrients, and are filling and satisfying at a relatively low cost in calories. Serve with whole-grain bread and a salad.

try it... **The George Foreman grill** Although many kitchen appliances probably sit in a cupboard gathering dust, the George Foreman grill may become the one appliance that occupies a permanent spot on your kitchen worktop. This device allows you to barbecue inside your house. The health bonus: a drip pan catches the grease, reducing the fat content of cooked meat, which also makes it easier to clean. One of these grills gives you the convenience of low-fat barbecuing during the winter months, when it's too cold to barbecue outdoors.

● **Invest in a slow cooker and/or a breadmaker** Imagine popping a few ingredients – chicken, a few vegetables, barley and stock – into a slow cooker before you leave the house in the morning and coming home to a satisfyingly healthy home-cooked meal, or waking up to the delicious aroma of bread in the timed breadmaker.

● **Plan which night you'll eat out – and stick to it** Rather than eating out whenever you lack the inspiration – or provisions – to cook at home, eat out on a designated night. This makes eating out what it should be – a treat. You'll enjoy the restaurant more and eat more healthily through the week.

● **Avoid alcohol before dinner** In a study conducted at the University of Liverpool, men who drank a glass of beer 30 minutes before a meal ate more during the meal than men who had a soft drink. They also ate more fatty, salty foods and felt hungrier after the meal than men who didn't drink.

Alcohol stimulates the appetite, so, if you don't want to eat too much, avoid alcohol or enjoy one glass with, not before, your meal.

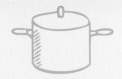

● **Have breakfast for dinner** A great option for dinner is an omelette. It's quick and easy to make, a good protein source and relatively low in calories. Fill it with vegetables instead of cheese.

● **Relax to combat night-eating**
People who eat more than 50 per cent of their calories after 6pm tend to suffer from insomnia, gain weight more easily and feel more stressed than people who spread their food intake through the day. One solution to this condition, known as night-eating syndrome, is relaxation.

Sit in a chair or lie on your back. Then progressively tense and relax various muscles in your body, starting at the top of your head, moving down through your body and ending at your feet. Tense as you inhale. Slowly release as you exhale. When you reach your toes, it's time to eat.

FAMILY MEALS ARE BEST

Children who eat dinner at the table with other family members at least three times a week are more likely to enjoy a healthy diet than those who do not, according to research by the National Family and Parenting Institute.

• To simplify healthy eating, make use of tried-and-trusted standbys. Choose three low-fuss, nutritious recipes that you and the family enjoy and serve them every week.

• Turn off the television during dinner. A study has found that the more television and videos students watched, the fewer fruits and vegetables they ate. They tended to reach instead for soft drinks and crisps.

• If your children don't eat what you give them, say nothing. Hassling children over their eating habits during dinner actually causes children – and their parents – to eat less well, according to one study. Both the children and their parents consumed more fat during meals when they argued over eating behaviour. The stress from the argument may have led to cravings for fatty comfort foods.

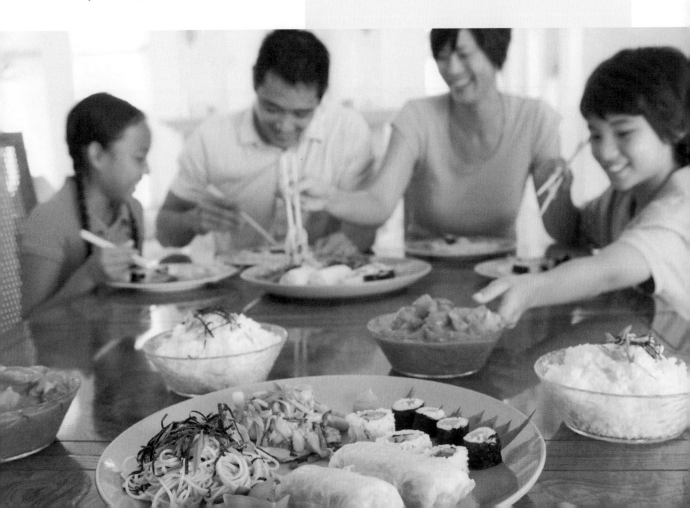

DIETARY SUPPLEMENTS

Daily multivitamin and multimineral supplements can help to fill gaps created by less-than-perfect eating habits and metabolic changes that occur naturally with age. Research indicates that there are also good reasons for using a variety of supplements, including herbs, for both prevention and healing.

● **Get enough iron** Do you feel lethargic most of the time? You could have iron-deficiency anaemia, a common cause of fatigue. Iron is essential for producing haemoglobin, which carries oxygen to your body's cells, where it's used to produce energy. Good food sources of iron are red meat, iron-fortified breakfast cereal, green leafy vegetables, beans and pulses. You may also need a supplement – check with your doctor.

● **Boost your immune system with echinacea** A natural antibiotic and infection fighter, echinacea can help to prevent the two most common ailments – colds and flu. The herbal supplement acts by stimulating immune-system cells that are key weapons against infections. It is most effective when taken at the first hint of illness. It is also useful if you are already suffering from the aches, pains, congestion or fever of colds and flu.

● **Take vitamin D** Also called the sunshine vitamin, because it's produced in the skin on exposure to light, vitamin D can protect against more than a dozen types of cancer, help to maintain strong bones, reduce the risk of developing Type 2 diabetes and multiple sclerosis, and improve immunity and brain function, among other benefits, according to research. People who are not exposed to much sunlight should get an extra 1,000 IU (international units) per day from food or supplements. Others should aim to have at least 400 IU a day.

● **Check your calcium source** Getting enough calcium throughout life is a central factor in preventing osteoporosis, the bone-thinning disease that leads to a higher risk of fractures, spinal deformities and loss of height. We need around 700mg a day of elemental calcium from food or supplements to maintain good health – but many modern diets are severely lacking in calcium.

When taking supplements, choose calcium citrate, which is better absorbed than calcium carbonate. But as calcium citrate contains less elemental calcium, you may need to take more of it.

● **Calm yourself with ginseng** Derived from a slow-growing root, ginseng has been used in Chinese medicine for thousands of years to

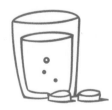

Take supplements with food and plain water

enhance both longevity and the quality of life. It has antioxidant properties and stimulates the production of specialized immune cells called 'killer-T cells', which destroy harmful viruses and bacteria.

Ginseng is also prized for its ability to protect the body against the adverse effects of stress. Many long-distance runners and body-builders take ginseng to boost physical endurance.

● Ease joint pain with fish oils
The fat in fish contains a class of polyunsaturated fatty acids called omega-3s. Omega-3s play an important role in a range of vital body processes, from regulating blood pressure and blood clotting to boosting immunity, and they appear to reduce the risk of heart disease. Omega-3s are also effective anti-inflammatories, useful for joint problems, lupus and psoriasis.

If you eat oily fish at least twice a week, supplements may not be necessary, but people with rheumatoid arthritis have been shown to experience less joint swelling and stiffness when they take fish-oil supplements.

● Take peppermint for indigestion
Peppermint is a traditional remedy and it works for all kinds of intestinal disturbances, from indigestion to flatulence. Peppermint oil stimulates the secretion of digestive juices and improves the flow of bile, so helping the body to digest fats. But don't take peppermint supplements if you have heartburn or reflux disease – it could make symptoms worse.

● Combat memory loss with ginkgo biloba
Extracted from the leaves of an ancient tree, ginkgo biloba appears to benefit both the circulatory and central nervous system. It increases blood flow to the arms and legs and the brain by regulating the tone and elasticity of blood vessels.

The fact that ginkgo aids blood flow to the brain is particularly important to elderly people whose arteries may have narrowed with cholesterol build-up or other conditions. Diminished blood flow has been linked to Alzheimer's disease and memory loss, as well as to anxiety, headaches, depression, confusion, tinnitus and dizziness. All may be helped by ginkgo supplements.

● Get wise to zinc
Zinc is critical for hundreds of processes that take place in the body, from cell growth to sexual maturation and immunity – even for taste and smell. Consequently, everyone who takes a daily multivitamin and mineral supplement should make sure that it contains zinc – but an excess can be harmful, so don't take too much.

Taking zinc can help to prevent colds, flu and other infections, and also helps to treat a wide range of chronic ailments, from rheumatoid arthritis and underactive thyroid to chronic fatigue and osteoporosis.

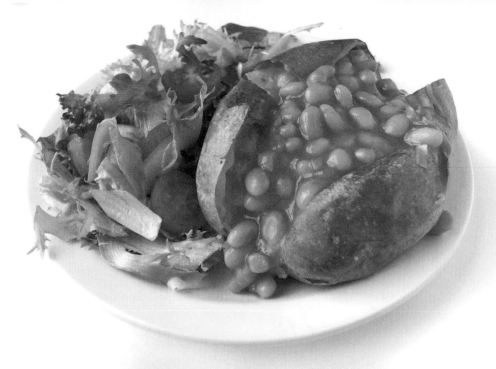

GOOD AND BAD
CARBOHYDRATES

Complex carbohydrates form a crucial part of a balanced diet, but eating too many simple carbs, such as white flour, refined sugar and white rice, is bad for you. 'Bad' carbohydrates are digested so fast that they cause blood-sugar surges, leading to weight gain and other health problems.

● **Eat potatoes boiled with the skin still on** The effect of potatoes on blood sugar depends on how the potatoes are prepared. There's no need to avoid them completely, but keep your portion size modest. Also, new potatoes tend to have fewer simple carbohydrates than other types of potatoes.

● **Choose brown rice** Brown rice hasn't been processed and it retains its high-fibre nutrients. Limit the amount you eat to 180g.

● **Make a healthy snack** Cut up 30g (1oz) portions of cheese and measure out 30g (1oz) portions of nuts, then put one of each into snack bags.

● **Don't let yourself get too hungry** Eat every 3 to 5 waking hours, and only until you're satisfied but not stuffed. You should never reach the point where you feel ravenous. Not only is that a recipe for overeating, but your body will want sugary, quick-to-digest bad carbohydrates to satiate your need for fuel quickly.

● **Buy your snacks in child-sized bags**
Crisps, tortilla chips and biscuits
are mostly bad carbohydrates, made
primarily from refined flour, sugar, salt
and/or oil. You want to remove as many
of these foods from your daily eating as
you can. But if you can't live without
them, buy them in small bags – 30g (1oz)
is a typical 'lunch box' size – and limit
yourself to one bag a day.

● **Eat plenty of good carbohydrates**
Good carbohydrates are foods such
as whole grains and beans which are
composed largely of complex sugar
molecules that require lots of time and
energy to digest and break down into
the simple sugars that our bodies need
for fuel. Among the benefits of these
foods is that they provide energy and
large amounts of dietary fibre, which is
vital for good health. In addition, whole-
grain products such as wholemeal bread
are much better sources of vitamins and
minerals than refined cereals.

● **At the cinema, skip the popcorn**
Popcorn isn't a bad food – it contains
useful fibre, for example. But it's a simple
carbohydrate with little other nutritional
value and, when bought at the cinema,
it's often drowning in salt and fat. Better
snacks are small bags of nuts or seeds and
fresh or dried fruit.

● **Start the day with a bowl of
porridge** Choose porridge rather than
eggs and bacon for breakfast. It is a
tasty, high-fibre way to start the day.
Sweeten it with sugar-free sweetener
or sugar-free muesli.

● **Wrap your food in lettuce leaves**
Yes, skip the rolls, tortillas and bread
slices and instead make a sandwich inside
lettuce leaves. Go Mexican with a sprinkle
of Cheddar cheese, salsa and chicken; or
Chinese with sesame seeds, peanuts, bean
sprouts, sliced green beans and prawns
with a touch of soy sauce; or deli style
with turkey, cheese and mustard.

● **Find pasta alternatives** Almost
everyone loves a big bowl of pasta topped
with rich tomato sauce. The tomato sauce
couldn't be better for you; spaghetti,
however, is pure carbohydrate with a high
glycaemic load – and if you eat too much
you are liable to put on weight. If you
want to cut back on your pasta intake,
here are some healthier alternatives.
• Switch to wholemeal pasta. It's denser
than traditional pasta, with a firm, al dente
texture similar to what you'd find in Italy.
• Grill vegetables such as aubergines,
courgettes, peppers and onions and slice
into long, thin pieces. Mix up and pour
your spaghetti sauce over the vegetables
for a tasty and immensely healthy meal.
• Try healthy whole grains instead of
pasta. Spaghetti sauce goes better than
you'd expect with brown rice, pearl
barley, chickpeas, and so on.

did you know?

**How to lighten your glycaemic
load** The terms 'glycaemic index' and 'glycaemic load'
are applied to individual foods to indicate how much,
and how fast, the carbohydrate in that particular food
raises the level of sugar in your blood. The glycaemic-
load measurement also takes account of the quantity
of carbohydrate in a food. Foods with a low glycaemic
load – such as beans, bran cereal, brown rice, wholemeal
bread and nuts – have less impact on your blood sugar
than foods with a high glycaemic load – including white
rice, spaghetti, potatoes, cornflakes and sugary juices
and drinks. Eating more low-glycaemic-load foods will
help you to keep your blood sugar steady and avoid
the lightheadedness and 'shakes' associated with blood-
sugar drops, which usually follow rises.

12 top ways to stabilize your blood **sugar**

Diabetes, a disease reaching epidemic proportions, is directly linked to blood-sugar levels. Whether you already have diabetes, are overweight, or simply want to prevent future problems, there is a lot you can do to make sure your blood-sugar and insulin levels are as healthy as can be.

1 SERVE A SPINACH SALAD FOR DINNER

Spinach is high in magnesium, which a large study suggests can help to prevent Type 2 diabetes developing. One study in women found that higher intakes of magnesium (also in nuts, avocados, other leafy greens and fish) reduced diabetes risk by about 10 per cent overall, and by about 20 per cent in overweight women.

2 EAT BEANS EVERY DAY

These high-fibre foods take longer to digest, so they release their glucose more slowly. Studies find just 75g (3oz) a day can help to stabilize blood-sugar and insulin levels.

3 HAVE AT LEAST TWO SERVINGS OF LOW-FAT DAIRY PRODUCTS A DAY

One serving is a 200ml/⅓ pint glass of skimmed or semi-skimmed milk, or a 150g/5½oz pot of yoghurt or fromage frais. A study of 3,000 people found that those who were overweight but also ate a lot of dairy foods were 70 per cent less likely to develop insulin resistance (a precursor to diabetes) than those who didn't. It turns out that the lactose, protein and fat in dairy products improves blood sugar by filling you up and slowing the conversion of food sugars to blood sugar.

4 SPRINKLE A FEW WALNUTS OVER YOUR SALAD

Walnuts are a great source of monounsaturated fat, which won't raise your blood sugar as many other foods do. And some researchers suspect that this fat even makes cells more sensitive to insulin, helping to combat high blood sugar.

5 DISCOVER THE POWER OF CINNAMON

Sprinkle cinnamon over your porridge, yoghurt, coffee and tea. Researchers from Pakistan, where cinnamon is widely used, asked volunteers with Type 2 diabetes to take either 1g, 3g or 6g of cinnamon or a placebo for 40 days. Those taking the fragrant spice saw their blood-sugar levels drop by between 18 and 29 per cent depending on how much cinnamon they took.

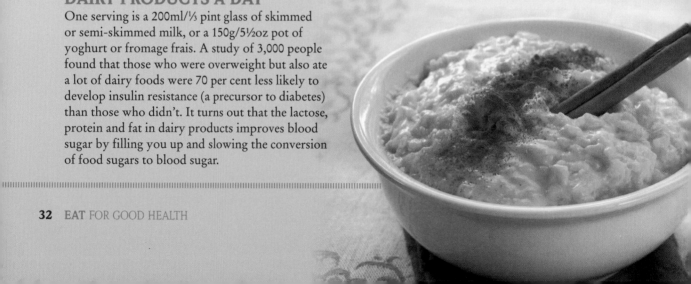

6 DON'T SKIP A MEAL

Your blood sugar drops like a rock when you're very hungry (hence the headache and shakiness). Then, when you do eat, you flood your system with glucose, forcing your pancreas to release more insulin and creating a dangerous cycle.

7 HAVE A GLASS OF WINE

One study found that women who had a glass of wine a day cut their risk of diabetes in half compared to teetotallers. Not a wine lover? The study found the same effects for beer. But cork the wine bottle once dinner is over. An Australian study found that drinking a glass of wine immediately after eating can result in a sudden drop in the insulin in your blood, meaning the glucose from your meal hangs around longer, eventually damaging the arteries.

8 HAVE HALF A GRAPEFRUIT

American researchers asked 50 obese patients to eat half a grapefruit with each meal for 12 weeks and compared them to a group who didn't eat any grapefruit. Those patients who ate the grapefruit lost an average of 1.6kg (3.6lb). They also had lower levels of insulin and glucose after each meal, suggesting a more efficient sugar metabolism. (If you are on any medication, talk to your doctor first before eating grapefruit, as it can affect the way that medicines are processed in the liver.)

9 DIVIDE MEALS IN HALF

Prepare your breakfast, lunch and dinner, but then divide each meal in half. Eat half now and wait for a couple of hours before eating the second half. Eating several small meals rather than three large meals helps to avoid the major influx of glucose that, in turn, results in a blood-sugar surge and a big release of insulin.

slashing the **risk**

If you were to do only three things to maintain healthy blood-sugar levels and prevent diabetes, here is what doctors recommend. Together, they can slash your risk of the disease by nearly 60 per cent:

• **LOSE WEIGHT.** If you're overweight, losing 3kg to 3.5kg (7lb to 8lb) – and keeping it off – is all it takes.

• **ADD MORE FIBRE TO YOUR DIET.** Eat vegetables, fruits, whole grains, nuts, seeds, beans and lentils regularly.

• **BE PHYSICALLY ACTIVE.** All you need is 30 minutes a day.

10 CUT BACK ON SATURATED FAT

American scientists evaluated 3,000 people and found that those with the highest blood levels of saturated fats were twice as likely to develop diabetes.

11 GET PLENTY OF FIBRE & PROTEIN FROM BREAD

Buy bread products with at least 3g of fibre and 3g of protein per serving. Complex carbohydrates of this type slow down absorption of glucose and decrease possible insulin rises.

12 WALK ABOUT A MILE A DAY

That's all it took in one large US study to slash the risk of dying from diabetes by more than a third. If you walk 6 miles a week, you'll be nearly 40 per cent less likely to die from all causes and 34 per cent less likely to die from heart disease, the leading cause of death in people with diabetes. The reason? Walking makes your cells more receptive to insulin, which leads to better control of blood sugar. It also raises levels of 'good' HDL cholesterol.

BEST AND WORST **FATS**

All dietary fat was once regarded as bad for health. We now distinguish between 'good' fats (monounsaturated and polyunsaturated) and 'bad' fats (saturated and trans fats). Good fats are found in fish oils and plant oils, for example. If a fat is solid at room temperature, it should be eaten only in strict moderation. Trans fats should not be eaten at all.

● **Choose 'sat-fat-free' spreads** Butter-like spreads are now available that are low in or even free from all saturated and trans fats – and they actually taste good. Good brands to try include Benecol and Flora pro.activ (which will also help to lower your cholesterol when used regularly).

● **Use avocados in place of butter and cream** There's a reason why these green fruits are called butterfruit in Mexico. It's because the texture of a mashed-up avocado resembles that of butter. Try them in soups as a thickening agent, and in mashed potatoes to provide a creamier texture.

Interestingly, avocados and olives are the only two varieties of fruit that are high in fat – yet both are rich in heart-healthy monounsaturated fat.

● **Mist your fat** Use an olive-oil spray to coat pans and foods before cooking. You'll use much less oil than you otherwise would.

● **Eat the right meats** Meat is one of the primary forms of saturated fat – but meat, red or white, is also an excellent source of protein and trace minerals such as zinc and iron. Choose lean cuts and trim off visible fat before cooking. For instance, 100g/3½ oz of lean topside of beef contains 2.7g of fat and lean sirloin steak contains 4.5g, but 100g of fatty beef silverside contains 14.8g and 100g of pork loin chops contains a mighty 21.7g of fat.

> Use an olive-oil spray to coat pans and foods. You'll use much less

try it... **Find an alternative to great slabs of steak** Slice the raw beef and sauté it with peppers and onions, fajita-style. Or cook strips of steak in a wok with plenty of vegetables. Or top a large crunchy salad with steak slices. Or make shish kebab with steak cubes and chunks of vegetable. Why? Because you almost always eat less meat when you've prepared it as part of a nicely integrated dish. Reserve a whole steak for very special occasions.

● **Eat an exotic meat occasionally**
How about emu, venison, wild boar or ostrich? All have less than 1g of saturated fat per 100g (3½oz) serving, are super-rich in protein and taste extremely good.

● **If you can plainly see fat on your food, remove it**
• If there's fat on the meat, trim it off.
• If there's skin on the chicken, remove it.
• If there's oil pooling on the top of the pizza, mop it up with a paper towel.
• If there's leftover dressing at the bottom of your salad, pour it off.
• If there's a pool of fatty juice under a piece of cooked meat, drain it.
• If there's fat at the top of a bowl of stew or soup, skim it off.

● **Have mayonnaise in small doses only** Stick to mustard, ketchup and other non-creamy condiments in place of mayonnaise and tartare sauce. Mayonnaise is particularly dense with fat.

● **Try soya milk on your cereal**
Be sure to look for brands with added calcium. You can also substitute soya milk in baking and other recipes.

● **Look for key words on labels**
Although manufacturers in the UK are not required to list the amount of trans fats in their products, it is still possible to identify the bad stuff with a bit of careful label reading. Look for the words 'partially hydrogenated' or 'hydrogenated'. If you see these, put the item back on the shelf.

● **Put salsa on your baked potato**
Make it a substitute for butter or soured cream. You not only avoid the fat but also add in a healthy, low-calorie serving of vegetables.

great idea!

Buy a pretty bottle, fill it with olive oil and top it with a pourer Keep the bottle in plain view and use the oil every time you fry some food or make a salad dressing. Olive oil contains high amounts of monounsaturated fats and low amounts of saturated fats. Buy the deepest green extra-virgin olive oil you can find – the darker the colour, the greater the quantity of phytonutrients, potent plant-based cancer fighters, to be found in the product. If you want an alternative to olive oil, rapeseed oil is one of the healthiest options.

CHOOSE **REDUCED-FAT AND LOW-FAT PRODUCTS**

Don't believe the argument that reduced-fat and low-fat products don't taste as good as the standard versions. Low-fat products may lack some of the flavour you are used to, but after a week or two you'll stop noticing the subtle decline in richness.

• **Milk** you needn't jump all the way to skimmed; use semi-skimmed as a stepping stone from whole milk, but don't stop there – 35 per cent of the calories still come from fat in semi-skimmed milk.

• **Ice cream** most 'light' versions taste as rich and creamy as the full-fat versions.

• **Yoghurt** given that most people eat their yoghurt flavoured, it's hard to notice the difference between standard and low-fat or fat-free versions.

• **Minced beef** don't think that buying fatty minced beef and pouring off the grease makes it healthy. Much of the fat is bound in with the meat. Buy extra-lean mince – but bear in mind, even that can contain up to 10 per cent fat, so keep portions modest and bulk it out with vegetables or beans.

• **Cheese** choose reduced-fat or low-fat, particularly with mozzarella cheese for pizza. Low-fat versions still have all the taste and texture you could want.

HEALTHY **WEIGHT LOSS**

Carrying too much weight increases your risk of heart disease, diabetes, stroke, high blood pressure, cancer and other illnesses. Plus, if you do fall ill or need surgery, being overweight can make treatments riskier. Successful weight loss requires a mixture of well-informed strategies, clever tactics and practical calorie-reduction measures.

● **Make a plan** You know the drill by now when it comes to losing weight – and you probably also know that most weight-loss diets are very hard to sustain. The key to reaching and maintaining a healthy weight is to combine plenty of physical activity with a carefully devised eating plan that is tailored to your individual needs.

● **Check your weight every day** One study of 40 obese people found that those who carefully monitored their diet and fluctuations in weight lost nearly twice as much as those who didn't. Other studies have found that those who check their weight daily lose more and keep it off better than those who don't.

> **try it...**
>
> **Dine only when you hear your stomach rumbling** It's surprising how often we eat out of boredom, nervousness, habit or frustration – so often, in fact, that many of us have actually forgotten what physical hunger feels like. Next time, wait until your stomach is rumbling before you eat. If you're hankering after a specific food, it's probably a craving, rather than a genuine hunger. If you'd eat anything you could get your hands on, the chances are that you're truly hungry.

● **Hypnotize yourself** Several studies have shown that adding self-hypnosis to weight-loss programmes improves the results. Every night, just before falling asleep, repeat four or five times out loud, 'I am in the process of becoming thinner and thinner.' If you repeat this for 30 consecutive nights, it will become your automatic subconscious thought – and you should soon begin to see results.

● **Accept your body** If you accept your body for the way it is, you're more likely to eat better and may even lose weight unintentionally, according to researchers at Ohio State University, who carried out studies on the eating habits of more than 500 female students. They discovered that those who were broadly happy with their body shape were more likely to choose a diet that was well balanced and in tune with their nutritional needs than the ones who were unhappy with their looks.

● **Take a walk before dinner** Going for a short walk does more than burn calories. Like most exercise, it also lessens appetite. In a study of ten excessively overweight women conducted at Glasgow University, 20 minutes of walking reduced appetite and increased the sensations of fullness as effectively as eating a light meal.

● **Keep a food diary** Buy a notebook and use it to record what you eat. Each day for two weeks, write down everything, especially snacks, and note when you ate, where you were, what else you were doing at the time and how you felt. You will soon have a clear picture of your eating habits, which may help you to plan better ways of balancing your food intake. Your food diary will reveal your 'danger' times and the conditions that trigger your urge to reach for that biscuit or chocolate bar.

● **No-nibble cooking** About an hour before you start to prepare an evening meal, have a small healthy snack – a pot of low-fat yoghurt or some raw vegetable crudités. Many cooks consume as many calories while making the evening meal as they do while eating it. If you're hungry and tired before you start cooking, you are far more likely to nibble on what you're preparing.

● **Get a good night's sleep** An uninterrupted 7 or 8 hours of sleep a night can help to prevent obesity. In a study of more than 15,000 adults, researchers from the University of Warwick found that sleep deprivation is linked with almost twice the risk of being obese. They also found that the less you sleep, the more your body mass index and waist size increase over time. This is probably due to hormonal changes produced by sleep deprivation.

● **Limit your hours at work** If you work more than 9 hours a day (and lunch is included, whether you work through it or not), you are more likely to be overweight and will often be less productive. Consider looking for a less stressful and less demanding job.

did you know?

The pernicious effect of television There's probably no simpler way to lose weight than to cut back on the time you spend in front of the television. One US study involving 486 people in Boston, two-thirds of whom were overweight or obese, found that every hour of television viewing was associated with 144 fewer steps walked. Researchers have estimated that the ideal level of daily activity is around 10,000 steps a day, measured with a pedometer. So, for each hour of television the study participants watched, they were 16 per cent less likely to achieve the 10,000-steps goal. And, because watching television encourages snacking, you'll probably consume far fewer calories if you limit your viewing.

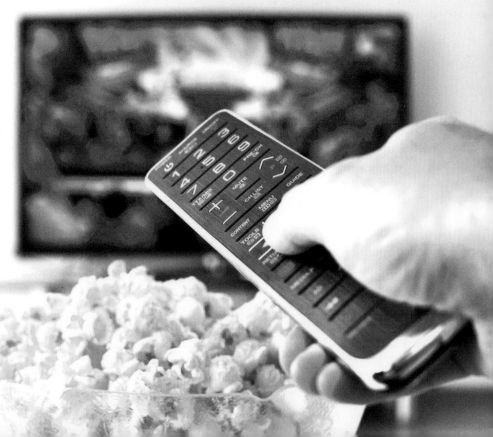

● **Passionately kiss your partner ten times a day** According to the 1991 Kinsey Institute New Report on Sex, a passionate kiss burns 6.4kcal per minute. Ten minutes a day of kissing equates to about 23,000kcal – or 3.5kg – a year!

● **Hang a mirror opposite your seat at the table** One study found that eating in front of mirrors reduced the amount people ate by nearly a third. It seems that having to look yourself in the eye reflects back some of your own inner standards and goals, and reminds you of why you're trying to lose weight in the first place.

● **Get the blues** There's a good reason why you won't see many fast-food restaurants painted blue: the colour blue functions as an appetite suppressant. So serve up dinner on blue plates, dress in blue when you eat, and have a blue tablecloth. Conversely, avoid red, yellow and orange in your dining areas. Studies find they encourage eating.

● **Wash something thoroughly once a week** It could be a floor, a couple of windows, the shower cubicle, a car. A 68kg (10½ st) person who exerts some elbow grease will burn about 4kcal for every minute spent cleaning. If you scrub for 30 minutes, you could work off 120kcal – the calories in two digestive biscuits.

● **Spend 10 minutes a day walking up and down stairs** That's all it takes to help you shed as much as 14.5kg (2st 4lb), assuming you don't start eating more.

● **Clear your wardrobe of 'fat' clothes** Once you've reached your target weight, throw out or give away every item of clothing that doesn't fit. The idea of having to buy a whole new wardrobe if you regain the weight will be a strong incentive to maintain your new figure.

● **Once a week, indulge in a treat** A treat that tastes high in calories even though it isn't should stop you feeling deprived and therefore bingeing on higher-calorie foods. Examples include olives (only 39kcal in five stuffed olives), prawns (58kcal in 75g/2¾ oz) and smoked salmon (58kcal in 50g/1¾ oz).

● **Consume one fewer biscuit a day** Or go without that daily can of fizzy drink, or take three bites fewer of a burger. Doing any of these saves you about 100kcal a day. That's enough to prevent you from gaining the kilo or so (2lb) that most of us put on each year.

● **Eat cereal for breakfast** Studies find that people who eat cereal for breakfast every day are significantly less likely to be obese and have diabetes than those who don't. They also consume more fibre and calcium – and less fat – than those who eat other breakfast foods. But be sure to choose a high-fibre, low-sugar variety.

● **Eat 90 per cent of your meals at home** You're likely to eat more high-fat, high-calorie foods when you eat out than when you eat at home.

● **Eat slowly and calmly** Put your fork or spoon down between every bite. Sip water frequently. Intersperse your eating with stories of the interesting things that happened during your day. Your brain lags behind your stomach by about 20 minutes when it comes to satiety (fullness) signals. If you eat slowly enough, your brain will catch up and tell you that you no longer need food.

● **Beware of hidden sugars** Avoid any prepared food that lists sugar, fructose or corn syrup among the first four ingredients on the label. You should be able to find a lower-sugar version of the same type of food. Look for sugar-free varieties of foods such as ketchup.

● **Eat equal portions of vegetables and grains at dinner** A medium-sized portion of boiled rice (150g/5½oz) and a medium-sized portion of cooked pasta (230g/8oz) both contain about 200kcal, whereas a portion (80g/3oz) of cooked vegetables contains around 30kcal. To avoid a calorie overload, eat a 1:1 ratio of grains to vegetables. The high-fibre vegetables will help to satisfy your hunger before you overeat the grains.

● **Serve your dinner restaurant-style** Serve the food on individual plates rather than putting bowls and dishes on the table and letting people help themselves. When your plate is empty, you've finished; there's no reaching for seconds.

Serve the food on individual plates rather than ... allowing people to help themselves.

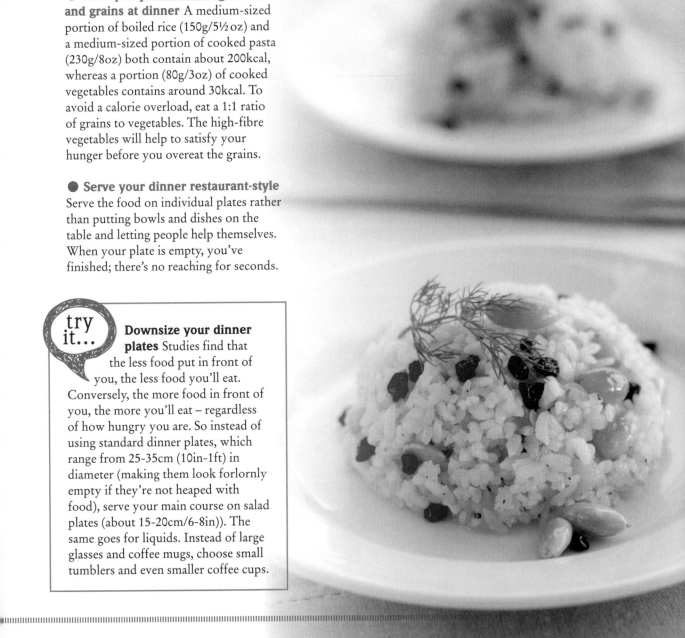

try it...

Downsize your dinner plates Studies find that the less food put in front of you, the less food you'll eat. Conversely, the more food in front of you, the more you'll eat – regardless of how hungry you are. So instead of using standard dinner plates, which range from 25-35cm (10in-1ft) in diameter (making them look forlornly empty if they're not heaped with food), serve your main course on salad plates (about 15-20cm/6-8in)). The same goes for liquids. Instead of large glasses and coffee mugs, choose small tumblers and even smaller coffee cups.

● **Get real** Maintain a realistic expectation of what's considered to be a 'healthy' rate of weight loss; about 0.5kg to 1kg (1lb to 2lb) a week is ideal.

● **Revise your calorie estimate upwards** Add 10 per cent to the number of calories you think you're eating daily, then adjust your eating habits accordingly. If you think you're consuming 1,700kcal a day and don't understand why you're not losing weight, add another 170kcal to your estimate. The new number is probably more accurate.

● **Eat five small meals throughout the day** This is instead of three large meals. You might think you should eat less often if you want to lose weight, but that's just not the case. By eating every few hours, you keep your metabolism fired up and ensure it doesn't slow down between meals in order to hang on to calories. A 'meal' can be as small as a cup of soup.

> Walk on grass, sand or a gravel path instead of the road. It takes more muscle power to glide smoothly over these uneven surfaces

try it...

Improve your walking technique
• Walk with intent – and intensity. Burn more calories in the same amount of time with these strategies:
• Swing your arms when you walk. You'll burn 5 to 10 per cent more calories.
• Walk on grass, sand or a gravel path instead of the road. It takes more muscle power to glide smoothly over these uneven surfaces (especially sand) than over tarmac.
• Use walking poles. A US study found that you get a much more intense workout than you would without the poles.
• Walk along the shoreline of a beach, lake or pond with your ankles in the water. The resistance burns more calories and gives your muscles an added workout.

● **Don't worry about yo-yo dieting**
There's a myth that if you've spent your life losing and gaining 5kg to 9kg (11lb to 20lb), your metabolism gets out of kilter and ends up slowing right down. Don't believe it. When researchers reviewed 43 studies, they found no difference in the metabolic rates of yo-yo dieters compared to those of everyone else.

● **Use interval training to rev up your workout** Walk for the same amount of time at the same intensity every day and your body will get as bored with your workout as you do. Introduce some variety with interval training, which involves changing the intensity of your workout throughout your exercise session. Every 5 minutes of your walk, jog for 1 minute. Every 5 minutes of your bike ride, shift into a higher gear and pedal hard for a minute. If you swim, speed up every other length. You'll burn more calories in the same amount of time.

● **Sip a couple of cups of coffee throughout the day** Studies find that the caffeine in coffee increases the rate at which your body burns calories. This does not mean, however, that you should order a fancy calorie-packed frappuccino. And skip the espresso if it makes you toss and turn at night.

● **Exercise outside** Maybe it's the fresh air, maybe it's the sunshine, but something about exercising out in the open makes you walk or run faster than doing the same exercise in the gym.

● **Keep a small squeeze ball with you** Grip and squeeze it often during the day. It's one of the few exercises you can do at any time. You'll build up the muscles in your hands – and muscle, wherever it is, burns a lot of calories.

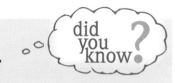

Best ways to boost your metabolism
The more weight you lose, the harder your body fights to hold on to the calories it gets and the fewer calories it burns. Eventually you reach what's called a weight-loss plateau. This is normal and easily explained.

Your basal metabolism, the energy your body uses to survive, accounts for about 70 per cent of all the calories you burn – and it depends on your weight. The less you weigh, the lower your basal metabolic rate (BMR). As you lose weight, your metabolism slows down until you hit the weight-loss plateau.

The only way to lose more weight is to cut the number of calories you take in, increase the number you burn, or both. You can boost your BMR by building up muscle. Muscle tissue requires more energy than fat does, even at rest. In fact, every pound of muscle burns another 30 to 50kcal a day. Walking helps a bit, but resistance training helps even more.

● **Don't starve yourself** Cutting out too many calories can backfire in more ways than one. If you try to subsist on morsels, your metabolism will slow down so much that you'll not only stop losing weight, but you'll be lucky to be able to drag yourself away from the sofa.

● **Increase the protein in your diet** There is some evidence that if you increase your protein intake to the upper end of the recommended range (roughly 20 per cent of overall calories), the amount of energy you expend at rest will remain the same even while you're losing weight. Normally, as you lose weight, your body adjusts and you burn fewer calories at rest.

● **Fidget** People who drum their fingers or bounce their knees burn as much as 500kcal a day. That could help you to lose 0.5kg (1lb) a week.

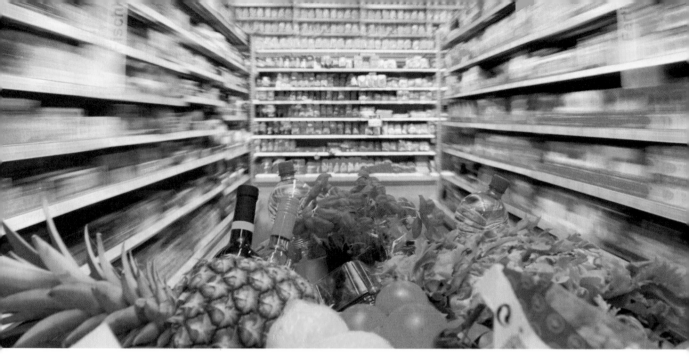

SHOPPING **KNOW-HOW**

Healthy eating starts with wise shopping. Aim to keep your fridge and larder well stocked, so that there is less temptation to resort to fast food and takeaways, and learn what to look for on a product's nutrition label to ensure that you're getting the healthiest ingredients.

● **Spend some time in the condiment aisle** With the following ingredients you have the basis for tasty sauces, low-fat marinades and low-salt flavourings – and you can stay away from the less-healthy ingredients such as mayonnaise, butter and creamy salad dressings: relishes, chutneys and barbecue sauces (look for sugar-free varieties), horseradish, mustards, flavoured vinegars, extra-virgin olive oil and pesto sauces, jars of olives, capers, sun-dried tomatoes, anchovies, roasted red peppers, Worcestershire sauce, chilli sauce, hot pepper sauce, soy sauce, sesame oil, walnut oil, teriyaki sauce and jars of salsa.

● **Buy rapeseed oil instead of vegetable oil** It's rich in healthy monounsaturated fatty acids and contains the essential fatty acids (EFAs) alpha-linolenic acid (ALNA) and linoleic acid (LA). It also costs less than olive oil.

● **Shop with a list** Organize your shopping list to reflect the different areas of the supermarket. This will allow you to progress quickly through the shop. By sticking rigidly to a well-planned shopping list, you can resist the seductive call of junk-food aisles, thereby saving your family and yourself from an overload of empty calories.

● **Choose wholemeal bread** Studies show that people who eat three or more servings of whole grains a day are less likely to suffer from diabetes. If your family will eat only white bread, choose a fibre-enriched variety.

● **Buy low-fat natural yoghurt and flavour it at home** Pre-flavoured yoghurts contain sugars that destroy any healthy benefits. If you add fruit at home, it will still taste good, plus you'll consume far fewer useless calories.

● **Buy fresh food** If more than half your usual shopping consists of pre-prepared foods, you need to redress the balance by opting for more fresh vegetables, fruit, seafood, unsweetened juices and dairy products.

● **Shop for food on a full stomach** Walking through a supermarket when you're hungry can have unhealthy results. If you can't arrange to shop shortly after a meal, eat an apple and drink a large glass of water before entering the shop.

● **Stock up on frozen vegetables** Frozen vegetables, which are often cheaper than unfrozen ones, can also be more nutritious. This is because they're flash-frozen within hours of picking, whereas some 'fresh' vegetables – particularly out-of-season varieties – have travelled hundreds or thousands of miles.

● **Try something new** Green soya beans (edamame), available frozen in most supermarkets, are nutritious, low in fat, high in protein and much easier and quicker to prepare than dried soya beans. A small 80g (3oz) helping counts as one of your 5-a-day portions. They can be used like peas in risottos and stir-fries, or as a tasty vegetable accompaniment.

THE LABELLING LINGO

Understanding the information on food packaging will make you better equipped to make healthy choices.

• **Fat** Low fat: less than 3 per cent fat (for example, 3g of fat per 100g/3½oz). Reduced fat: must contain at least 25 per cent less fat than the standard equivalent product.

• **Sugar** Reduced sugar: must contain at least 25 per cent less sugar than the standard equivalent. No added sugar: no additional sugars added as an ingredient. Remember that this doesn't necessarily mean a food will have low sugar as it may contain ingredients (such as fruit) that have a naturally high sugar content.

• **Fibre** High fibre: has at least 6g of fibre per 100g serving. Source of fibre: contains at least 3g of fibre per 100g serving.

• **Energy** Reduced calorie: must contain at least 25 per cent fewer calories than the standard equivalent. Be aware that reduced calorie doesn't necessarily mean the item in question is low in calories.

QUICK GUIDE TO FOOD LABELS

Labelling regulations stipulate that information must be given per 100g or 100ml, although many manufacturers now give information per serving. A note of caution: a manufacturer's idea of what constitutes a serving may be different from your own.

	High	Low
Fat	more than 20g	less than 3g
Saturated fat	more than 5g	less than 1.5g
Sugar	more than 15g	less than 5g
Salt	more than 1.5g	less than 0.3g

● **Stock up on tinned tomatoes** Crushed and stewed tomatoes contain higher amounts of the antioxidant lycopene than fresh ones. Warm up some tinned tomatoes with crushed garlic for a chunky pasta sauce; pour over chicken breasts and simmer; add to stews to provide flavour and extra nutrients.

READY MEALS **WISDOM**

These days, many of us stop at the supermarket on our way home, not for raw ingredients but for ready-prepared or 'home-cooked' meals that simply need to be put in the microwave for a few minutes. They are called 'ready meals', and they come in all varieties and qualities. Here are some guidelines for making healthy choices.

● **Look for sandwiches made from whole-grain bread** When choosing sandwiches, check the ingredients before buying. A particularly healthy choice is whole-grain bread, chicken or turkey filling, with lots of vegetables such as tomato, lettuce, peppers and cucumber, and just a small amount of spread.

● **Grab a tin of beans** When you get home, add the beans to the selection of salads you've just bought. You'll have made an economical choice (because beans are so filling) while adding valuable fibre and other nutrients to the salad.

● **Pick up a rotisserie chicken** Serve it with a salad, some instant brown rice and a couple of sliced tomatoes – and you've got a healthy, easy, barely-have-to-cook it meal.

● **But remove the skin . . .** Much of the internal fat from a rotisserie chicken drips out in the cooking, but the skin still holds quite a bit of fat.

● **Turn your pasta salad into a main meal** Grill some skinless chicken breasts, cut them into strips and add to a ready-made pasta salad. Toss in some fresh broccoli, peppers and tomatoes with low-fat dressing, and you've got an easy and healthy main course.

● **Go for sushi** Low in fat, sushi is one of the healthiest choices you can make when popping into your supermarket to buy dinner, and many shops now stock a good selection. If you can't stand the thought of raw fish, all is not lost. Plenty of shops offer cooked-fish sushi or even vegetable-only sushi.

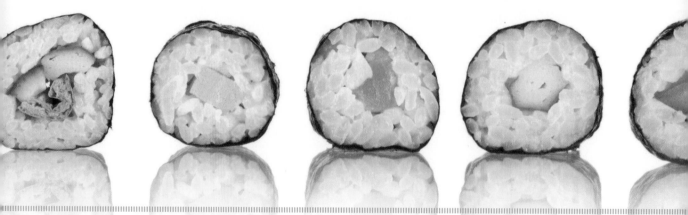

Go Mediterranean
Buy two packets of wholemeal couscous for cooking in the microwave (put boiling water in a Pyrex measuring jug, add the couscous, cover with a plate and let it steam). When the couscous is ready, add pre-prepared roasted vegetables, a tin of chickpeas, a sprinkling of feta cheese, sliced black olives and a drizzle of olive oil. Now you've got a gorgeous Mediterranean salad that's great for outdoor eating in summer.

● **Buy prepared foods that you don't have time to make** If you buy pre-prepared food to save time, buy only those things you don't have time to make. The less you buy pre-made, the more control you have over what you're eating.

So choose a low-calorie stew, by all means, but also go to the fresh food department for a potato to microwave instead of using fried or roast potatoes, and add some spinach that you can quickly steam or some colourful fresh salad ingredients.

● **Always think vegetables** How are you going to get vegetables into your meal? If you don't want to cook, pick up a selection of ready-prepared raw salad vegetables. But remember that while pre-washed leaves make salad preparation as complicated as finding a bowl, it's always better and tastier to prepare your own from fresh.

● **Get two meals at a time** Again, you're trying to save time. So that whole roasted chicken you got for tonight can double as a chicken Caesar salad tomorrow night. If you're making a bowl of couscous to go with your takeaway dinner tonight, double the amount and pick up some extra vegetables and feta cheese for a Mediterranean salad the following night. Or perhaps for lunch tomorrow.

● **Choose prepared soups made with vegetables** Minestrone, lentil soup and black-bean soup are good examples of prepared soups to which little fat is added. However, avoid creamy or cheesy soups such as broccoli and cheese or cream of asparagus. If you're not sure, check the composition of the soup stock. The best soup base is vegetable broth, followed by chicken broth, then beef stock and, finally, cream.

● **Go easy on the mayonnaise** Instead of buying ready-prepared coleslaw that is drenched in mayonnaise, buy a packet of shredded vegetables used to make coleslaw and drizzle on fat-free Italian dressing when you're ready to eat. For a lower-fat alternative to mayonnaise for summer salads, simply mix equal quantities of mayonnaise with fat-free Greek yoghurt.

great idea!

Have an indoor picnic for dinner
For a fresh take on healthy eating, buy a loaf of whole-grain bread, a punnet of strawberries, a favourite low-fat cheese, some thinly sliced roast beef or turkey, a small tub of olives, pre-cooked prawns, cherry tomatoes, pre-sliced green or red peppers and bite-sized carrots. When you get home, put it all on the table and – after cleaning the fruit and veg as necessary – declare that dinner is served. This type of 'grazing' dinner is fun, easy and makes an enjoyable change.

8 great ways to make cooking fun & easier

Healthy eating depends on knowing the ingredients of your meals and how they have been prepared. This is much simpler if you do your own cooking rather than relying on prepared food, but many of us need to go back to basics to regain the cooking habit.

1 MAKE YOUR KITCHEN A PLACE YOU LIKE TO BE

Is there music playing? Is the evening sun shining through the window? Are the knives sharp, the vegetables fresh, the pots good quality, the worktops clutter-free? All of these factors will contribute to your desire to make good food.

2 ENJOY COOKING

Cooking is a pleasure – and far easier than many non-cooks realize. For the sake of your health, your pleasure and your wallet, aim to learn – or relearn – the joys of cooking. Spend time with your friends and family while they cook so that you can absorb the methods and routines. Consider taking a class, or buy an introductory cookbook. Most of all, lose your fear. It is harder to be a bad cook than a good cook, particularly if you use good ingredients.

3 KEEP YOUR KITCHEN TIDY

Families tend to congregate in the kitchen, bringing with them newspapers, schoolwork, post, toys and other things. Don't allow it. Set a new policy: the kitchen is for cooking and eating only. Why? It's hard to get motivated about cooking if you have to clean up a mess first, not to mention what it does to your mood.

4 PLAN A WEEK'S WORTH OF DINNERS

Planning ahead takes just a few minutes. Every Friday night or Saturday morning, sit down with a pad of paper and your favourite cookbooks or cookery magazines. Think about what's in your freezer and fridge, what your family likes to eat, what the coming week entails. Then plan out a week's worth of menus (you can always leave one night for takeaway pizzas). At the same time, write out your shopping list.

5 DELEGATE, DELEGATE

If you have children aged ten-plus or another adult who gets home before you do, get them started on dinner. For example, you might ask your teenager to start chopping vegetables for the salad and fill the pasta pan with water, and your younger child to gather ingredients for a given recipe and put them on the worktop for you. Involving your children from a young age will make them more interested in nutritious food and encourage them to try new things.

6 STOCK YOUR FREEZER

Stews and soups freeze wonderfully, so it's worth cooking them in bulk for the freezer so that you always have a few meals in reserve.

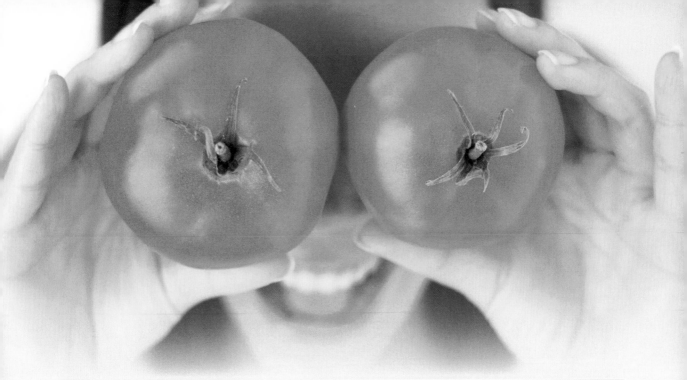

7 ADD EXTRA FRUIT AND VEGETABLES

Here are two simple ways to increase your and your family's intake of fruit and vegetables:

• Purée a few handfuls of lightly sautéed mixed vegetables, such as onions, celery, red peppers, cauliflower or carrots. Then stir this into sauces, stews and soups to add extra flavour, along with a healthy dose of vitamins and antioxidants.

• Replace half the fat in cake recipes with apple or prune purée. Allow about 5 tablespoons of water for every 100g (3½ oz) cooked apples or soaked, pitted prunes, and blend to make the purée. Or, to create a quick dessert, simply add the purée to yoghurt.

8 REPLACE THE CREAM IN SAUCES

When you're making beef stroganoff or a creamy pasta sauce, use Greek yoghurt or fromage frais instead of cream. Either option will provide the same rich taste for far fewer calories and much less fat.

creative ways with **vegetables**

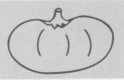

Cooking is always more fun when it involves a bit of creativity, and it's especially rewarding when your know that the meal you've cooked is healthy as well as delicious. Here are three slightly unusual vegetable dishes to inspire you.

• **SERVE CELERIAC** instead of mashed potatoes or white rice as a side dish. Peel it and slice it into chunks, drizzle with olive oil, then roast in a hot oven until soft. Or boil it and mash with seasoning and a little olive oil.

• **SUBSTITUTE SWEET POTATOES** for potatoes. Peel them, slice into bite-size chunks, then boil until soft and mash with seasoning and olive oil. Alternatively, roast them (as for celeriac above), or make sweet potato wedges as a healthy change from chips — peel and slice the sweet potatoes into wedges, parboil them, then drain and coat with a little olive oil and fajita or spicy seasoning before baking in a hot oven for 15 to 20 minutes.

• **CUT AN AUBERGINE** in two down the middle and stuff each half with tomatoes. Top with slices of Parmesan, drizzle with olive oil, wrap in foil, then bake or grill until softened.

RESTAURANT CHOICES

For all-round healthy eating, you need to control what you eat when you're not at home. Whether you are dining out at a major national chain or a locally owned family restaurant, following a few tips will guarantee you an enjoyable meal while keeping your health goals firmly in view.

● **Drink water throughout the meal** Drinking water slows down the rate at which you eat, helps you to enjoy the food more, and gets the message to your brain that you're full – before your plate is empty. If you are not given a jug of water automatically, ask for one as you order.

● **Be assertive** It's no time to be meek when you are dining out. Assert yourself by requesting changes to what's on the menu. For instance, if an item is fried, ask if you can have it grilled or baked. If it comes with chips, request a side order of vegetables instead.

● **Skip dessert** You can always have some fruit or even a small piece of chocolate at home. That's much healthier than a rich chocolate Black Forest gateau or a mountain of ice cream topped by a second mountain of whipped cream. Plus, it will save you money.

Read between the lines
Any menu description that uses the words creamy, breaded, crisp or stuffed is likely to be full of hidden fats – much of it comprising saturated or even trans fats. Other words to beware of include buttery, sautéed, pan-fried and au gratin.

did you know?

● **Try to be the first to order** Studies show that people are often unduly influenced by their companions' choices when they eat out. If you order first, you're not as likely to be tempted by the less healthy options on the menu.

● **Ignore the bread basket** Don't fill up on bread while waiting for other food to be served.

● **Order a salad first** American scientists found that volunteers who ate a large salad before the main course ate fewer calories overall than those who didn't have a first-course salad.

● **Choose two starters** Before ordering, look around at what others are eating. If portions appear to be huge, why not go for two starters rather than a main course? You'll cut back on both calories and cost.

● **Keep an eye on wine-glass refills** If you're drinking wine, don't let the waiter fill up your glass before it's empty. If your glass is constantly being topped up, you can't keep track of how much you've had.

● **Order fish** Fish is a good low-fat, low-salt option, but it should be cooked as plainly as possible – steamed, baked, barbecued or grilled, but preferably not fried. Avoid sauce, if possible.

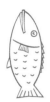 Fish is a good low-fat, low-salt option, but it should be cooked as plainly as possible – steamed, baked, barbecued or grilled, but preferably not fried

LEAN CUISINE **ITALIAN**

• Split and share. One order of pasta is often enough for two people, especially if you also have a salad.
• Dine on pasta rather than pizza – it's much less calorie-dense. You can increase the health benefits by ordering a side dish of fresh vegetables or spinach and mixing it in with your pasta dish.
• Pick tomato-based sauces such as marinara, bolognese or puttanesca. Avoid cream-based sauces such as alfredo and primavera.
• Do without garlic bread. Instead, ask for a dish of olive oil and plain bread, and dip.
• Order antipasti with extra chickpeas, olives, fagioli (beans), lettuce, tomatoes and other vegetables, and fewer meats and cheeses.

LEAN CUISINE **CHINESE**

• Order fewer dishes than there are people at the table. Chinese starters are designed for sharing.
• Eat with chopsticks. You'll get less of the high-calorie, high-salt sauce that way.
• Start with soup to fill you up.
• Avoid fried starters, such as spring rolls.
• Choose steamed rice rather than fried.
• Use the 2:1 ratio. Eat twice as much rice as main dish.
• Avoid menu items described as crispy, golden-brown or sweet and sour. They are all deep-fried.

LEAN CUISINE **INDIAN**

• Skip the starters – most are fried.
• Avoid chapati, naan and roti breads. They've all been fried or soaked in fat. A better bet is poppadoms, which are often made from lentil flour – but check that they have been baked rather than deep-fried.
• Order side dishes with vegetables, beans or peas, such as dhal or chutney.
• Look for the healthy dishes: chicken masala, prawn bhuna, fish vindaloo and tandoori (baked) options. Avoid dishes made with ghee (clarified butter).
• Choose a vegetarian main course.
• Ask what kind of oil is used in cooking. If it's coconut, ask if they can use rapeseed oil instead. Coconut oil is nearly all saturated fat.

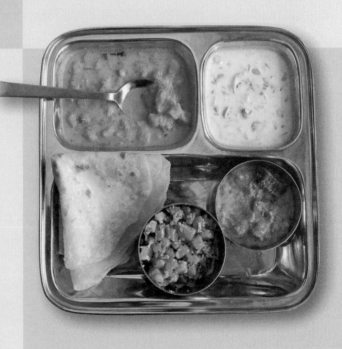

FAST FOOD &
TAKEAWAYS

The amount of fat in a fast-food meal can be stunning. Burgers, chips, 'special sauces' made from mayonnaise, even salads swimming in dressings – all of them are your worst dietary enemies. Some producers are changing their approach, however, offering salads that actually fill you up, smaller portions and healthier options.

● **Never supersize** Even McDonald's is now phasing out some supersized items.

● **In fact, order a child's meal** A small burger, a small serving of chips and an orange juice is a surprisingly filling meal for most adults and has many fewer calories than the adult version.

● **Avoid sweet-and-sour dishes** These meals should be a rare treat – one portion may contain as much as 8 teaspoons of sugar. That includes lemon chicken and some spicy beef dishes. Chicken with cashew nuts or peppers, stir-fried noodles and seafood dishes are all healthier, especially if you have boiled rice or noodles rather than egg fried rice.

● **Choose diet drinks** If you want a fizzy drink, choose a diet one. A large non-diet cola contains 210kcal, so making this one change could save you the same number of calories as the meal you're about to eat.

● **Go for salad, minus fried toppings** Although most fast-food restaurants offer decent-sized salads, if you top them with fried chicken, cheese and lots of dressing, you end up with as much artery-clogging saturated fat as if you'd had the double cheeseburger and chips. Instead, choose grilled or roast chicken as your protein source, skip the croutons, and ask for the low-fat dressing – then use only half.

● **Say no to the 'special' sauce** Many takeaway sauces consist of dressed-up mayonnaise, overflowing with fat and calories. The healthiest topping for your chicken, fish or burger is mustard (few calories, lots of flavour). The second best is ketchup (no fat, but plenty of sugar). Other good choices include vinaigrette (in moderation) and spicy sauces.

● **Ask for extra onions, lettuce and tomatoes** Whatever sandwich you choose, it'll now be healthier, crunchier and more filling. And it adds one more serving of vegetables to your day's quota.

● **Skip the cheese** Craving a burger? Then just get a plain one without the cheese. For instance, at McDonald's that will save you 50kcal, 40 of them from fat, including 2g of saturated fat.

● **Look for ways to add fibre** That means a baked potato including skin and chilli (but no cheese), bean burritos and tacos instead of meat (a bean burrito has 12g of fibre – roughly half your daily needs), and baked beans and corn on the cob (without butter) as side dishes.

● **Look for the words 'grilled', 'baked' or 'chargrilled'** If something is cooked in one of those ways, it's not fried – and you'll automatically be reaping some savings in terms of fat and calories.

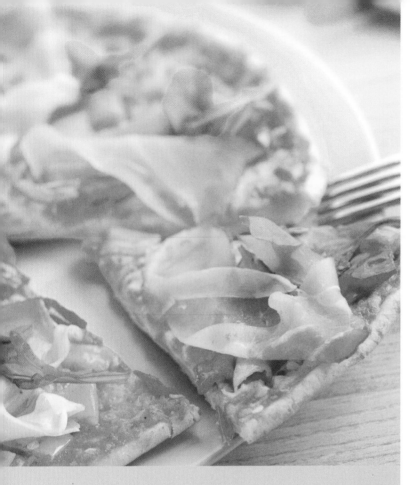

A HEALTHIER **PIZZA**

Although pizza is not the healthiest food you could choose, there's no reason to cut it out of your life entirely. It offers a quick, easy, tasty way to get loads of vegetables and fibre. But pizza, like any other takeaway food, has its negative aspects. An American scientific study that evaluated pizza slices from the top chains found fat levels approaching, and sometimes surpassing, a fast-food cheeseburger. The main culprit was far too much cheese. Add to that fatty meat such as sausage and pepperoni and you are in the unhealthiest reaches of the food world. Here's how to make pizza a healthier delight:

• Order half-fat cheese or no cheese.

• Ask for extra vegetables.

• Avoid pizzas with names such as Meat Feast or Pepperoni Special. In fact, order your toppings individually.

• Instead of the same old pepperoni and onions, do your health and digestion a favour and ask for the artichoke hearts, broccoli, hot peppers and other exotic vegetables that many takeaway pizza places now offer.

● **Stay away from coconut milk** Some cuisines, such as Thai, use a lot of coconut milk as a base, which is high in saturated fat. A healthier option at a Thai takeaway is to start with a soup such as tom yam, beef or chicken satay or Thai fish cakes, and follow up with a chicken, pork or fish-based noodle dish.

● **Try a drier style of curry** Some of the drier Indian takeaway options, such as tandoori, tikka and bhuna dishes, are usually the lower-fat options on the menu. Other healthier choices include vegetable and shellfish-based curries and dishes such as sag aloo (spinach and potato) and mutter paneer (peas with cheese) and baltis.

● **Go for skinless chicken** By not eating the skin, you'll save 240kcal and 16g of fat.

● **Choose chicken, not doner** Research by Dr Tom Sanders, Professor of Nutrition at King's College, London, showed that, of nine types of takeaway foods tested, doner kebabs were the outright loser. These kebabs were found to contain far more trans fats than any other takeaway meal. If you fancy a kebab, choose a chicken skewer instead and pile on the salad.

● **Avoid processed or cured meats** These include hot dogs, salami and ham. These heavily processed meats are often full of fat, salt, chemical additives and, in some cases, sugar. At a deli or sandwich shop, go for turkey breast, chicken breast or roast beef instead.

● **Have a snack before you order** Have an apple, banana or fat-free yoghurt before you go for your takeaway. That way, you won't arrive starving.

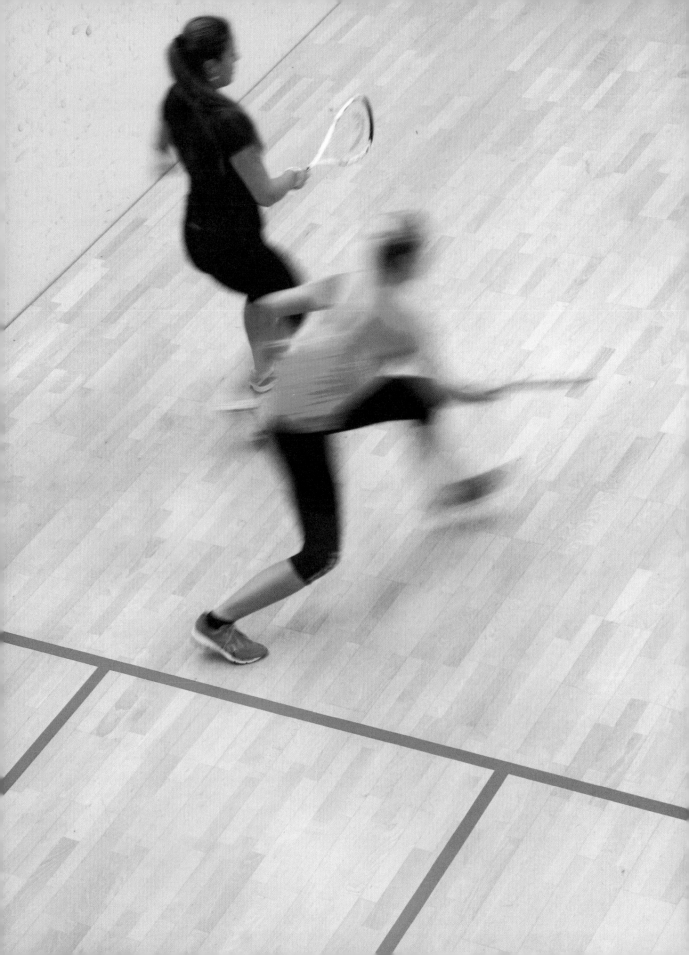

MOVE
your body

Our bodies were made to move and so it's not surprising that getting active is one of the very best things you can do for your health and wellbeing. Simply by increasing the number of steps you take each day, you can improve your blood-pressure and cholesterol levels and cut your risk heart disease and diabetes.

Building stronger muscles brings other benefits, too, as muscle burns up to 15 times more calories per day than fat; strong muscles also protect your joints and back. Then there's the mental boost – all in all, every reason to read on and kick-start your get up and go.

BEST WAYS TO **GET FIT**
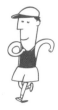

If you want to be fitter, the first step is to devise an exercise programme that suits your needs. Consider how you can integrate calorie-burning activities into your daily life and get the most benefit from them. Tell your friends and family about the fitness goals you are setting yourself and encourage them to check up on how you're doing.

● **Walk to control your body weight**
It may seem unlikely that such a low-key exercise as walking would have much effect on weight. But, in one major study, a group of sedentary people were given a daily goal of 10,000 steps of brisk activity, as measured by their pedometers. They improved their fitness levels as much as a group that followed a traditional gym-based aerobic routine. Overall, studies find that getting 8,000 to 10,000 steps a day (about 5 miles or 8km) helps you to lose weight, while adding to that another 2,000 steps (an extra 1 mile or 1.6km a day) helps you to maintain your current weight and stop gaining weight.

try it... **Develop the activity habit** Here are a few ways to be more active, and burn more calories, in everyday life.
• Stand up and walk around whenever you are speaking on the phone.
• Always take the stairs rather than the escalator or lift.
• When you take the stairs, try striding up two steps at a time.
• Stand up and move around during every television ad.
• Routinely stretch your arms, legs and back at intervals during the day.
• Carry more things more often – garden plants and supplies, groceries, washing. But be careful not to lift too much and strain your muscles.

● **Talk to your doctor** Busy GPs are more likely to want to discuss immediate ailments than ways to improve your general health, so you may have to be bold and ask for advice about getting fit. Surveys have shown that just 3 hours of counselling by GPs or other healthcare professionals over a period of two years can help to transform the physical health of many former couch-potatoes.

● **Exercise with a friend** Many people find it more fun to exercise with a friend than to go it alone. You can support each other and offer mutual encouragement. You could run, walk, cycle or go to the gym or a dance class together. The important thing is that the fitness activity becomes a regular commitment that you both want to sustain.

● **Measure what's important**
There are so many ways to measure fitness that it's hard to decide what matters. Weight? Body mass index (BMI)? Pulse? Is it mileage covered, calories burned or minutes of activity? For maximum motivation, focus on what concerns you most. Do you look or feel better than you used to? Do your clothes feel looser? Can you see a difference? Have other people noticed improvements?

Intensity is key to success

A study by exercise gurus at McMaster University in Ontario, Canada, found that intense exercise for a total of 6 minutes a week could provide the same physical benefits as longer periods of more moderate exercise. The 6 minutes were spread over three exercise sessions that also included some recovery time.

The researchers compared 'sprinters' – who did up to seven 30-second bursts of all-out cycling on exercise bikes three times a week for two weeks – with 'moderates', who did 4 minutes of regular cycling three times a week over the same period. All-in-all, the 'sprinters' achieved similar results to the 'moderates' but spent around 20 per cent less time exercising to achieve it (about 1¼ hours compared with 5¼ hours).

● Use music to pump up the pace

Programme your iPod or other portable music player to start with slow-moving music, followed by something a little faster and more vibrant, gradually building up to a burst of rapid-fire dance music. Studies show that this can help you to work harder and for longer than if you listen to either fast or slow music, or if you move from a fast piece to something slower paced. Research has also revealed that listening to music while walking can help people to cover more miles in a given timespan.

● Do it in the morning

Don't think about it. Just roll out of bed, brush your teeth, put some clothes on and get going. Extensive research has shown that you are far more likely to get serious exercise if you do it first thing. Later in the day, exercise may be over-stimulating and you may find it harder to sleep that night.

● Begin with a warm-up

Before you stretch or do any other exercise, warming up should be an integral part of your routine. It increases blood flow, bringing oxygen and nutrients to the working muscles and joints, and makes them looser, more pliable and less susceptible to injury. It also prepares your mind and body for activity.

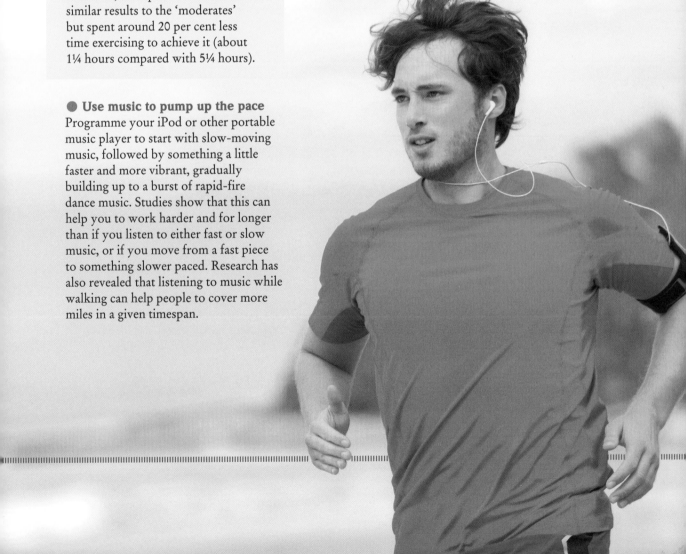

WOMEN AND WORKOUTS

Most hints and tips relating to exercise apply to both sexes – but, when it comes to getting more out of workouts, there are certain issues that are particularly relevant to women.

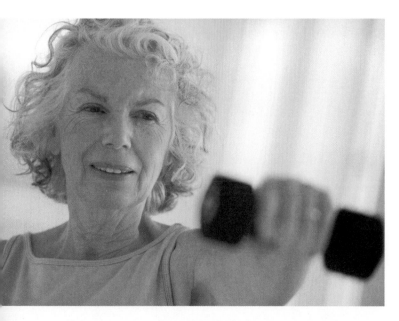

● **Time your exercise to your menstrual cycle** If you're in the latter part of your menstrual cycle, that's an excellent reason for an energetic work-out on the step machine. A study by the University of Adelaide in Australia found that women who exercise at this time of the month, when levels of oestrogen and progesterone are at their highest, burn more fat for energy, which leads to weight loss and less exercise-related fatigue.

● **Ignore the mirrors at gyms** The designers of fitness clubs often install mirrors in exercise rooms. These may be useful to monitor your technique, but looking at yourself can have a negative effect. One study found that women who exercised in front of a mirror felt less calm and more tired after 30 minutes of working out than those who exercised without mirrors.

● **You can be both healthy and heavy** Many women think they are too heavy to benefit from exercising; others get discouraged when they don't see significant weight loss after weeks of exercise. But the most important benefit of exercise is keeping your heart healthy. And research shows that the amount of activity you get, not your weight, is the chief predictor of heart disease.

● **Check your iron levels** A study at Cornell University in the USA found that women with low levels of iron in their blood – but not low enough to be classified as anaemic – find it harder to maintain an exercise regime than women with normal levels. If you suspect that this applies to you, consult your GP, who may prescribe a daily supplement of 100mg of iron, which can double the exercise endurance level of women who are slightly deficient in iron. But note that this is prescription-strength iron, which should be taken only on medical advice. Good sources of dietary iron include red meat and eggs. Drinking citrus juice with meals will improve absorption from iron-rich foods such as green leafy vegetables.

● **Find the right teacher** If you want a motivating exercise class, find a teacher with whom you feel relaxed – someone who, like most of us, looks as though they need to exercise to look their best.

6 essential warm-up exercises

Warming up before exercise is an important first step that is sometimes ignored. It prepares your body for the demands of activity – muscles and joints will not respond as easily while cold. This routine should take no more than 5 minutes and, if you are in a hurry, you can choose just a few of the exercises.

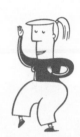

1 SIDE STEP

Stand tall with your feet together and your arms by your sides. As you sway gently to your right, step your right leg to the side and allow your left leg to follow, so that you are standing with your feet together again. Repeat the movement on the other side: sway gently to your left, with your left leg stepping and your right leg following. Continue stepping in this way for at least 2 minutes.

2 ANKLE CIRCLES

Stand with your feet together and your weight evenly distributed over both legs. As you push the toes of your right foot into the floor, lift your right heel. Using your toes as a pivot, circle your ankle ten times in a clockwise direction and ten times in an anti-clockwise direction. Repeat the exercise with the left foot.

3 KNEE CIRCLES

Bring your feet together, bend slightly forward and gently place your hands just above your knees. Bend your knees a little and slowly circle the knees ten times in one direction, using your hands for support. Repeat the exercise ten times in the opposite direction.

4 HIP CIRCLES

Bring your feet together, bend slightly forward and gently place your hands just above your knees. Bend your knees a little and slowly circle the knees ten times in one direction, using your hands for support. Repeat ten times in the opposite direction.

5 ARM RAISE AND TWIST

Stand with your feet together and your arms hanging down in front of you with the fingers of your two hands interlocked. Inhale and raise your arms above your head, turning the palms upwards as you do so. Twist your torso smoothly from the waist to face to the right. Take three or four normal breaths before turning to face forwards again. Repeat the exercise by twisting to the left.

6 SHAKE

Gently shake your hands, keeping your wrists and fingers loose. Do this about 20 times. Then, keeping your hands, elbows and shoulders relaxed, shake your whole arms about 20 times. Finally, let your whole body bounce up and down around 20 times, keeping the limbs loose and relaxed.

HOW TO GET THE EXERCISE HABIT

As with other health benefits, effective exercise depends on making subtle changes to your daily lifestyle and then sustaining them. There are many different ways to do this. Isometric exercises, for example, can be extremely helpful, particularly for people who have a limited range of motion – and you can do them any time and anywhere.

● **Practise proper posture** By making an effort to stand 'tall', you contract dozens of muscles from your legs up to your neck. This burns calories and builds muscle. Whether you're ironing, doing dishes or queuing at the bank, concentrate on keeping a solid foot stance, a slight bend in your knees, an open chest, with shoulders depressed and head up. Another secret workout: imagine you're squeezing a pencil between your shoulder blades and you have to hold the muscles tight so that the pencil doesn't fall. It doesn't take long before the muscles in your back start to tire.

Every time you realign your posture, or sit or stand a bit taller, you are exercising your back and core muscles.

● **Get outdoors** One of the best indications of a fit lifestyle is how much time you spend outdoors. Even if you are just walking, gardening or washing the car, you are likely to be more active than you would be indoors. So step outside for at least 3 hours every weekend. Best of all, once you get used to spending time outdoors, you'll soon be hankering after more active pursuits.

try it...

Office workout
If you spend most of your working life sitting at a desk, devote 10 minutes each day to building up your physical resistance. Here are some arm exercises to try.

• **Desk curl** Place your palms against the underside of your desk with your elbows bent. Push up into the desk with your palms, as if trying to lift the desk off the floor. Hold for a count of five, release, then repeat.

• **Desk push** Place your palms against the top of the desk with your elbows bent. Press into the desktop with all your might. Hold for a count of five, release, then repeat.

• **Desk push-up** Stand half a metre away from the desk. Keep your feet in place and lean forward from your ankles, placing your palms on top of the desk. Your body should form a straight line from ankles to head. Bend your elbows as you lower your chest towards the desk. Straighten your elbows as you push away. Keep your elbows close to your sides all the time.

● **Lengthen and speed up your stride while walking** You should aim to do this not just occasionally, but all the time. Become a high-energy walker – fast, confident, with good posture and healthy arm swinging. This small adjustment will burn extra calories and give you stronger legs and a shapelier bottom.

● **Squeeze hard** Your gluteus maximus is the biggest of the three gluteal muscles in your buttocks. Exercise it. Whether you're standing or sitting, an invisible buttock squeeze (tighten, hold for 2 seconds, release) repeated 10 to 15 times, one to three times a day, tightens the muscle and burns calories.

● **Exercise as you do the laundry** Whether waiting for the cycle to end or folding clothes, fit in some leg work. Try performing ten or so plié squats (think ballerina). Place your heels shoulder width apart and rotate your toes out to a 45-degree angle. Drop into a squat, keeping your knees in line with your toes and make sure your head, shoulders and hips are aligned. Return to the starting position, squeezing the muscles in your buttocks as you stand tall.

● **Play games with your children** Instead of always watching your kids play sports, join in. Chasing and catching games can be great fun; your children will love it and you'll burn plenty of calories.

ISOMETRIC **EXERCISES**

In isometric exercises, muscles are tensed without movement. For example, pushing as hard as you can against a brick wall is an isometric exercise, because neither you nor the wall moves. The rule is to hold the tension for 5 to 10 seconds, then relax for a few seconds. Repeat five to eight times. Here are some examples

• Tense your abdominal muscles.

• Hold your hands in front of you, as if praying, and press firmly together.

• Stand with your legs apart about a foot from a wall. Push against the wall with your hands as if you were trying to move it.

• Stand inside a doorway and, starting with your arms straight down by your sides, put the backs of your hands against either side of the door frame. Push your hands against the doorway as hard as you can, as if trying to widen the space.

• While still inside the doorway, lift up your arms above your head and put your palms against the frame on either side. Push your palms against the frame, as if you were trying to lift the building.

• Sit down in a chair, feet flat on the ground. Push your legs into the ground as hard as you can.

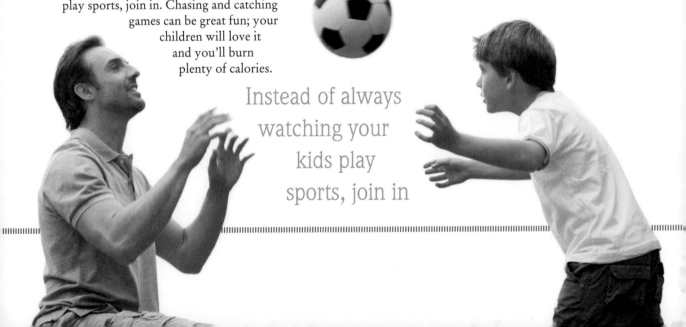

Instead of always watching your kids play sports, join in

WALKING YOUR
WAY TO FITNESS

It's so simple and convenient that it couldn't possibly count as exercise, right? Wrong. Study after study shows that regular moderate walking can help you to lose weight and reduce your risk of heart disease. This section of the book offers a wonderful variety of ways both to get more walking into your life and to reap the benefits from every step.

● **Walk for entertainment once a week** Instead of walking around your neighbourhood, walk around a zoo, an art museum, or a shopping centre. You could even try walking around them twice – first at a brisk pace and then more slowly to take in the sights.

● **Make a commitment** If you have a friend to meet, you're more likely to get out of bed on cold winter mornings or skip the cafeteria for a lunchtime walk. If one of you backs out for any reason, put £1 in a kitty. If you manage to build up a substantial sum, donate it to charity.

● **Explore on your walks** You can walk anywhere at any time, from your neighbourhood to your local shops to a local nature trail. But rather than walking the same old route every day, use your walks as a way to experience and explore the great outdoors. Varying your route and terrain will do more than keep you mentally engaged. It will also help you to target different leg muscles.

● **Aim for 10,000 steps a day** Don't let that number scare you. Most people walk about 5,500 to 7,500 steps during an average day as they amble to and from meetings, to the water cooler, to the postbox. In fact, researchers in the field consider 5,000 steps a day a 'sedentary lifestyle'. Studies have found that you should be able to cover 7,499 steps a day without participating in formal sports or exercise. If you reach 10,000 steps a day, you're considered 'active', while 12,500 steps a day earns you the title of 'highly active'.

Using a pedometer, find your baseline of how many steps you normally take in a day. Then, increase that amount by at least 200 steps a day until you reach 10,000 to 12,500 daily steps.

great idea!

Use a pedometer
These nifty gadgets measure how far you've walked in steps and miles or kilometres. They provide motivation by spurring you to meet a particular goal and showing you if you've met it. And research shows that they work. In one American study of 510 people, those who wore a pedometer automatically increased the amount of steps they took in a day. Most pedometers hook onto your belt and are small and easy to use.

Walking can reduce the dangers of obesity In a study published in *Diabetes Research in Clinical Practice*, Japanese researchers tested obese men before and after they joined a one-year modest walking plan. All they did was increase the number of steps they took during their daily activities. The result: their blood pressure and cholesterol levels improved and the amount of body fat around their abdomen – the dangerous kind that leads to higher rates of heart disease and diabetes – significantly decreased.

● **Take your dog with you (or get a dog)** There's nothing more effective than a set of puppy-dog eyes to get you out of your armchair and through the door. Once dogs get used to walks, they look forward to them and will give you a gentle nudge (or annoying whine) on the days you try to get out of it. If you don't have a dog, offer to walk a neighbour's dog twice a week. The commitment will keep you motivated.

● **Discover dog-agility classes** In addition to walking locally, consider signing up for a dog agility class. Try the Kennel Club for more information. During the class, you and your dog will circumvent a course with see-saws, hurdles, tunnels and other obstacles. (Your dog tackles the obstacles. You run or walk alongside and issue commands.) Both you and your dog will get a great workout and you'll end up with a better-behaved and calmer dog as a result.

LEARN **THE BASICS**

For walking to count as exercise, you need to walk at a pace that has you breathing heavily but still able to speak without too much effort.

● Your goal, first and foremost, is to walk five days a week, 30 minutes a walk. Do that, and you are getting the base-level amount of exercise that research says should maintain your health and vigour.

● Don't assume you can reach that goal quickly. During the first week, walk for as long as feels comfortable, even if it's just to the postbox and back. Each subsequent week, increase that amount by no more than 10 per cent.

● Start every walk with 5 minutes of easy-paced walking, about the same pace at which you'd do your grocery shopping, to get your body warmed up. Then, cool down at the end of each walk with another 5 minutes of easy-paced walking. This allows your heart rate to speed up and slow down gradually.

● When you reach your target of 30 minutes a day, five days a week, set a new target. Either increase further the time you spend walking or consider whether your are ready for new activities, such as strength-building exercises twice a week.

● **Pump up the volume** In a study published in the journal *Chest*, people with severe respiratory disease who listened to music while walking covered 4 miles more during the eight-week study than a similar group who walked without listening to music. Researchers speculate that the music made the participants less aware of any shortness of breath and distracted them from possible boredom and fatigue. It's something everyone can enjoy. Carry an iPod and play your favourite tunes, or invest in a portable DAB radio.

TOP TIPS FOR IMPROVING YOUR WALKING POSTURE

Proper posture will reduce discomfort as you walk and help you to burn more fat and calories.

• Stand tall with your spine elongated and breastbone lifted. This allows room for your lungs to expand fully.

• Keep your head straight with your eyes focused forward and shoulders relaxed. Avoid slumping your shoulders forward or hunching them towards your ears.

• Roll your feet from heel to toe. As you speed up, take smaller, more frequent steps. This protects your knees and gives your bottom a good workout.

• Allow your arms to swing freely.

• Firm your tummy and flatten your back as you walk to prevent lower back pain. Hold in your lower stomach around your waistband. Make sure that you continue to breathe normally.

● **Periodically increase the pace** Boredom can quickly bring a walk to a premature end. Keep your mind and your body engaged by increasing the pace or challenging yourself by trudging up a hill from time to time. Every 10 to 15 minutes, complete a 2 to 3 minute surge. During your surge, try to catch a real or imaginary walker ahead of you.

great idea!

Walk to fund-raise There are many charities in the UK, including the Samaritans and Marie Curie Cancer Care, that regularly stage fund-raising walks. You'll need to find sponsors but you'll take pride in the fact that you're walking for something beyond yourself, which will motivate you to go longer and faster. After every walk, mark the amount that you've raised on a chart: it will encourage you to do more.

● **Take the family** If you take the family with you on your daily walks, not only will you be exhibiting good fitness habits for your children, but you'll also be able to supervise them while you walk rather than getting a babysitter. If your children walk too slowly, ask them to ride their bikes or roller skate beside you. To keep everyone entertained, play your usual repertoire of long car-trip games such as I Spy. You can also try a treasure hunt, where you start out with a list of items to check off during your walk.

● **Walk and talk** Use a cordless phone and walk around the house or up and down the stairs as you chat with friends or conduct your business. This is a also a good way to make use of those long periods when you're left on hold. You get some heart-healthy exercise, and the exercise will help you to maintain your mental cool. Use your pedometer to count your steps and you will enjoy the added bonus of feeling as if you have accomplished something rather than wasting time.

● **Head for a pleasant area** Walking in the nicest part of town (or country) will encourage you to walk more often. When researchers from the University of Wollongong in New South Wales, Australia, asked people about their walking habits, they found that men who perceived their neighbourhood as 'aesthetic' were much more likely to walk there regularly. Other studies have found that localities with well-kept pavements and well-lit pedestrian areas encouraged more walking than localities that were badly maintained and poorly lit. In fact, one study found that people living in pleasant walkable areas walk an average of 70 minutes more each week than people in less attractive surroundings.

● **Walk around the office or house**
Are you stuck at your desk all day long, practically chained to your computer screen? Get up and walk around for 5 minutes every 2 hours at least. A brisk 5-minute walk every 2 hours adds up to an extra 20 minutes walking by the end of the working day. And getting a break will make you less likely to eat compulsively at your desk.

It's also a good idea to get up and walk around for a few minutes every hour or so if you are sitting for long periods of time at home reading, watching television or pursuing any other sedentary hobby.

● **Pick a charity and pledge to contribute a small sum for every mile that you walk** You will take pride in the fact that you are walking for something beyond yourself, which will motivate you to walk faster and for longer. After every walk, mark the amount you owe on a chart, then, when you reach your target amount, send off a cheque.

Alternatively, consider training for a charity event. Check at your local sports shop or on the internet for details of walks being held in your area. Generally fun runs ands sponsored walks raise money for good causes.

● **Walk when you shop** Online shopping is marvellous in terms of convenience, but it is pretty useless when it comes to burning calories.

By contrast, making the effort to go out shopping, walking to the shops if they're close enough and carrying your shopping back home, can burn about 200kcal an hour, which is much more than what you'd burn while sitting at your desk surfing the internet. You can increase the effectiveness of your walk by doing a circuit of the shopping centre between shop visits.

> **try it...**
>
> **Carry light weights on your walk**
> Take 1–2kg weights with you and periodically try some arm exercises as you walk. This will do more than increase the benefit of the workout. Carrying weights also builds muscle, and each pound of muscle burns about 30 to 50kcal more a day, even when you're relaxing.
>
> Another option is to try isometric exercises of the arms, chest and abdominal muscles using weights. For instance, as you walk, go through the action of throwing a punch in slow motion. As you extend your arm, tense the muscles along it and do the same as you retract it. You should feel tension in your triceps, biceps, deltoids and pectoral muscles. Then repeat with your arms going straight up and down, or out to the side. You can also tense your chest muscles by bringing your hands together in front of your body and contracting across the chest and shoulders. Do this rhythmically to match your gait.

● **Breathe deeply as you walk, to a count of three** Many of us hold our breath during exercise, without intending to, then suddenly feel breathless and tired. Oxygen is invigorating and muscles need it to create energy. So as you inhale, bring the air to the deepest part of your lungs by expanding your ribs outwards and your tummy forwards and inhale for a count of three. Exhale fully through your mouth, also to a count of three.

● **Learn your mph (miles per hour)**
Monitoring your speed will help to keep you motivated. A leisurely pace is 2mph, a healthy, brisk pace is 3.5mph, and going over 4mph is fast. A pedometer will measure this for you, but if you don't have one, you can simply count your steps during 15 second periods. For a normal adult stride, if you walk 15 steps in 15 seconds, you're walking at 2mph. At 23 steps, you're walking at 3mph. At 30 steps, you're walking at about 4mph.

Walking after dinner will take you away from the television

● **Walk faster earlier in your walk** If you want to increase the amount of fat you burn, add some bursts of faster walking near the beginning of your walk, rather than going for a final spurt.

A study in the *European Journal of Applied Physiology* found that people exercising burned more fat and felt less tired when they inserted their faster segments towards the beginning of a workout. You'll speed up your heart rate early and keep it elevated for the rest of your walk.

● **Don't cancel** When you feel like cancelling your walk, promise yourself you'll do just 10 minutes. You might end up doing more. 'Even if you don't walk for longer, 10 minutes is better than no minutes at all,' says Steve Nance, performance director at Pure Sports Medicine and Leeds Rugby Union Club.

● **Walk in the evening** After-dinner walks take you away from the television, they keep you from eating too much at dinner, they give you a chance to chat to your neighbours and it's often a lovely time of day.

Don't let bad weather stop you, though – that's what jackets, boots and umbrellas were invented for. There's something childlike and fun about a walk in the rain or snow.

try it...

Walking poles The lightweight walking poles sold at many sports shops can help you to feel steadier and safer when walking on rough ground. The poles encourage you to bend your elbows and use your arms as you walk, which will prevent swelling in your hands. The movement also provides a great upper-body and lower-body workout, which burns more calories as well as strengthening your muscles. Finally, the poles take stress off your knees.

● **If you're over 60, walk on soft surfaces** As you age, the fat padding in your feet deteriorates. The absence of this natural shock absorber can make walking on pavements and other hard surfaces feel like foot torture. Flat grass and dirt paths will provide more cushioning for your feet than roads or pavements.

● **Climb stairs** Five times a day, climb up and down a flight of stairs for 2 minutes. You'll get the same heart rate-enhancing results in those 10 minutes as you would get from 36 minutes walking on a level surface.

● **Sign up for a new parents' walk** If you're a new mum or dad, you know how hard it is to make time for keeping fit. The good news is that you can take your infant with you on your walks. A growing number of community groups and fitness centres organize buggy walks for new parents. Use the internet to make contact with a local group.

● **Split it up** When you're too busy for a 30 to 60 minute walk, think about going for 5 or 10 minutes at a time. That may be as simple as taking a 5-minute walk break around the building after completing a project at work. Such short walking breaks will refresh your mind, so that you can return to work with more vigour. Research shows that most people can focus at top capacity for only 30 minutes at a time; after that, concentration begins to sag – so your intermittent walk breaks may actually make you more productive.

● **Apply some Vaseline** If you're a long-distance walker or a bit overweight, chafing clothes can make you want to call it quits. You can solve the problem by wearing skin-hugging clothing and applying Vaseline to your sensitive areas.

TURNING UP THE ENERGY

There are plenty of other energetic, health-promoting activities that offer enjoyable alternatives to walking – from cycling to swimming to team games.

THE MOST EFFICIENT CALORIE-BURNERS

Activity	Calories (kcal) burned per hour*	Special benefits
Bicycling	544	you feel like a child again
Swimming	544	low impact; eases joint pain
Scuba diving	476	scenic and serene
Tennis	476	builds strong bones
Hiking	408	communing with nature
Ice skating/roller skating	408	great family fun
Golfing	374	improves flexibility
Gardening	340	pleasures of cultivation
Kayaking/canoeing	340	builds upper-body strength
Volleyball (casual)	204	improves hand–eye coordination

*Based on a 67kg person. Lighter people burn less; heavier people burn more.

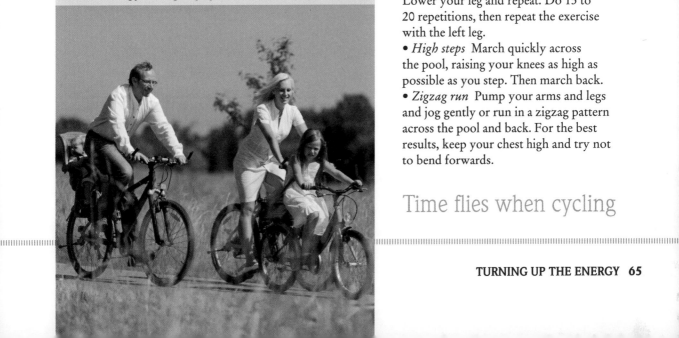

● **Get in the game** Resolve to take up one active hobby this year. Sporting hobbies such as tennis, cycling and golf include short bursts of heart-pumping effort – and they're fun, so time flies when you're absorbed in them.

● **Head for the hills** Cycling burns more calories than almost any other sporting activity. Riding a bike uphill means working harder against gravity – an added challenge for your muscles, heart and lungs.

● **Dance, dance, dance** Whether it's country dancing, salsa or ballroom, dancing burns 480kcal an hour, uses your muscles in new ways – and makes you feel full of the joys of life.

● **Make a splash** Water is 800 times denser than air, so moving your body in water can provide an unrivalled level of exercise intensity. Get into the habit of visiting your local pool once or twice a week for some sustained lane swimming – as many lengths as you can comfortably manage – or, during an off-peak period, try the following exercises.
• *Side kicks* Bend your right knee and then, without lowering it, kick out to the side, leaning towards the left as you kick. Lower your leg and repeat. Do 15 to 20 repetitions, then repeat the exercise with the left leg.
• *High steps* March quickly across the pool, raising your knees as high as possible as you step. Then march back.
• *Zigzag run* Pump your arms and legs and jog gently or run in a zigzag pattern across the pool and back. For the best results, keep your chest high and try not to bend forwards.

Time flies when cycling

8 effective ways to stretch yourself

Your body was made for movement. If you spend a lot of time sitting, regular stretching will help keep you lithe, active and free from injury.

1 DANCE YOUR WAY TO FLEXIBILITY

In a Swedish study, 20 cross-country skiers were tested for flexibility. Half the skiers took a weekly dance class, and the other half served as a control group. Within three months, the skiers taking the dance class had improved spine flexibility compared with the control group and consequently also increased their agility and skiing speed.

2 STRETCH DURING TV TIME

Lie on the floor and go through the stretching routine described on page 68. If you feel good, do the stretches a second and third time. If you do these stretches late in the day, your muscles will already be warmed up from your daily activities.

3 STRETCH AFTER DRIVING

Even short periods of driving can cause back pain if tension is not released. When you get out of the car, lean backwards. Stand with your feet shoulder-width apart, put your hand in the small of your back and lean backwards using your hand to support your lower back. Then bend forward and place your hands on your knees. Exhale as you round your back and tuck in your chin. Then flatten your back, inhaling as you go. Hold each position for a count of two, repeating in both directions ten times.

4 STRETCH YOUR LEGS AS YOU WAIT IN A QUEUE

If you're standing in a queue, stand on your toes, as high as you can, for as long as you can. Then, with your feet back on the ground, lift the toes of your right foot as high as they can go without lifting your heel, and hold for 20 seconds. Do the same with your left foot.

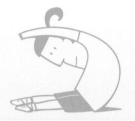

5 REST YOUR LEGS UP A WALL

Sit with one hip as close to a bare wall as you can get it. Then lie on your back and extend your legs up the wall, so that your bottom, the backs of your thighs and your heels touch the wall. You'll feel a mild stretch in your legs as gravity encourages fluids to drain out of your legs, back up to your heart. Hold the position for 5 minutes.

6 RELEASE YOUR NECK DURING PHONE CALLS

The next time someone puts you on hold during a phone call, use the opportunity to do some neck rolls.

7 STRETCH AFTER EVERY WALK, RUN OR BIKE RIDE

Your muscles are at their most flexible and pliable after exercise, making stretching more effective. After any activity designed to increase heart rate, spend 5 to 10 minutes cooling down and bringing your heart rate back to normal.

8 HANG FROM A BAR

Grab a pull-up bar and just hang from it – no pulling or swinging – for a minute or two. It's surprisingly refreshing and can do a lot of good for your spine, as well as your arm, shoulder and chest muscles. If you haven't exercised for a while, or have a history of shoulder problems, consult your doctor before trying this stretch.

good stretching technique

- **FEEL THE MUSCLE YOU ARE TARGETING.** As you proceed gradually through the movement, you should feel a stretching sensation in your muscle as it lengthens and relaxes. If you feel a sharp pain in a joint, you have either gone too far or your technique is at fault.

- **RELAX.** Many people tense up as they stretch – hunching their shoulders towards their ears, for example. If you notice a clenched muscle, gently allow it to release as you exhale.

- **BREATHE INTO A STRETCH.** If you breathe slowly and deeply, you'll increase blood flow and make your stretching more effective. Always exhale as you move into the stretch. As you hold, inhale by expanding the abdomen, rib cage and chest, then exhale as you visualize your breath flowing through the tension you feel in your muscle.

- **STRETCH EACH AND EVERY DAY.** When it comes to flexibility, what you don't use you lose – and quickly. It is much better to stretch a little every day than to do a long stretching routine once or twice a week.

- **KNOW YOUR TIGHTER SIDE.** Hold a stretch on the tighter side of your body twice as long as on the more flexible side. Prevent muscle imbalances by training the major muscle groups equally. If you are tighter on one side of your body, stretch that muscle for twice as long or repeat a stretch on that side to even things out.

- **USE PROPER BODY ALIGNMENT.** The most common fault when stretching is rounding the back. In 95 per cent of all stretches, you should aim to keep your spine long and flat. Before bending forward into any stretch, first inhale and extend upwards, creating as much space as you can between each vertebra in your spine. When you bend forward into a stretch, bend from the hips, not the waist. As you bend forward, your pubic bone should move forward while your tail bone (coccyx) moves back and up.

GREAT EARLY MORNING MOVES

To get your day off to the best possible start, try some gentle stretching first thing in the morning just after getting out of bed. These simple exercise routines are safe to perform even with cold muscles.

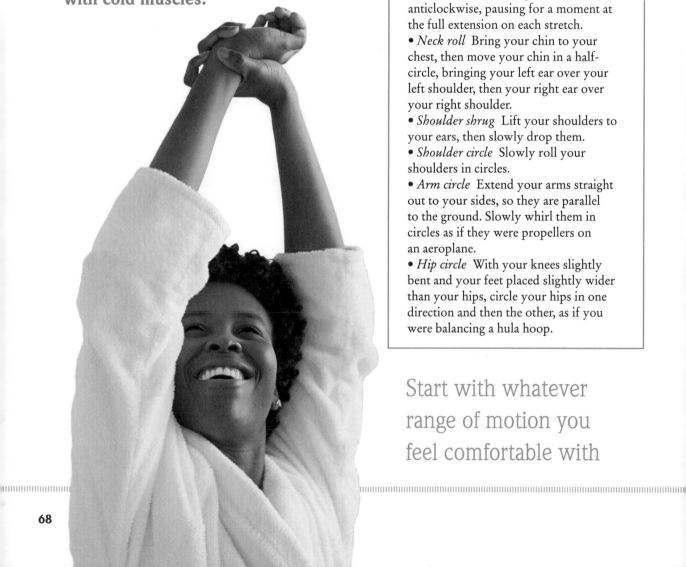

try it...

Relieving stiff joints This 3-minute routine consists of simple, natural moves, and is good for anyone with stiff joints or mild arthritis. It gently warms your muscles and moves your shoulders, knees, elbows, wrists and neck through a full range of motion, stimulating the release of synovial fluid, a thick secretion that lubricates and cushions your joints.

Do the following stretches in a standing position, starting with whatever range of motion you feel comfortable with, gradually increasing it as your joints warm up. Do 10 to 12 repetitions of each stretch, moving clockwise and anticlockwise, pausing for a moment at the full extension on each stretch.

• *Neck roll* Bring your chin to your chest, then move your chin in a half-circle, bringing your left ear over your left shoulder, then your right ear over your right shoulder.

• *Shoulder shrug* Lift your shoulders to your ears, then slowly drop them.

• *Shoulder circle* Slowly roll your shoulders in circles.

• *Arm circle* Extend your arms straight out to your sides, so they are parallel to the ground. Slowly whirl them in circles as if they were propellers on an aeroplane.

• *Hip circle* With your knees slightly bent and your feet placed slightly wider than your hips, circle your hips in one direction and then the other, as if you were balancing a hula hoop.

Start with whatever range of motion you feel comfortable with

Pelvic tilts boost blood flow to your abdominal region and help to realign the sacrum

● **Keep your hands nimble** Regular finger stretches keep your hands nimble and strong. Stretch one hand at a time for best effect.
• *Finger stretch* Place a hand on a table top or on your thigh, with your palm facing down. Spread your fingers as wide as you can and hold for 20 to 30 seconds.
• *Thumb touch* Place your hand, palm up, on a table with your fingers open and relaxed. In a smooth movement, touch the tips of your thumb and index finger together. Hold this for a second, then return to the starting position. Then touch the tip of your thumb to all of your other fingertips.
• *Spider walk* Place your hand, palm down on a table top. use your fingers to pull your palm across the table as far as you can reach.

● **Stretch your hamstrings** Lie on your back with your knees bent and your feet on the floor. Lift your right knee in towards your chest and thread a rope (or a tie or towel) round the arch of your right foot. Hold the ends of the rope with your left hand. Extend your leg towards the ceiling. Place your right palm against your right thigh and press into it as you use the rope to increase the stretch. Hold for 30 seconds, release and repeat three times. Switch legs and repeat.

● **Tilt your pelvis** Pelvic tilts help to increase blood flow to your midsection, relax your back muscles and realign your

sacrum, one of the large, flat bones that form your pelvis. Lie on your back with your knees bent and feet on the floor. Lift your right thigh towards your chest, grasping the back of your thigh with both hands. Bring your knee as close to your chest as you can. Hold for 2 seconds, release, then repeat ten times. Switch legs and repeat.

● **Try a trunk extensor stretch** Prepare your back for the challenge of sitting for hours at a desk with this stretch, and repeat it periodically during the day to release tension.
   Sit on the floor with your knees bent and feet flat on the floor. Lift your toes until only your heels touch the floor. Sit tall with your back straight and spine long and extended. Place your hands on your shins. Tuck your chin into your chest, bend forward from the hips, and pull your torso as far down as you can. Hold for 2 seconds, release, then repeat ten times.

BEST NECK AND SHOULDER EXERCISES

Whether the cause is bad sleep, bad posture or too much stress, neck and shoulder pain is among the most common everyday complaints. And weak shoulders increase the stress on elbows and wrists. Regular stretching is a preventive measure, but neck and shoulder-strengthening exercises may be even more effective.

● **Shrug your shoulders** The action of lifting your shoulders up to your ears will strengthen your neck and shoulder muscles. For a fuller workout, do three sets of ten shrugs.

● **Retract your shoulder blades** Do this while watching television for example. Sit on the edge of your chair and lengthen your spine, as if trying to grow taller. Place your hands in your lap. Bring your shoulders as far back as you can, pinching your shoulder blades together. Hold for the length of an entire advertisement. Relax, then repeat once more during the course of the evening.

A spicy remedy When you get home from work, loosely fill a knee-high sock with white rice, 2 cinnamon sticks and 1 tablespoon of cloves. Seal the end tightly with a rubber band. Heat for 2 minutes in the microwave, then drape the sock around your neck for a luscious aromatherapeutic remedy for sore shoulders and neck. There's no need to empty the sock when you've finished. You can use it over and over again, until the spices lose their fragrance.

● **Every hour, drop your chin to your chest** Then roll your neck to the left, back, to the right and down again in a circular motion. Repeat five times, then switch direction, starting with a roll to the right.

● **Turn turtle** Whenever you spend more than 45 minutes driving a car, do the 'turtle' exercise, which is designed to counteract stress on the back of the neck. As you drive, pretend you're a turtle retracting its head into its shell. Keeping your chin level, bring your head back, flattening the curve in the back of your neck. Hold for a count of five, release, and repeat ten times.

● **Go rowing or kayaking** Take your partner for a romantic jaunt on a lake or pond. As you row or paddle out onto the water, you'll strengthen the area of your shoulders between the shoulder blades. When these muscles are weak, your shoulders slump forward.

● **Exercise your rotator cuff** Your rotator cuff is a group of muscles and tendons that holds your shoulder joint in place. Strengthening this area of the body can do much to prevent shoulder problems in later life. You can do the following exercises at home.

• Stand with your elbows pressed into your waist and your upper arms close to your ribs, elbows bent at 90 degrees, and palms facing each other. Pull your shoulder blades together behind your back. Keeping your elbows touching your waist, open your hands slowly out to the side. You should feel the tension between your shoulder blades. Hold for a count of five, bring your palms together, and repeat ten times.

• Stand with your feet under your hips and your arms at your sides. Raise your arms out to the sides and forward at an angle of 45 degrees to your torso, as high as you can, with little fingers facing up. Keep your shoulders relaxed and away from your ears as you raise your arms. Lower, and repeat 10 to 20 times.

BUILDING NECK AND SHOULDER **STRENGTH**

To relieve the physical tension caused by office work, try these simple exercises while sitting at your desk.

• Lean forward and place your elbows on the desk. With your head centred over your shoulders, press your forehead into your palms, using your palms to resist the pressure of your head. Hold this position for 3 to 5 seconds, release and repeat three to five times.

• Sit up straight and place your palms on the back of your head with your elbows out to the sides. Press your head back into your palms as you use your palms to resist the pressure of your head. Hold for 3 to 5 seconds, release, then repeat three to five times.

• Place your palms on the edge of your chair and press down into your hands, lifting your hips and bottom a few centimetres into the air. Hold for 5 seconds, lower and repeat five times for a great shoulder-muscle strengthener.

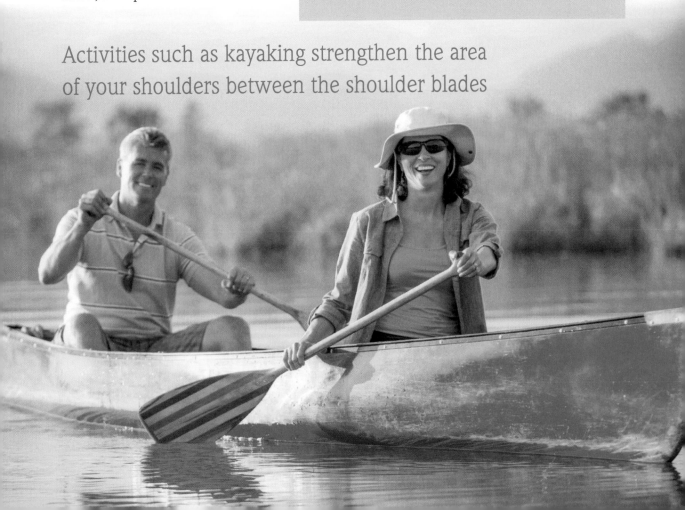

Activities such as kayaking strengthen the area of your shoulders between the shoulder blades

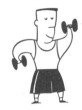

ARM **STRENGTH**

Before the advent of mod cons, the strength of our arm muscles was maintained by physical labour such as washing clothes by hand, chopping wood and scrubbing floors. To achieve the same effect today, we either have to replicate these activities or do special exercises.

● **Biceps curl** Grasp a dumbbell in each hand. Extend your arms at your sides with palms facing forward. Exhale as you curl your hands towards your shoulders, keeping your elbows close to your sides. Inhale as you lower the weights. This exercise strengthens the biceps, the muscles along the front of the upper arms.

● **Scrub floors on your hands and knees** Not only will you have cleaner floors than a mop provides, but you'll strengthen your arms at the same time.

● **If you have a garden, stop using weedkiller** This will encourage weeds to grow with wild abandon. That's good, because your job is to get down on your hands and knees once a week and get weeding. Leaning onto your hands as you weed will build arm, shoulder and upper-back strength, and pulling up the weeds provides an extra dose of arm-building strength. Just remember to alternate hands as you reach and pull so that you are working both arms equally.

● **Trade in your electric mixer for a whisk and wooden spoon** You'll build arm strength as you use your own elbow grease to mix batter. Be sure to use both hands to work your arms evenly.

● **Try a cleaver** Have a large cleaver available for everyday kitchen chopping. Professional chefs love cleavers for their weight and super-sharp, slightly rounded edge. Using one will give your hand and arm a great workout while you cook.

● **Make a breakfast omelette rather than a fried egg** Fill it with at least three different vegetables, such as spinach, mushrooms and onions. You'll not only use your arms to whisk the eggs and chop the vegetables, but you'll also improve your health by incorporating vegetables into your morning meal.

● **Use cast-iron pots for cooking** And store your pots and pans on low-level shelves. That way, you need to lift the heavy pots onto the hob each time you need them – building more arm strength with every meal.

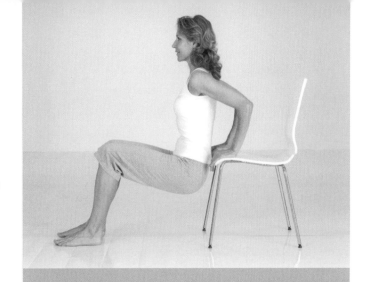

● **Exercise your arms at least once a week** Aim to do three slow sets of ten repetitions, with 20 seconds of breathing time between sets. For the biceps curl, beginners should use 2kg (4lb) dumbbells, while more active adults can try 5kg (10lb) or 7kg (15lb) versions.

● **Make your own pizza dough and pastry** The forward and back action of using a rolling pin is a great arm and shoulder workout. And your family will thank you for your effort later, as no shop-bought product compares to the home-made alternative.

● **Pour water out of a large jug** Bearing the weight of a large jug of water may do wonders for your arms (2 litres/3½ pints) of water weighs nearly 2kg/4lb). Curl your jug five times – bending your elbow and bringing your hand to your shoulder – before pouring.

● **Cut your own wood** If you have a real fire, the chances are you're burning pre-cut logs. If you have the option, though, go out and chop your own wood. Do 30 minutes of log chopping every weekend. If you do too much at once, it will be bad for your back, but a short session of wood-cutting is amazingly good exercise.

● **In autumn, plant bulbs on three consecutive weekends** Make each planting session last at least an hour. Congratulations – that's your arm workout for the week. Digging in your garden will strengthen your hands, wrists, forearms, upper arms and shoulders. Your hard work will pay off in spring, when your daffodils and tulips bloom.

THE CHAIR DIP

This exercise strengthens your triceps, the muscles along the back of your upper arms, and your chest muscles. Make sure that the chair is firm and won't slide, or place it against a wall.

Sit on the edge of the chair. Place your palms on the seat of the chair, either side of your bottom, with fingers facing forward. Place your feet flat on the floor with knees bent. Press into your hands and lift your bottom about 3cm (1in) up and forward, until you can clear the seat of the chair. Inhale as you bend your elbows, lowering your bottom towards the floor. Keeping your elbows close to your sides, exhale as you extend your arms and return to the starting position. Be careful you're not cheating by pushing yourself back up with your legs rather than your arms.

● **Bake bread once a week** You'll strengthen your arms, shoulders and hands as you simultaneously soothe away stress. Nothing is more calming than the repetitive motion of kneading dough, nor more pleasing than the smell of bread in the oven. Plus, home-baked bread tastes better than anything bought from the shops or made in a breadmaker.

Everyday tasks can help to strengthen your arm muscles

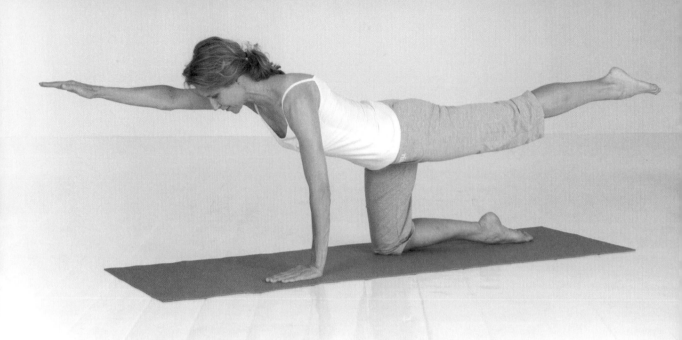

ABDOMINAL AND BACK **STRENGTH**

Your abdominal muscles and back are the core of your body, the power centre from which all movement originates. Strengthen them and you'll move with more power and grace. Strong abdominal muscles also help to support and move your spine, protecting your back from injury.

● **Fly like Superman** This simple exercise will strengthen your lower back. Lie on your tummy with your legs extended. Extend your arms in front. Inhale as you lift your shoulders and feet, reaching your hands and feet away from each other. Hold for 10 to 20 seconds. Lower and repeat once or twice.

● **Calm your nerves** If you're nervous, tighten and release your abdominal muscles over and over again. You will strengthen your abs at the same time as taking your mind off your anxiety.

● **Check your posture regularly** Your abdominal muscles support your spine; strengthening them will help to improve your posture, which will in turn help to strengthen your abdominal muscles. So do a regular posture check.

Every hour, stop and extend your spine and neck, stretching the top of your head towards the ceiling. As you do so, your lower abdomen should pull up and in towards your spine and your lower back should flatten slightly as your tail bone reaches down towards the floor.

● **If you walk for fitness, squeeze your bottom** As you walk, imagine someone is poking you in the bottom with a sharp instrument. Tighten your bottom muscles but don't squeeze them together. As you firm and lift your bottom muscles, you'll strengthen them.

You can also work your abdominal muscles as you walk by imagining you have a zip along the midline of your abdomen. Picture yourself zipping up a tight pair of jeans. As you pull the zip up your abdomen, feel your torso lengthen and your abdomen firm up.

Keep your abs zipped up and your bottom tucked under throughout your walks and you'll strengthen your core even as you burn fat.

try it...

Do the reciprocal reach
The reciprocal reach helps to strengthen the abdominal muscles and back at the same time. Get on all fours with your hands flat on the floor directly under your shoulders and your knees under your hips. Extend your left leg behind, placing the ball of your left foot against the floor. Tuck in your tail bone (coccyx) and try to keep it tucked in throughout the exercise.

Lift your left foot off the floor as you lift your right arm, reaching your right hand and left foot away from each other. Keep your hips level. Don't let your back arch. Imagine you have a large glass of water standing on your lower back as you do it. As you move your arms and legs, your back must stay stable so as not to spill the water. Hold for 10 to 20 seconds, release, then repeat on the other side. Work up to two to three sets.

great idea!

Pretend to be a scaredy cat Once in the morning and once at night, pretend that you are a scared cat. Get on the floor on your hands and knees. Exhale as you curl your spine towards the ceiling, tucking in your tail bone and bringing your chin to your chest. As you do so, bring your navel up and in towards your spine. Inhale as you gently flatten your back, raise your head and push up your hips, letting your back dip in the other direction to mobilise your spine really effectively. Continue to curl and flatten your spine as you breathe, doing ten repetitions.

● **Do a simple back stretch** For a simple, effective back stretch, lie flat on your back. Lift one knee to your chest, then the other, keeping your lower back on the floor. Wrap your arms behind your knees, using them to support your legs and, if necessary, pulling them so that your bottom rises off the floor. Hold for 30 seconds, then release.

● **Strengthen your pelvic floor**
Tighten your abdominal and pelvic-floor muscles, the lowest part of your core. Starting with your pubic area, begin to tighten from the bottom up. Once you have squeezed your pelvic floor, suck in your lower belly and then your upper belly towards your spine as you exhale. Hold for a count of five, then release and repeat 10 to 20 times. Doing this exercise regularly helps to prevent incontinence and may even improve your sex life.

● **Make the most of having to queue**
Whenever you find yourself standing in a queue, lift one foot off the floor and try to hold your balance. You'll feel the myriad muscles in your abdomen and back firing up to help to steady your body. Be sure to alternate your feet.

Your abs and back are the core of your body, the power centre from which all movement originates

● **Use an exercise ball** Whenever you perform abdominal-strengthening movements on a large air-filled ball (see opposite), you use more of your core muscles for every movement.

● **Try a handbag or briefcase side bend** Stand upright with your briefcase or bag in your right hand, palm facing in, your feet about shoulder-width apart. Slowly bend to your right, allowing the item to drop directly down your right leg until you feel a stretch along your left side. Keep your body facing forward the whole time. Once you've gone as low as

possible, slowly return to upright, repeat for a set of 10 to 20 repetitions, then switch hands and repeat on the other side.

● **Adapt gym exercises for home use** Among the many gym activities that can be adapted for home use is the simple exercise known as captain's chair.

Most gyms have an abs-strengthening device which allows you to sit with your forearms on padding, grip handholds and, while pressing your lower back against the back pad, lift your legs off the floor, drawing your knees up towards your chest. You can do this at home in a sturdy, armless chair. Sit up straight, grabbing the chair's edges just in front of your hips. Don't let your back arch or move. Supporting yourself with your hands, slowly draw your knees up towards your chest, keeping your lower back against the chair. Hold, slowly lower, then repeat.

● **Get into crunches** Some of the most effective abdominal exercises are crunches, including the ball crunch and the reverse crunch shown opposite. Another variation is the extended leg crunch, described below.

Lie on your back. Extend your legs towards the ceiling and cross one ankle over the other. Place your fingertips behind your head with your elbows open to the sides. Tuck in your tail bone. Slowly lift your shoulders off the floor as you exhale. Lower and repeat.

● **Do the bicycle** Lie on your back. Tuck in your tail bone and press your lower back to the floor. Place fingertips behind your head and elbows out to the sides. Bend your knees and lift your feet off the floor, keeping a 45-degree bend in your knees. Begin to pedal your legs, bringing your opposite elbow to the opposite knee as you extend your leg.

did you know?

Shapelier abdominals
It takes a lot of targeted exercise to create shapely abdominal muscles. While most of us imagine a simple band of muscles across the top of the abdomen, there are in fact many separate abdominal muscles, and a thorough abs workout could involve ten different exercises. Is all this necessary? For athletes or models perhaps – but not for you. What matters is that your muscles are conditioned well enough to support your back and allow you to twist, turn and lift without a problem. If you are a healthy weight but have a little fat covering your abs, consider yourself well ahead of the game.

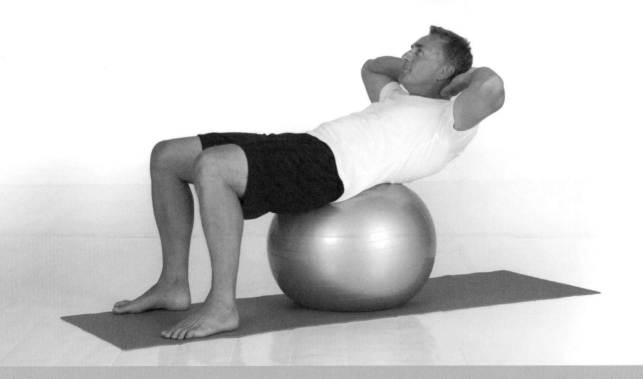

ABDOMINAL CRUNCHES

Ball crunch and reverse crunch are among the most effective exercises for abdominal strength.

▲ **Ball crunch** Sit on the ball with your feet on the floor. Walk your feet away from the ball as you recline onto it. The ball should rest against your lower back. With your fingertips behind your head, open your elbows to the sides. Tuck your tail bone in and exhale as you lift your shoulders. Lower and repeat.

▼ **Reverse crunch** Lie on your back. Bend your knees and lift your feet off the floor, forming a 90-degree angle between thighs and calves. Place your fingertips behind your head with elbows open to the sides. Cross your ankles. Press your lower back into the floor, tuck your tail bone in and press your shins towards the ceiling. Lower and repeat.

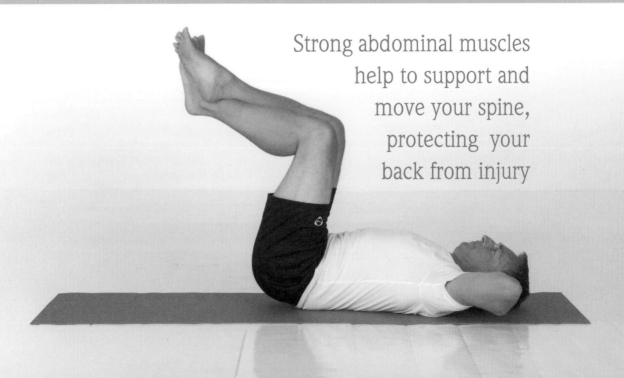

Strong abdominal muscles help to support and move your spine, protecting your back from injury

LEG **STRENGTH**

A stronger pair of legs will help you to accomplish more every day. You'll climb stairs more easily and be able to bend your knees and squat down to pick up heavy objects, protecting your lower back from strain. To strengthen your legs and avoid injury, you must work all of the muscles in your legs equally.

● **Master the 'lunge walk'** During each step forward, bend your knees and sink down until both legs form 90-degree angles. Then press into your front heel to rise. Lift your back leg and knee all the way into your chest before planting it in front of you for the next lunge. This takes a little practice, but if you 'lunge walk' for 20 or 30 steps a day, your legs will be far stronger and shapelier.

● **Exercise while driving your car** Whenever you stop at traffic lights, tighten your thighs and bottom, over and over again. You will firm your leg muscles, boost blood flow (preventing the pins-and-needles sensation that tends to attack your bottom when you've been sitting in a car seat for too long) and give yourself something to focus on.

great idea!

Get a stronger bottom If you feel drowsy at work, get up, place your palms against the desk and do some donkey kicks. Bend one knee, flex that foot and kick your leg back, as if you were a donkey kicking out at someone behind you. Alternate legs for 15 kicks in total. You will return to work refreshed – and with a stronger bottom.

● **Do the twist** Next time you find yourself at a wedding or other function with a dance floor, do the twist. Or, do it in your living room tonight. Bend your knees and squat down as far as you comfortably can as you shimmy from side to side. You'll burn calories, have a few laughs and strengthen your legs – all at the same time.

● **Do the clam** This exercise should be done before you get out of bed in the morning. Lie on your back, bring your feet together, and open your knees out to the sides. Then, as you exhale, lift your knees, bringing them together. Lower and repeat this exercise 10 to 15 times and you'll strengthen your inner thighs.

● **Try leg lifts as you cook dinner** Flex your foot and lift your leg out to the side, lower it, then repeat 10 to 15 times. Make sure you move only at the hip – don't let your waist move. Then swap legs. You'll finish your leg workout before dinner time.

● **Mount the stairs two or three at a time** This strengthens the gluteal muscles in your bottom and revs up your heart rate, boosting your cardiovascular fitness.

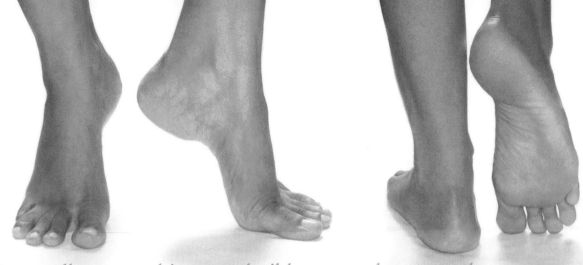

Hop, walk, run and jump to build up your leg strength

● **Try toe-walking** Challenge your children, grandchildren, partner or colleagues to a toe-walking competition every other day. Rise onto the balls of your feet and walk across the room. Whoever lowers his or her heels to the floor first loses. You'll have plenty of laughs and strengthen your arches, ankles and calves.

● **Exercise your calf muscles while you brush your teeth** Place your feet flat on the floor, then rise up onto the balls of your feet, hold for 2 seconds, and sink down. Repeat this sequence 20, 30, 50 or more times. You can do this not only while brushing your teeth, but any time you are waiting.

● **Play leapfrog** You'll get a good leg and cardiovascular workout – and lots of fun – from playing leapfrog with your children. To start the game, everyone squats down low, imitating a frog on a lily pad. To leap over the person in front of you, place your hands on his or her back, then spring forward and up. Keep your legs and feet wide, in case you need to take two hops to clear your obstacle. Land with your knees soft and slightly bent to protect whoever's in front.

try it... **Jump into the pool once or twice a week – literally** The next time you find yourself entertaining your children or grandchildren at the local swimming pool, try the following routine in the shallow end to see if they can keep up with you:
• **Hop** With your legs together, hop the width of the pool from one side to the other and back. Rest for up to a minute, then repeat twice.
• **Exaggerated running** Run the width of the pool slowly with an exaggerated motion, lifting your knees into your chest and pushing off with your rear foot just enough to lift your entire body off the bottom of the pool. When you reach the other side, turn round and run back. Rest for up to a minute, then repeat twice.
• **Hop on one foot** Hop on the spot on one foot for 30 seconds, trying to get as high as possible. Then switch legs. Rest for up to a minute, then repeat twice.

● **Always squat to pick things up** Bending over from the waist to pick something up puts stress on the lower back, especially if you're lifting a heavy item. But a squat forces you to use your legs, building up your leg strength.

Keep your feet hip-distance apart or wider, your knees bent and your bottom stuck out as you squat down. Then bend forward and pick up your object. Bring your torso upright, then rise by pressing up through your heels.

● **Perfect the full squat** Stand with your feet slightly wider than hip distance apart. Tuck in your tail bone (coccyx), flatten your back and firm up your abdominal muscles. Inhale and slowly bend your knees as you sit back, as if you were going to sit back into a chair. Your upper body will lean slightly forward, but don't allow your lower back to arch or your spine to round. Bend your knees until your thighs are parallel with the floor. Exhale as you press up through your heels and extend your legs in a fast, explosive motion. Repeat 10 to 15 times. Do this two or three times a week.

● **Try some squat variations** If you lack the leg strength to do a full squat or, more importantly, if you feel pain in your knees or back, try one of two variations.
• Hold on to a doorknob with both hands as you squat. This removes some of your body weight from your legs and helps to keep your torso upright.
• Squat with your back against a wall and a small 20cm (8in) diameter ball between your thighs. The ball keeps your thighs and knees in good alignment, and the wall provides more support for your back.

● **Do a quarter-squat** For this exercise, you'll do the same motion and use the same technique as the full squat, but you won't bend your knees quite so far. Rather than lowering your thighs to parallel, bend your knees only a quarter of the distance of the full squat before rising to the starting position. Repeat 10 to 15 times, two or three times a week.

● **Extend your quadriceps** Sit in a chair with your knees bent and feet on the floor. Lift and extend your right leg, until your calf is parallel with the floor. Lower and repeat 15 times. Change legs. For extra resistance, use ankle weights.

● **Do the lunge** Stand with your feet together. Take a large step forward with your right foot. Bend your right knee until the thigh is parallel with the floor. Exhale as you straighten your legs and step back to the starting position. Repeat with the left leg. Alternate stepping forward with your right and left leg for a total of 10 to 15 repetitions on each leg.

● **Practise 'hot seats' as you watch TV** Television time doesn't have to be couch-potato time. Pledge that you won't sit down in your favourite chair until you've done 15 to 20 hot seats during the adverts. To do a hot seat, stand with your feet slightly wider than your hips. Sit back into a squat, just until your bottom touches the seat of the chair. As soon as you feel the seat of the chair under your bottom, spring up to a standing position, as if the seat were 'hot'.

try it… **Perform the 'lunge walk' in your garden** Your neighbours might laugh if they see you, but you'll have the last laugh when – by investing just a few minutes each day in the exercise – you are able to show off a finely sculpted and toned pair of legs.

During each step forward, bend your knees and sink down until both legs form 90-degree angles. Then press down into your front heel to rise. Lift your back leg and knee all the way into your chest before planting it in front of you for the next lunge.

This takes a little practice, but if you do the 'lunge walk' for 20 or 30 steps a day, your legs will be far stronger and more shapely.

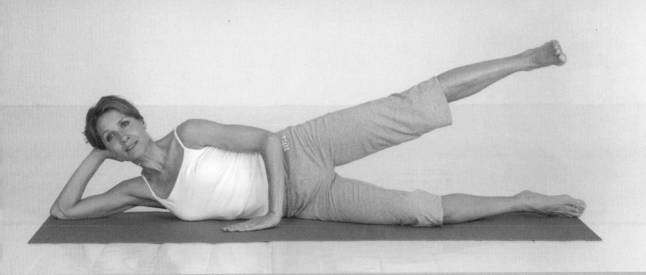

GREAT LEG EXERCISES

Combine these leg-strengthening exercises with squats for a satisfying twice-weekly workout.

▲ **Leg lift** Lie on your right side with your legs extended, supporting your head with your right hand. Lift your left leg towards the ceiling, keeping your foot flexed and the edge of your foot level (don't lead with your toes). Lower and repeat 15 times. Then bend your left knee and rest your lower left leg on the floor in front of your torso. Flex your right foot and lift your right leg, feeling the effort in your right inner thigh. Lower and repeat 15 times. Then change sides. Once 15 repetitions begins to feel easy, strap an ankle weight on each ankle for extra resistance.

Choose ankle weights that let you add weight as you get stronger, with Velcro straps for easy access and removal. Many of these weights contain small pockets into which you can insert weighted bags.

▼ **Hamstring curl** Lie on your front with your legs extended. Bend your right knee, lifting your right foot towards your bottom. Lower and repeat 10 to 15 times. Then change sides. Again, once 15 repetitions begins to feel easy, strap an ankle weight on each ankle for extra resistance.

Practising a variety of leg exercises will not only strengthen your muscles but also balance them

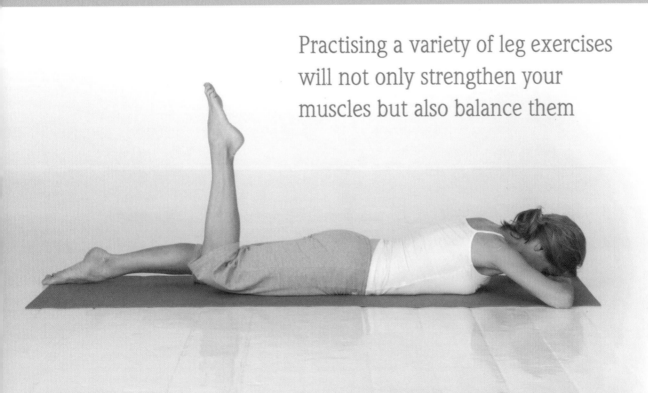

10 ways to have more fun at **the gym**

If you are one of the minority of people who regularly go to a gym for exercise, congratulations! You have the right priorities and excellent self-discipline. But even committed gym-goers sometimes need some inspirational ideas for making their workout more enjoyable.

1 THINK YOU CAN – AND YOU WILL

So simple, yet so often disregarded, positive thinking can help you to power your way through a workout. In one study, exercisers who thought positively were more likely to stay active than those who were full of self-doubt. Whenever you find yourself making excuses, replace negative thoughts with positive messages such as: 'I feel great.'

2 TRY AROMATHERAPY

Aromatherapy oils known to enhance energy, such as rosemary, can make a workout more productive. Dilute the essential oil of your choice and store it in a squirt bottle in your gym bag. Give your gym clothing a few squirts before leaving the dressing room so you can smell the oil as you work out. If you're in the midst of a more meditative, slower paced workout, such as Pilates or yoga, try lavender oil rather than rosemary.

3 DRINK WATER OR JUICE ON YOUR WAY TO THE GYM

If you're already dehydrated when you arrive at the gym, you'll feel very tired during your session. When you're dehydrated, you can't work as hard, you don't feel as good and your mental function is compromised.

4 LISTEN TO YOUR FAVOURITE MUSIC

Create your own personal gym-mix CDs or digital recordings, and listen to them as you work out. Researchers have found that people who listen to fast-tempo music get more out of their exercise-bike workouts. They pedal faster, produce more power and their hearts beat faster than when they listen to slow-tempo music.

5 WORK OUT WITH A FRIEND

If you are getting fed up with your gym workouts, ask a friend to meet you for a gym date. As you walk or run on the treadmill, you can share stories of your day and encourage each other to work a bit harder. Your friend can also help you to find the courage to approach unfamiliar gym equipment, as it's easier to laugh off your foibles when you have a trusted companion nearby.

6 GIVE VENT TO YOUR IRRITATIONS

Think of someone who irritates you, then step on the treadmill, exercise bike or elliptical machine and sweat out your aggression as you exercise. You'll achieve a better workout – and blast away anger and stress at the same time.

7 WEAR THE RIGHT SHOES

Resist the urge to wear the old trainers you found in the back of the cupboard. Various fitness disciplines require specific types of footwear. The wrong shoes will not only make your workout feel harder, it could cause an injury.

8 SET A SHORT-TERM WORKOUT GOAL

Goals motivate us to work harder, and the best exercise regimes include measurable goals to be achieved weeks or months in the future. Sometimes, though, when your motivation is weakening, you need a goal focusing on what you can complete in the next 30 minutes. So pick something achievable: maintain a sweat for 20 minutes, give your arms a good workout, or cover 2 miles on the treadmill.

9 WORK OUT DURING OFF-PEAK HOURS

You'll squeeze in a more effective workout in less time if you are able to visit the gym during the slowest period of the day, which is often the middle of the afternoon. You won't have to wait in a queue for equipment or feel hassled in the changing room.

10 PUT YOUR MIND BEHIND EVERY MOVE

Rather than daydreaming through your workouts, put as much mental emphasis on what you do at the gym as you do at work. For example, when doing a strength exercise, feel the muscle contract as you lift. This will help you to tune into your technique.

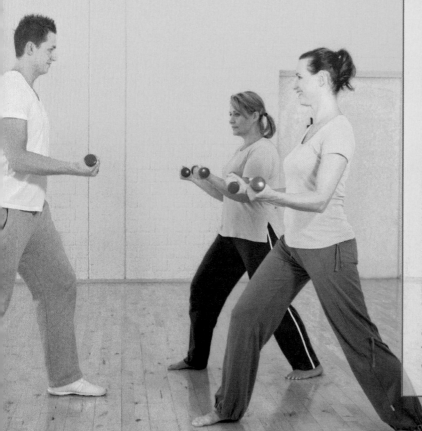

Warning: DVDs can be bad for you

A study by McMaster University in Canada found that exercise videos featuring super-skinny models with amazing muscles made participants feel less confident about their fitness and less inclined to exercise in the future. Videos featuring an ultra-slender host surrounded by plumper, more normal-looking women reduced motivation even more. The researchers realized that seeing a slim instructor surrounded by fleshier participants intensified the participants' awareness of the slimness of the instructor.

To choose a motivating exercise DVD or class, look for a teacher you can trust, who has a fitness background – and who clearly needs to exercise to look great.

HEALTHY AND **HAPPY FAMILIES**

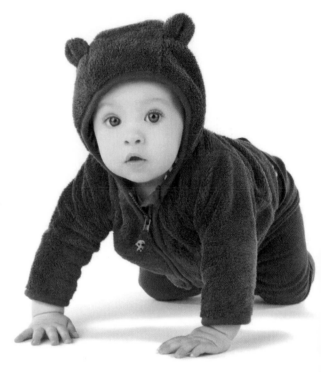

If you are a parent or grandparent of infants or young children, or if you look after children professionally, take every opportunity to get some high-quality exercise by playing with the kids. You should also teach them about the joys and importance of exercise – but, if you want fit and healthy children, you must set them a good example.

● **Crawl with your baby**
Too often, once babies start to crawl, they are confined to a bouncy chair. Crawling helps to develop upper-body strength for both you and your baby, and it's a great aerobic activity. So get down on all fours and crawl round the room with your baby. To add to the challenge, take a large, air-filled ball (perhaps your exercise ball) and push it with your nose as you crawl.

● **Play 'chase my shadow'** The children have to jump and run to catch your shadow, then vice versa.

● **Move like an animal** If you have young children aged between three and eight, organize an animal race. Let everyone in the family pick an animal, such as a snake, monkey or crab. Then race across the room as you imitate

how that animal might move. For example, if you choose a monkey, race using your hands and feet, but not your knees or torso. If you are imitating a snake, slither across the room. Add some animal noises for extra fun.

● **Act like a child** Remember Blind Man's Buff, Hopscotch and What Time Is It, Mr Wolf? You probably thought of these games as just that, children's games. But they also require movement and count as exercise. Teach them to your children and play along. As you laugh, you'll burn extra calories.

● **Organize a playgroup** Get together with other parents and children in your area and organize a playgroup. As the toddlers actively play together, the adults can exercise around the periphery.

● **Let infants discover the world**
We often keep small children in one place, preventing them from getting the exercise they need. For example, have you ever placed your baby in a swing to give yourself some free time? Ever settled your children in front of the DVD player or television when you needed a break?

Instead of finding a stationary occupation for your children when you need a break, encourage more activity. For toddlers and crawlers, find a safe space on the floor where you can plop them down and let them move. Suggest that older children play in the sandpit or climb a tree in the garden as you keep an eye on them.

● **Waltz with your baby** If your baby is crying for attention, don't simply stick a dummy in his or her mouth or go for a drive. Instead, take your baby in your arms and waltz around the room. The more exaggerated and smooth your movements the better.

The waltzing will give your baby new sights to focus on, soothing the crying. Meanwhile, you'll burn extra calories and tone your arm muscles.

● **Play follow-my-leader** If you have two or more children in your care, line up in single file and weave your way through the house or garden. Every few steps, hop, skip, jump or do some other movement that your followers must imitate. Once the children get the hang of it, let them take turns as leader. Their naturally creative minds will come up with all sorts of imaginative movements for the followers to imitate. You'll be out of breath before you know it.

● **Go on a treasure hunt** Take a group of older children to a local park and set an expedition course on a map,

LIMITING **SCREEN TIME**

Increase your children's physical activity and decrease their sedentary behaviour with a few simple actions.

• Remove TVs and computers from children's bedrooms. According to US research, a child's weight increases in proportion to the number of hours he or she watches TV.

• Put activity toys such as skipping ropes, mini-trampolines and hula hoops within easy access in children's bedrooms or playrooms.

• Encourage your children to exercise during TV ad breaks.

• Put a curfew on electronics. For instance, nothing that requires batteries or electricity may be used until 5pm on school days.

• Create a like-for-like rule. For every 30 minutes spent watching TV or surfing the internet, your child must do 30 minutes of physical activity.

circling various 'checkpoints'. Take turns navigating to each point on the map and leading the team to each destination. If this sounds too complicated, go hunting for insects, animals or flowers instead.

● **Walk your children to and from school** By walking with them, you not only get peace of mind that they're safe, but you also get to hear about their upcoming day on the way there, and how their day went on the way home.

● **Give your children a list of indoor chores** Then join in. Younger children often like to feel helpful and will enjoy helping you with household chores. Ask them to help you to make the beds, join in with the dusting, fold the laundry and put it away, and set the table – all are physical activities that can help to get your heart rate up, stretch your body and build your muscles.

great idea!

Play a family-friendly game of 'flag rugby' Buy some table napkins in two colours. Divide your family into two teams and ask everyone to tuck one of the coloured napkins into his or her waistband. When an opposing team member pulls a napkin from the ball-carrier's waistband and places it on the ground, the play has ended. Allow only 20 seconds to prepare for the next kick-off. Switch positions every 15 minutes to keep the entire family active. Not only will you get in some family fitness time, but you'll also be teaching your children valuable lessons about practice, perseverance, cooperation and teamwork.

● **Try aerobics DVDs** Purchase some family-friendly aerobics DVDs to use on cold or rainy days. Choose ones that describe the workout as 'low intensity' or 'low impact'. These types of aerobic exercise are better for children's developing bodies.

● **Create an obstacle course** Set out hula hoops, pillows and other objects that you can imagine as 'rocks'. Then ask your children to imagine that the different objects are rocks in a turbulent river. You must all jump from rock to rock to avoid falling in and getting swept away, or eaten by a crocodile.

● **Try out the hula hoop and other toys** You and your children will bond, and you'll be the coolest parent around if you can master the hula hoop.

● **Play tug-of-war** You'll develop upper-body and lower-body strength as you tug on the rope. To keep it fair, place two children on one side of the rope and yourself on the other. Bend your knees and bring your legs into a lunge position to get a leg workout as you tug the rope.

● **Hold a sports party** As a change from the usual cakes-and-games event, hold your child's birthday party in an activity-based location, such as a roller-skating or ice-skating rink, a climbing centre, or an indoor 'soft play' area. You don't have to limit this to parties. A growing number of indoor playgrounds offer structured games every week.

● **Plan 10-minute bursts of activity** Each period of activity should be followed by a 5-minute rest period. Trying to foist an adult exercise programme on your children is likely to turn them off exercise later in life.

Instead, take advantage of their natural tendency to participate in intermittent and sporadic play. A game of 'it' is a perfect example. Children's bodies are designed to sprint and rest, sprint and rest.

● **Sign up for a race** Check your local paper for a list of 5k and 10k walks or runs in your area. Many of these events also raise money for charity, which can inspire your children to train with you. Don't worry if at first you can't finish; the training brings its own reward.

● **Play volleyball** Set up a net, get a ball and invite other children and their parents over for a game.

● **Dance with your children** Vigorous dancing burns just as many calories as brisk walking. And children love it – particularly when the adults pick them up and swing them round every now and then. Don't just leave dancing to chance, or until you happen to be in the mood – make sure you have one or two family dance sessions a week. Let everyone take turns to choose some music, and let yourself go.

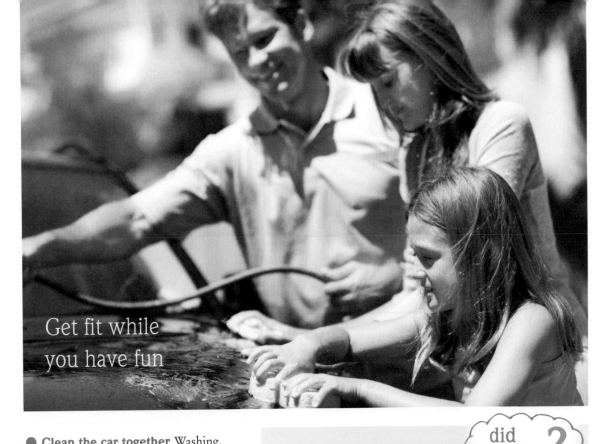

Get fit while you have fun

● **Clean the car together** Washing, drying and polishing is good exercise, but everyone getting wet and soapy is the most enjoyable part for children.

● **Walk around the world** Place a city, country or world map somewhere prominent in your home. Ask your children to help you to reach a certain destination. Then, based on family walks, plot your progress on the map using drawing pins. There are about 2,000 steps in a mile, so you can plot progress using a pedometer. To add some incentive, why not promise to take a trip to your actual destination once you complete the number of steps it takes to get there?

● **Throw a ball to one another or play Frisbee** It may seem more like relaxation than structured exercise, but you'll get your heart rate up every time you have to run or leap for an errant ball or Frisbee. Plus, you'll both improve your hand-eye coordination.

did you know?

An epidemic of obesity

More than 2.3 million children in the UK are overweight or obese. Even more alarmingly, many under-12s already show signs of high blood pressure, high cholesterol and liver disease. More and more young people are developing Type 2 diabetes, a disease that once occurred exclusively at or beyond middle age. Unless there is a sea change in behaviour, today's children will have a shorter life expectancy than their parents, as they eat themselves into an early grave.

Among the strongest predictors of childhood obesity is family environment. According to one study, children of sedentary parents were more likely to gain weight and become overweight than children of active parents. Don't forget that you and your child burn more calories while standing than you do while sitting, and more while walking than that you do while standing. The more you move, the more you burn. And it doesn't really matter what type of activity you choose. If you are moving and having fun, you are burning calories and getting fitter.

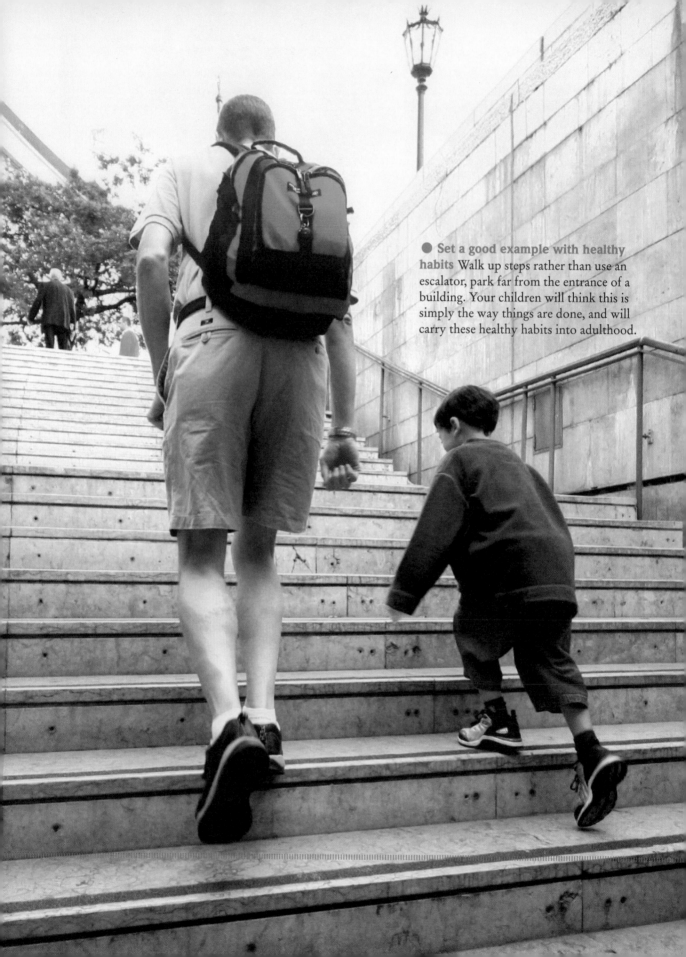

● **Set a good example with healthy habits** Walk up steps rather than use an escalator, park far from the entrance of a building. Your children will think this is simply the way things are done, and will carry these healthy habits into adulthood.

try it...

Spend an hour working in the garden together
Raking leaves, pulling up weeds and spreading out mulch all help to build strength and endurance. Plus, when your children help, it doesn't take as long or seem as much of a chore (depending on the age of the child, of course). As an added bonus, children are more likely to eat the vegetables they help to grow, which means that your gardening experiences will help your child to follow a more nutritious diet. There are numerous ways to make gardening more fun for children. For instance, when you finish raking a pile of leaves, you get to jump in them.

● **Design your garden for activity**
What you put in your garden helps to determine how fit your children become. If they see it, they will play. If they don't, they will watch television or play computer games. Older children enjoy climbing on ropes or ladders and playing in forts. If you can, get a trampoline, a swing, slide or climbing frame, a net for practising netball or basketball, and other outdoor sports equipment.

● **Play active computer games**
Although most computer games exercise only the muscles in the fingers and eyes, a few can produce a decent workout. At the video arcade, challenge your child to one of the dance-mat games where you step on floor squares in the order they light up. At home, consider investing in a Wii games console. Wii games require players to move around as they compete against one another. It's great fun and it will get everyone in the family moving more as you play together.

● **Patronize your local health club** Many fitness clubs offer fitness programmes for families, ranging from aerobics to swimming to roller skating. Don't just sign everyone up and hope for the best, though. For best results, sit down with your family and go over your options together.

● **Learn a sport together** How about roller skating or golf? Or plan a winter-sports holiday where you can all take lessons together. Or try martial arts. Many local community colleges and fitness centres offer martial arts classes designed for adults and children, and many forms of martial arts provide aerobic, strength and flexibility training. These classes will give your children the chance to learn self-control and discipline as well as improving their self-esteem, balance and posture.

● **Plan a pedometer competition**
Decide that there will be a week in which each member of the family wears a pedometer – and all of you will compete to see who can achieve the most steps.

Children are more likely to eat vegetables they helped to grow

great idea!

Go on a walking adventure
Equip yourselves with small backpacks, plenty of water (everyone should aim to drink 250ml/ about ½ pint every half-hour) and a light lunch, and make your way to a local area of countryside for a walking expedition. Wear walking boots for rough terrain or trainers for smoother paths, and pack sunscreen and insect repellent. To make it more fun, get children to focus on something else, such as looking for a particular animal, climbing to see a lake or pond, or seeing how many rocks they can scamper over without touching the ground. Make your picnic in advance – this is a great opportunity to share a delicious but healthy meal.

9 ideas for active holidays

Active holidays can be more relaxing than lazy ones. The idea is to spend 2 to 4 hours a day doing things: walking the city streets, exploring a nature reserve, going to a zoo. Such activities will improve your physical and mental health as well as making your holidays more memorable.

1 GET INTO THE WATER AS MUCH AS YOU CAN

Don't allow yourself to spend all your time sitting in front of the water. Whether it is the sea, a swimming pool or a tree-lined lake, make sure you get into the water for swimming or games or even walking. Merely standing in waist-high water is a good workout, thanks to the action of the water.

2 GET ON THE WATER AS MUCH AS YOU CAN

Paddle boats are fun. Rowing boats are romantic, powerboats exhilarating, sailing boats serene – and kayaks pure adventure. Even standing at the rail of a steamboat is exciting. Boats make you feel young and, whether you are propelling them or not, being on a boat burns calories and engages your muscles more than being on dry land.

3 CHOOSE A CRUISE

It's amazing how active you can be while stuck on a boat in the middle of the ocean. Most cruise ships offer numerous options for seaworthy exercise. Many have pools, golf simulators, climbing walls, fitness centres, jogging and walking areas and instructor-led fitness classes – and that's just what's on board. During any sea and land excursions you can burn calories as you snorkel, hike, scuba-dive and horse ride.

4 SCHEDULE AN ACTIVITY-BASED HOLIDAY

Ready to commit to more action? Plan your entire holiday round an activity, such as sailing, hiking, cycling or swimming. No expertise is necessary – just a willingness to take on a new challenge. There are any number of holiday packages targeted at novices to experts, adolescents to older people, singles to whole families. A skiing holiday with lessons for different ages and ability levels is perfect.

5 MAKE MORNING TIME YOUR ACTIVITY TIME

The weather will probably be friendlier, your energy levels higher and your agenda emptier than later in the day. Forget about cooking if you have to clean up a mess first, not to mention what it does to your mood.

6 GET OUT OF THE CAR

Many of us spend a large part of our holidays on the road, either getting to and from our destinations, or using the car for sightseeing. But, no matter how beautiful the scenery is, great, memorable trips don't happen in a car seat. Get out at least every 2 hours and stretch, walk, picnic, shop, visit and have fun. It's important for your health and energy, and it makes travel a lot more interesting.

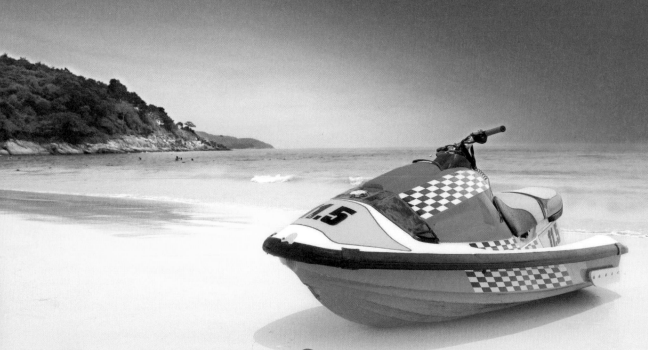

7 FLY A STUNT KITE

If there's a good wind blowing, buy a stunt kite and take it to the beach or other large open space. These kites can be easily assembled, then taken apart, making them perfect for travelling. You'll give your upper body a great workout as you struggle to control the kite. You may also have to run or walk to keep the kite in the air – or chase it down once it plummets to the ground.

8 EXPLORE ON FOOT

Of course, you can rely on your holiday rep, travel guides, maps or a tour bus to get you acquainted with a new location. But only by getting out and walking can you truly get the feel for a place. So how about spending the first few hours at your holiday destination walking round the area? If you're in a city, pick a few restaurants to try to make your reservations in person. Locate the parks, museums and shopping areas.

9 PLAY ACTIVE GAMES

When most people think of outdoor games, they think of team sports such as football, rugby or cricket, all of which can be both intimidating and excessively strenuous for adults who stopped playing such sports a long time ago. Opt instead for gentler games – badminton, table tennis, crazy golf, croquet. Your goal: to play an outdoor game every day while on holiday.

Don't over-indulge

When on holiday, many of us spend long, lazy days on a deckchair and socialize the night away drinking and eating delicious food. Too often, we return home flabbier than we've been since, well, our last holiday. A little moderation helps. Try limiting yourself to one or two treats a day. Any more and the uniqueness of the pleasure fades away – and you'll spend too much time recuperating.

MAKING THE MOST OF YOUR **WEEKENDS**

Are your weekends dominated by shopping, cleaning, cooking, ferrying children around and finishing work you didn't get done during the week? If so, for the sake of your health and wellbeing, you need to reassess your priorities and reclaim time for physical activities, relaxation and mental enrichment.

● **Shift weekend duties to weekday evenings** There's no need to wait until the weekend to go to the supermarket, clean the house or mow the lawn. Make, say, Tuesday and Thursday evenings your 'weekend duty' evenings and get the housework out of the way then. That way, come the weekend, you'll have free days to do as you wish.

● **Designate each Thursday evening for making weekend plans** Start by getting the weather forecast. Next, detail your 'must-do' stuff, such as taking your child to a class. Then, be creative and bold by filling in the blank spaces with interesting and new activities. Get on the phone – make reservations, call friends or family to arrange get-togethers.

● **Join a club** Many outdoors organizations arrange group walking expeditions and other outings at the weekends. In fact, all over the country, there are surprisingly large numbers of walking, cycling, birdwatching or running clubs that have regular weekend events. Enquire at your local fitness centre or search on the internet to find the right one for you.

● **If you must work, get it out of the way early** A good way to reclaim your weekend from your work is to get up an hour earlier than normal, set the alarm for 2 to 3 hours later, stay focused, then, when the alarm rings, turn off the computer. The rest of the weekend is yours – with no guilt.

● **Set aside one day for fun** Never allow errands and work to occupy both Saturday and Sunday. On one of the days, visit a park, go hillwalking or spend time playing tennis, badminton or other games with friends and family. You and your companions will come to look forward to this day, devoted not to formal exercise but to enjoyable activities that you can do together.

● **Spend as much time playing sports as watching sports** Many people have become addicted to watching sports on television. So take up this challenge: for every hour that you watch sport on TV, commit to 30 minutes of doing a sport or some other exercise. Gradually increase the ratio to one-to-one; that is, an hour watching, an hour doing. Nothing can be compared with taking part yourself.

● **Don't sleep in** You may have every intention to be active at the weekend – until you sleep late, that is. When you spend half the day under the covers, it's hard to find time for fun and exercise. Make it a habit to get out of bed at the same time at weekends as during the week. In addition to freeing up more time for your weekend fitness forays, you'll also regulate your body clock better. Once your body gets used to a regular wake-and-sleep schedule, you'll fall asleep faster, feel more refreshed when you wake up, and avoid that Monday morning 'hungover' feeling.

● **Go for a walk first thing in the morning** Before you become engrossed in the Saturday newspaper and your breakfast, go for a walk. Once you return, you'll feel invigorated and be more likely to be active during the rest of the day.

● **Combine physical work with pure indulgence** For instance, chop some logs or gather firewood as the physically active part of your day, then sit in front of the fire with someone special for the indulgent part. Or tidy up your garden by day, then have a barbecue for friends and family that evening.

● **If you cycle, go for a long ride** During the week you probably can't ride much, but weekends allow you the luxury of riding for half the day or more. Scout out a local route or put the bike in your car and drive to a great cycling location.

● **Take the family camping** There's nothing quite like the great outdoors to put your body in a calorie-burning state, or to create happy, memorable times for your children. After you've set up your site, you can look into other activities such as swimming, canoeing and hiking.

Rake the leaves rather than using a leaf blower

● **Spruce up the garden** Many types of gardening, from digging to mowing, build upper-body strength and burn excess calories. In fact, one major study found that gardening was the best physical activity for preventing osteoporosis. But don't make it too easy for yourself. Rake the leaves rather than using a leaf blower, for example. The more you use your own body, the more calories you burn.

● **Take calisthenics breaks** If you find yourself working at the office (or at home) over the weekend, take a 10-minute break every hour and do star jumps, lunges, push-ups and crunches. Over the course of the day, you'll have exercised for more than 60 minutes.

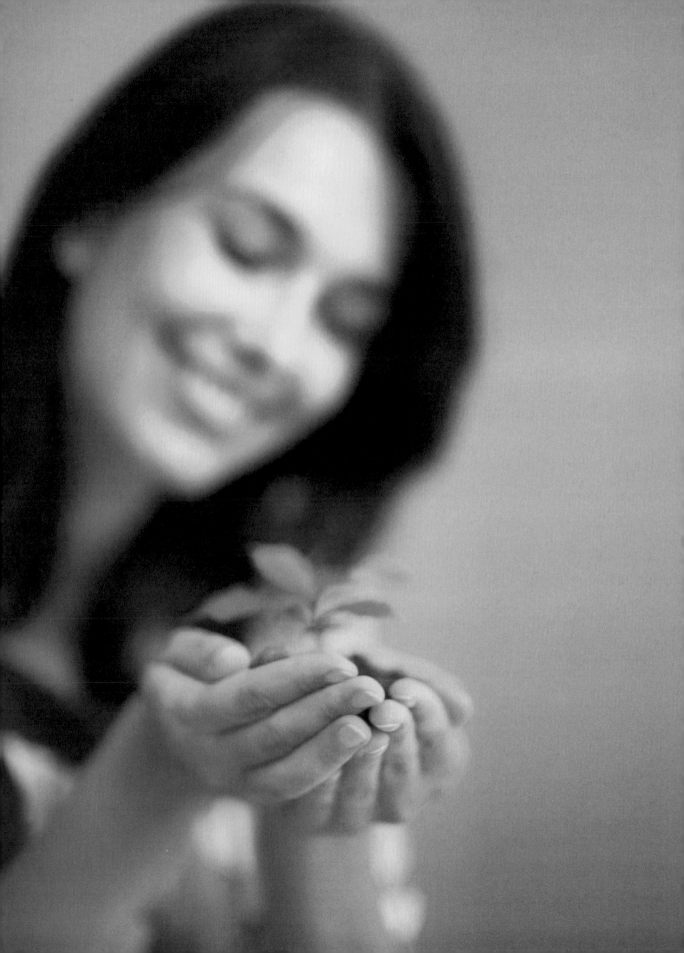

THRIVE:
beat and
treat illness

As we travel through life, each of us encounters unique health challenges and concerns. This section is your mini-health bible, helping you to look after yourself and your family – spotting early symptoms of minor and more serious problems, building immunity, treating long-term problems such as diabetes, and caring for babies, children and older loved ones.

Good health is also more than merely beating off illness; here are tips for keeping mobile, for boosting your sex life and for looking after your precious senses , savouring your capacity to enjoy your favourite sights and sounds.

BEST WAYS TO **LOOK AFTER YOURSELF**

Even if your lifestyle is supremely healthy, you may be afflicted by illness or injury. Since the human body has a huge capacity for healing and repair, most ailments resolve themselves quickly, but you need to know when, and how urgently, to seek medical help. You can also monitor your wellbeing with regular health checks.

● **Treat yourself** You can normally treat these ailments and symptoms at home, at least in the first instance: bites and stings; allergic or irritant skin rash; colds, coughs and flu; vomiting; constipation; diarrhoea; indigestion; fever; hay fever; headache; minor wounds; mouth ulcers; sunburn; thrush.

● **Check your blood pressure** Do it every six months, either at a local health clinic or at home with a home blood monitor. If the top number is more than 140 and the bottom number is higher than 90, wait a day, then check it again. If it's still high, consult your doctor.

● **Have a cardiovascular check** If you're over 40 and not on treatment for heart disease or high blood pressure, you can request a full cardiovascular screening on the NHS. You can also request one if you're under 40 with a strong family history of heart attack or stroke. Blood-cholesterol levels are one of several factors that need to be measured and assessed, including smoking status, blood-glucose level, ECG (electrocardiagram) results and blood pressure. Ask for advice at your GP's surgery.

● **Recognize emergencies** In the case of a medical emergency, dial 999 or get the person to the nearest hospital accident and emergency (A&E) department as fast as possible. Emergencies that need urgent medical intervention include:
• difficulty breathing or shortness of breath that interferes with speech
• sudden confusion, unnatural drowsiness or difficulty in waking someone
• inability to swallow
• chest pain, especially if it spreads to the neck, jaw or arms or is accompanied by sweating, shortness of breath, dizziness or vomiting
• paralysis or weakness, especially of one side of the face or body
• an asthma attack that lasts for more than 10 minutes despite the use of medication
• calf pain accompanied by chest pain, shortness of breath or coughing up blood
• sudden intensely severe headache
• sudden loss of vision or visual disturbances

● **Seek medical advice** You need a doctor's advice within a day for:
• dramatic worsening of any symptom not listed as emergencies
• increasing pain

- high fever
- vomiting for more than 24 hours
- unexplained bleeding from any orifice, or blood appearing in urine, faeces, sputum or vomit
- a skin wound that becomes hot, red and throbbing, is painful or leaks pus
- inability to pass urine
- constipation that is severe or sudden, especially if you are aged over 50
- significant unexplained weight loss over two months or longer
- hoarseness lasting more than two weeks
- sore throat with a raised temperature, swollen lymph nodes in the neck and pain on swallowing

● **Monitor the colour of your urine** Your urine should be a clear straw colour; if it's dark or smells strong, you may not be getting enough fluids. If it stays dark-coloured even after you increase your liquid intake, consult your doctor.

● **Do a head-to-toe skin check** Every three months, with the help of your partner or a close friend, conduct a head-to-toe skin check, looking for any new moles, changed moles, suspicious spots or rashes. Be sure to check your scalp, between your toes and fingers, and even on the underside of your arms. If you find anything worrying, see your doctor.

● **Measure your height every year after you turn 50** This is especially important for women as a way of assessing posture and skeletal health. A change in stature can reveal as much about your overall bone health as a change shown by a bone-density scan. Bone-density tests can identify bone loss even before your height changes.

SELF-MONITORING TIPS

Mainly for women: check your breasts

Check your breasts every month just after your period or, if you're postmenopausal, on the first of the month. Report any changes to your GP without delay. (This applies to men as well as women, even though men make up less than 1 per cent of breast-cancer cases in the UK.) Here's what to look out for:

- Size: has one breast become larger or lower? Is there any change in the outline or shape of the breast?
- Nipples: has a nipple become inverted or has it changed position or shape? Are there any rashes on or around the nipple, or moist reddish areas that don't heal easily? Is there any discharge?
- Skin changes: do you notice any dimples or puckering?
- Is there any pain or discomfort in one breast that seems abnormal, particularly if it is new or persistent?
- Is there a lump, thickening or bumpy area in one breast or armpit that seems to be very different from the same part of the other breast or armpit?

Men only: check your testicles

Follow these steps every month to become familiar with what's normal so you can recognize if anything feels wrong. If you find a lump on your testicle, see a doctor right away. It may be only an infection, but if it's testicular cancer, it will spread without treatment. The best time to check is after a bath or shower, when your skin is relaxed.

- Stand in front of a mirror. Check for any swelling on the scrotal skin.
- Examine each testicle with both hands. Place the index and middle fingers under the testicle with the thumbs placed on top. Roll the testicle gently between thumbs and fingers – you shouldn't feel any pain as you do it.

The human body has a huge capacity for healing and repair

COLDS AND FLU

In most cases, the only practical difference between colds and flu is that flu is likely to make you feel a lot worse for longer. Both types of infection are caused by viruses, so antibiotics are no help. But there are many things you can do to improve how you feel with a cold or flu, hasten your recovery – and prevent infection in the first place.

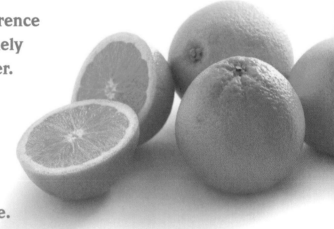

● **Take it easy** Your recovery will be faster if you take care of yourself rather than trying to tough it out. Don't struggle into work feeling dreadful. Instead, take it easy for a day or two, especially if you have a fever or a bad cough. Keep warm and stay in bed if you feel exhausted – sleep helps your immune system to combat infection. Eat a healthy diet, rich in infection-fighting nutrients, and avoid dusty or smoky atmospheres, which will aggravate your symptoms.

great idea!

Humidify the air One of the best ways to relieve a stuffy nose is to add water vapour to the air. You can do this by using a humidifier or by placing bowls of water on top of hot radiators. Alternatively, try sitting in a steamy bathroom for a while. Adding moisture to the air helps to reduce irritation and makes it easier for you to sleep. Dry air not only dries out mucous membranes, which makes nasal congestion, sore throat and coughing more likely, but also helps flu viruses to survive.

● **Do some gentle exercise** Exercise can boost your immune system and help to fight off the bugs. Gentle stretching exercises or yoga for 20 to 30 minutes a day are ideal. But avoid doing anything too strenuous – vigorous exercise, especially if you're not used to it, can set back your recovery.

● **Don't forget zinc** Some studies suggest that zinc taken within a day of the onset of symptoms may also help to shorten the duration of a cold. Use a supplement or lozenges, but avoid zinc nasal sprays, as these may damage your sense of smell. Research indicates that taking zinc combined with high dose (2g) vitamin C is even more effective.

● **Consume more fluids** Taking in plenty of fluids may help to keep mucus loose and avoid dehydration. It will also ease congestion and makes up for moisture lost in mucus production and by fever. Water, juices and soups are ideal, but avoid alcohol and caffeinated drinks as these cause dehydration.

● **Gargle with warm salt water**
Dissolve about half a teaspoon of salt in half a glass of warm water and gargle for 1 or 2 minutes, then spit out. A salt-water gargle soothes soreness and may also help to clear mucus.

● **For fast fever relief, pop a pill** If you have a fever, an over-the-counter painkiller such as paracetamol, aspirin or ibuprofen will help to lower your temperature and combat headache or general aches and pains. Take care not to exceed the maximum recommended daily intake of paracetamol (for adults 4,000mg or eight 500mg tablets) or you may suffer permanent liver damage.

● **Boost your immune system** You can kick-start the recovery process by including plenty of the following infection-fighting nutrients in your diet.
Protein Rebuilds strength and many sources also supply B vitamins, zinc and selenium, which are vital for a healthy immune system. Try to eat at least 50g of protein daily from lean meat, poultry, fish, eggs, pulses, nuts and seeds.
Antioxidants Health-boosting compounds, such as vitamins C, E and beta carotene, found in many plant foods. Try to eat at least five portions of fruit and vegetables every day. Lightly steam, rather than boil, vegetables when possible, to minimize the loss of their nutrients during cooking.
Bioflavonoids Nutrients that boost immune responses and hasten recovery from infections. Found especially in citrus fruits, such as oranges and grapefruit, which also contain the powerful immune-boosting nutrient vitamin C.
Zinc Important for healthy immune-system function and resistance to infections. Foods rich in zinc include eggs, seeds, nuts and whole-grain cereals.

● **Sip a lemon drink** There's science behind the traditional advice to sip a hot lemon drink. Lemons are rich in vitamin C, which improves the function of the white blood cells that destroy viruses. Lemon also reduces mucus production. Add some honey to the drink to coat your throat and help to ease soreness and to reduce coughing

● **Try an echinacea supplement**
Widely available in tablet or tincture form, echinacea cuts the duration of cold symptoms. What's more, taking the herbal supplement regularly could more than halve your chances of catching a cold in the first place.

WHAT IF I START TO FEEL WORSE?

If any respiratory infection makes it hard for you to breathe or you feel unusually drowsy, or if you have difficulty rousing someone else, seek immediate medical advice. Also, if the symptoms worsen or don't improve within a week or so, consult your doctor. Seek help for:

• prolonged hoarseness that persists for longer than two weeks

• pain or pressure in the region of the nose, eyes or forehead that persists for more than two weeks (indications of sinusitis)

• a worsening sore throat accompanied by fever, swollen lymph nodes in the neck, hoarseness and painful swallowing

• increased coughing with grey-green sputum and perhaps accompanied by fever, wheezing, shortness of breath and chest discomfort (indications of bronchitis)

• suddenly feeling very ill, perhaps occurring with persistent cough, shortness of breath, high fever accompanied by sweating or chills, chest pain, muscle aches and headaches (indications of pneumonia)

Fend off colds and flu with clever prevention strategies

try it...

Chocolate can protect you against coughs
A persistant cough is one of the most common reasons for visiting the doctor. But there is usually little on offer in the way of effective medicines, so try a regular dose of dark chocolate. Researchers in London and Budapest have proved that an ingredient in chocolate – theobromine – is highly effective in inhibiting laboratory-induced coughs in volunteers.

● **Don't blame yourself when things go wrong at work** Blaming yourself makes you more likely to catch a cold, according to a study of more than 200 workers over 3 months. Even those who had control over their work were more likely to begin sneezing if they lacked confidence or tended to blame themselves when things went wrong. Researchers believe that such attitudes make people more stressed on the job, and stress can challenge your immune system.

● **Carry hand sanitizer with you** Colds are typically passed not from coughing or kissing (although those are two modes of transmission) but from hand-to-hand or hand-to-object contact, since most cold viruses can live for hours on objects. If you put your hand in or near your mouth or nose after touching an infected object, you are likely to be infected. Carrying hand-sanitizer gel or sanitizing wipes with you allows you to clean your hands at any time, even if the closest water supply is miles away.

● **Wash your hands often – and do it twice** A US study of 40,000 naval recruits who were ordered to wash their hands five times a day found that the recruits cut their incidence of respiratory illnesses by 45 per cent. Every time you wash your hands, do it twice. Researchers who looked for germs on volunteers' hands found that one handwashing had little effect, even when using antibacterial soap.

● **Use your knuckles to rub your eyes** Your knuckles are less likely to be contaminated with viruses than your fingertips. This is particularly important given that the eye provides a perfect entry point for germs, and most of us rub our eyes or nose or scratch our faces between 20 and 50 times a day.

● **Have a weekly sauna** An Austrian study published in 1990 found that volunteers who frequently used a sauna had half as many colds during the six-month study as those who didn't use a sauna at all. It's possible that the hot air you inhale in a sauna kills cold viruses.

● **Sterilize your toothbrush** Once you're finished brushing your teeth, your toothbrush is a breeding ground for bacteria. Put it in the microwave on a high setting for 10 seconds to kill germs that can cause colds and other illnesses.

● **Get a flu vaccination** Annual flu vaccination is generally offered free of charge on the NHS to everyone over 65, and to anyone with a long-term medical problem that makes them more vulnerable (for example, heart or lung disease, being on immunosuppressant drugs, having diabetes or no spleen).

● **Take a garlic supplement** When 146 volunteers received either one garlic supplement a day or a placebo for twelve weeks between November and February, those taking the garlic were less likely to get a cold – and, if they did catch one, their symptoms were less intense and they recovered faster.

● **Eat yoghurt** A study by an American university found that people who ate a pot of yoghurt each day – whether live culture or pasteurized – had 25 per cent fewer colds than non-yoghurt eaters. Start your yoghurt-eating in the summer to build up your immunity before the cold and flu season starts.

● **Wipe your nose – don't blow** The force of blowing not only sends the phlegm out of your nose into a tissue but also propels some of it back into your sinuses, prolonging your cold symptoms. If you need to blow, blow gently, and blow one nostril at a time.

● **Reduce the heating in your home** The dry air of an overheated home provides the perfect environment for cold viruses to thrive. And when your mucous membranes (of the nose, mouth and tonsils) dry out, they can't trap those germs very well. Lowering the temperature by a few degrees and using a room humidifier helps to maintain a healthier level of humidity in winter.

● **Scrub your fingernails every day** Fingernails are great hiding places for all sorts of germs.

● **Sneeze and cough into a tissue** Whoever taught us to cover our mouths when we cough or sneeze got it wrong. That just puts the germs right on our hands, where we can spread them to objects – and other people. Instead, use a tissue whenever possible, and dispose of it hygienically – or hold the crook of your elbow over your mouth and nose when you sneeze or cough.

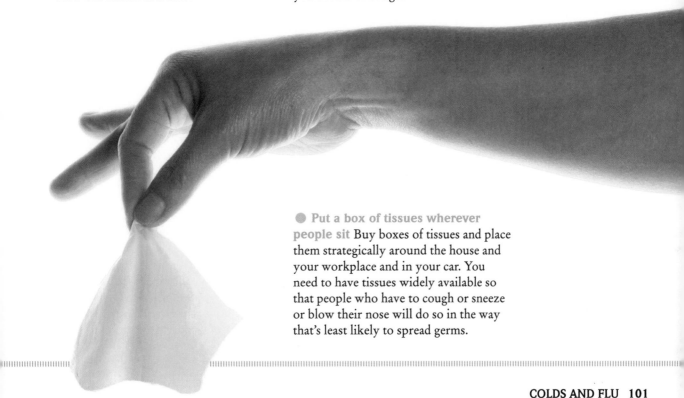

● **Put a box of tissues wherever people sit** Buy boxes of tissues and place them strategically around the house and your workplace and in your car. You need to have tissues widely available so that people who have to cough or sneeze or blow their nose will do so in the way that's least likely to spread germs.

DEALING WITH ASTHMA

Often triggered by an allergic reaction that leads to a narrowing of the airways, asthma is characterized by intermittent attacks of wheezing, coughing, and feeling short of breath and 'tight-chested'. If you or your child has asthma, make sure that you have appropriate medication (usually in the form of inhalers) to use in case of an attack.

● **Avoid fatty 'junk' foods** Researchers at the University of Newcastle in Australia fed 40 asthma patients either a high-fat, high-calorie meal of fast-food burgers and hash browns or a low-fat, low-calorie meal of yoghurt.

Those patients who consumed the high-fat meal demonstrated marked increases in inflammatory cells in their sputum (indicating that they had become more susceptible to an asthma attack) and responded less well than the other group to asthma medication.

● **Snack on nuts and seeds** Instead of cakes, biscuits and crisps, keep nuts and seeds available for between-meal nibbling (unless you are allergic to them).

As well as having a low sugar content, these foods are high in omega-3 fatty acids, which have been shown to relieve inflammation and are thought to reduce asthma symptoms. Walnuts and flaxseeds, in particular, are good sources of omega-3 fatty acids.

● **Beware of mould** Tiny mould spores released into the air can sometimes trigger asthma attacks. If you suffer from asthma, keep well away from compost heaps, piles of rotting leaves and damp woody areas. Make sure that your home is well ventilated; don't leave piles of damp clothes or towels lying around; wipe up condensation quickly; and treat any areas of mould as soon as you can.

● **Take exercise** If your asthma is well controlled and you take precautions, you should be able to take part in almost any physical activity. If symptoms start, stop exercising, use your 'reliever' inhaler and wait until you feel better.

Swimming While there is some evidence that prolonged exposure to chlorinated water in pools may increase asthma, swimming is a great exercise for people with asthma: it expands lung volume, develops good breathing techniques and improves physical fitness.

Yoga Yoga can improve your breathing technique as well as helping you relax.

Aerobic exercise If you want to do aerobic exercise, team sports such as football or hockey, in which the individual players are involved in only brief bursts of intense exertion, with short breaks in between, are less likely to provoke symptoms than those involving prolonged intensive effort, such as squash.

Golf and weightlifting Activities such as golf, weightlifting and walking are less likely to trigger symptoms than aerobic exercise that makes you breathe hard, such as running or playing football.

● **Avoid royal jelly** Supplements containing the bee product royal jelly may be dangerous if you have asthma. Royal jelly can provoke a serious – even fatal – respiratory reaction.

● **Keep away from pollution** A 2007 study in the *New England Journal of Medicine* found that 2 hours' exposure to diesel fumes in a busy urban street had a marked adverse effect on lung function, especially among asthmatics.

● **Control your weight** The typical Western diet is linked with a higher risk of developing asthma, worse symptoms and more attacks. What's more, such a diet – laden with unhealthy fats and processed carbohydrates, and low in fresh fruit and vegetables – causes obesity, which is itself linked to asthma in both adults and children. Losing a little weight, combined with making small adjustments to your diet, can improve lung function, reduce the need for asthma medication and lower the frequency of attacks.

The omega-3 fatty acids EPA and DHA in oily fish can reduce airway inflammation

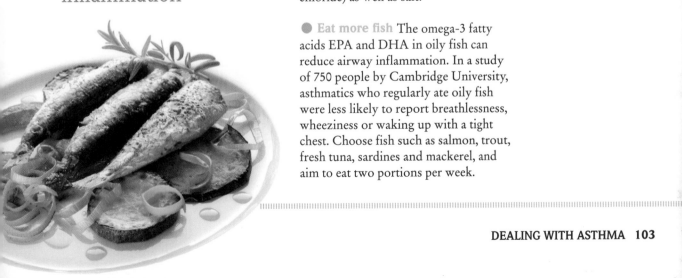

SIX KEY STEPS TO DEALING WITH **ASTHMA ATTACKS**

• **Use your reliever inhaler immediately** All asthma attacks need to be treated as soon as possible with a fast-acting inhaler. Take one or two puffs straight away. If you are using a Symbicort inhaler, follow the advice given by your doctor or asthma nurse.

• **Don't panic** Stress exacerbates symptoms. If you're helping someone who's having an asthma attack, remain calm and reassuring.

• **Sit down** Loosen any tight clothing. Don't lie down, as this will make breathing more difficult.

• **Repeat inhaler treatment** If there is no immediate improvement, take two puffs every 2 minutes for 10 minutes (up to ten puffs).

• **Seek medical help** If there is no improvement in your symptoms after 5 minutes, or if you are in any doubt, get medical help urgently – dial 999, if necessary. If you are the sufferer, do not attempt to drive yourself to hospital.

• **Keep using your inhaler** Continue to do this until an ambulance arrives.

● **Reduce your salt intake** Evidence suggests that high-salt diets are linked with asthma severity. Most salt in our diet comes from processed foods, so check the labels when you are shopping and look out for sodium content (salt is sodium chloride) as well as salt.

● **Eat more fish** The omega-3 fatty acids EPA and DHA in oily fish can reduce airway inflammation. In a study of 750 people by Cambridge University, asthmatics who regularly ate oily fish were less likely to report breathlessness, wheeziness or waking up with a tight chest. Choose fish such as salmon, trout, fresh tuna, sardines and mackerel, and aim to eat two portions per week.

9 top ways to fight allergies

Common allergies such as hay fever are not usually life-threatening, but they're nothing to sneeze at either, and an allergic reaction may trigger a more serious event such as an asthma attack. You can adapt your daily activities to protect yourself.

1 WARD OFF HAY FEVER WITH HONEY

If you are allergic to pollen, raw honey may be the answer. It contains traces of pollen, so eating a few tablespoons a day may help to accustom your immune system to pollen and stop it from triggering hay fever. Make sure the honey you use is raw and try to buy it from a source close to home so that it contains pollen from your area.

2 EAT ONE ORANGE EVERY MORNING

Oranges are rich in vitamin C, which acts as a natural antihistamine. Some studies have found a connection between allergies and low levels of vitamin C, so you may want to consider taking a vitamin C supplement too.

3 WATER HOUSEPLANTS SPARINGLY

Overwatering houseplants can contribute to the growth of mould in your home.

4 SPEND THE WEEKEND DECLUTTERING

Get rid of coats and other clothing you haven't used in the past year. Put sports equipment in the garage or attic where it belongs. When you finish, give everything a good vacuum to reduce significantly the amount of dust in your house.

5 AVOID FOODS CONTAINING MONOSODIUM BENZOATE

An Italian study found that the food preservative monosodium benzoate was responsible for triggering allergy-like symptoms, including sneezing and nasal itching, in adults without allergies. Monosodium benzoate is commonly found in juices, pie fillings, pickles, olives and salad dressings.

6 KEEP YOUR THERMOSTAT SET ABOVE 18°C IN WINTER

If you set your thermostat too low, you will encourage the growth of mould in damp air. Heat dries the air, preventing mould, though air that's too dry can also irritate your lungs and sinuses. An inexpensive humidity meter could help: the perfect level is about 50 per cent.

7 TAKE ALGAE FOR ALLERGIES

Try drinks or supplements that contain spirulina, a blue-green algae. Spirulina is a powerful anti-inflammatory agent and can help to quell an over-reactive response of the immune system to triggers such as pollen.

In a study that involved giving a group of hay-fever sufferers a daily dose of 2,000mg spirulina, researchers recorded a reduction of approximately 32 per cent in the severity of hay-fever symptoms.

best routes to **home hygiene**

If you're allergic to anything you encounter frequently – common triggers include house-dust mites, pet fur and dander, pollen and mould spores – life can be miserable. Implementing allergen-avoidance strategies at home can make all the difference.

Choose a doormat made of synthetic material
Doormats made of natural material (coir, etc.) can break down and become feeding grounds for mites, mould and fungus, which then get carried through the house on people's shoes.

Put a shelf by the front door for shoes Encourage your family and guests to remove their shoes before entering to reduce the amount of allergens carried in.

Keep animals out of your bedroom You spend more time in your bedroom than in any other room of the house, so keep it free of cat and dog dander, to which many people are allergic.

Prevent mould growth Always run the extractor fan and/or leave the window and door open when having a shower or bath. Or run a small portable fan (away from water sources) during and after showers. You're trying to keep surfaces dry and prevent mould growing.

Wash your shower curtain in hot water and bleach
Do this every month, or use a shower liner that you can replace every couple of months for just a few pounds.

Clean the tray under the fridge regularly The tray is a veritable mould magnet. Clean it with a bleach solution and sprinkle with salt. Adding salt reduces the growth of mould and bacteria. Also, clean under the fridge itself occasionally; food can get trapped there, become mouldy and the mould spores are blown into the kitchen every time the compressor kicks in.

Wash all your bedding in very hot water It's the best way to kill those nasty microscopic dust mites that love your bed even more than you do.

8 CLEAN OUT YOUR GUTTERS

Clogged gutters can result in water seeping into the house, leading to mould growth, which can exacerbate allergies. Next time it rains, check your gutters. If you see water leaking out of the end caps, flowing on the outside or dripping behind them, it's time to get out the ladder.

9 INSTALL HARD-SURFACE FLOORING

Carpets are breeding grounds for dust mites and mould, and do a wonderful job of capturing animal dander and pollen – only to release it every time you vacuum or even just walk on it. Wood, tile or laminate floors are the best for people with allergies.

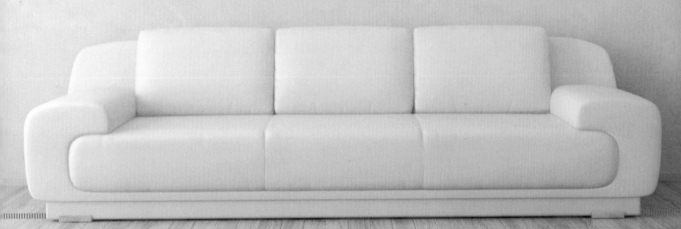

INDIGESTION AND UPSET STOMACH

Among the most common digestive complaints are indigestion and upset stomach. Indigestion involves discomfort or pain in the upper abdomen provoked by eating. Gastrointestinal infections or food poisoning from contaminated food or drink are characterized by nausea, vomiting, diarrhoea and abdominal pain or cramps.

● **Get checked for an underlying condition** If simple measures don't solve the problem, see your doctor in case there's an underlying condition that needs treatment. Your doctor may want to check whether you have a peptic ulcer, which has some symptoms in common with indigestion. Seek prompt medical advice if you also develop symptoms such as persistent vomiting, blood in your vomit, black tarry faeces, difficulty swallowing, unexplained weight loss or extreme fatigue.

Make sure you eat only soft, bland foods

● **Keep indigestion at bay** Fear of an attack of indigestion may start to spoil your enjoyment of meals, so it is worth learning how to control the problem.
• Eat little and often so that your stomach is never overloaded. And don't have your main meal too close to bedtime.
• Eat slowly and keep your mouth closed while you are chewing. This prevents you from swallowing air and ensures that food reaches the stomach in smaller pieces, helping the digestive process.
• Avoid alcoholic, fizzy or caffeinated drinks.
• It may be helpful to avoid drinking with meals.
• Don't smoke.
• Avoid spicy or greasy foods.
• Don't wear clothes with tight waistbands, which can constrict the stomach and inhibit digestion.
• Avoid aspirin and anti-inflammatory drugs that could irritate the stomach lining.
• Don't do anything energetic for an hour after a meal.
• If you are overweight, try to shed a few pounds as this will lessen pressure on the stomach and may reduce regurgitation and acid reflux.

● **Eat carefully** When you start to feel like eating normally, avoid fatty and fried foods, which can make you feel nauseous and worsen diarrhoea. Avoid citrus fruits, milk and milk products, including cheese and ice cream, and beware of sugar-laden foods or drinks (cakes, biscuits and cola-style drinks). Continue to base meals on bland, starchy foods. Try bananas, rice, boiled potatoes, toast and pasta.

● **Take peppermint** The menthol in peppermint helps to ease the pain and bloating of indigestion and dispel intestinal gas. It can also reduce the symptoms of irritable bowel syndrome. When trouble strikes, try sucking a peppermint or slowly sipping peppermint tea. Peppermint is also available in capsule form. However, if you have heartburn due to reflux of stomach acid, peppermint may make it worse, so be sure to test it out cautiously.

● **Try over-the-counter remedies** Products that contain loperamide will bring immediate relief from diarrhoea, but make sure you seek medical advice if symptoms aren't better within two days, get worse or if other problems develop.

● **Drink plenty of water** Even if you're feeling sick, take frequent sips of plain water, herb teas, diluted juice or clear soups. This is important for everyone, but especially for babies and young children, older people and those with existing illnesses, who are more susceptible to dehydration and its effects.

Those who are vulnerable should take a sip every 10 minutes or so. Specific rehydration fluids, available from pharmacies, that replace the correct balance of salts (electrolytes) in the blood are best. Encourage a baby to carry on feeding from the breast or bottle as usual.

INDIGESTION OR A HEART ATTACK?

Seek immediate medical attention if the pain is different or more severe than usual, comes on with exercise rather than after food, travels to anywhere else in the body, such as your arm or jaw, or is accompanied by shortness of breath, sweating or nausea. A sudden attack of belching, often with accompanying chest pain, is a common symptom of reduced blood supply to the heart, which occurs during a heart attack, and it requires emergency attention. If you are in any doubt, seek help at once by dialling 999.

● **Keep it bland** As symptoms improve, eat only soft, bland foods to maintain nutrition and reduce symptoms until you're feeling better.

● **Raise your head** If you tend to get symptoms of reflux – acid from stomach contents passing back up the oesophagus – then raising your bedhead slightly or using an extra pillow can often prevent or ease symptoms.

● **Try ginger or caraway** For many people, relief from indigestion is best provided by medicines that counter acid in the stomach, such as simple antacids and proton-pump inhibitors, but there are also natural remedies that have some proven benefits.
• Ginger can help to calm intestinal spasm and stimulate digestive secretions. It is best taken as a tea: steep about 0.25g of powdered ginger, or a few slices of ginger root, in water and sip either warm or cooled following each meal.
• Make a tea from caraway seeds or add a couple of drops of caraway oil to a glass of water.

CONSTIPATION AND IRRITABLE BOWEL SYNDROME

As well as infrequent bowel movements, constipation means having hard stools that are difficult to pass. Irritable bowel syndrome is a common problem affecting the large intestine. It is not serious but it does cause distressing symptoms such as abdominal cramps, bloating and flatulence.

● **Fill up on fibre** The indigestible, fibrous parts of plants add bulk to your stools, both softening them and stimulating the urge to defecate. Aim to eat between five and nine portions of fruit, vegetables or beans daily and choose wholemeal bread and pasta, and brown rice over the white alternatives. Try to drink more, as adding fluid to your digestive contents softens the stool and makes it easier to pass. Aim to drink at least six to eight glasses of fluids a day.

● **Keep a food diary** Many people find that certain foods make their symptoms worse. If you log everything you eat and drink, along with your symptoms, for three weeks, you may be able to identify suspect items and avoid them. Common culprits include alcohol, tea, coffee, chocolate, dairy products and sugar-free sweeteners such as sorbitol. If dairy products tend to provoke symptoms, you may be lactose-intolerant and need to avoid them altogether.

Get plenty of fresh air ... and make time to relax every day

● **Get into a regular habit** Your body becomes used to you opening your bowels at a particular time each day, so try to get into a regular habit. In the morning, just after breakfast, is often the best time, and at other times go when you feel the urge. But don't strain to defecate if you don't feel the need to do so; this can lead to the development of haemorrhoids (piles). If you can, become more active, since even gentle physical activity promotes bowel health and encourages intestinal contractions.

● **Monitor your fibre intake** Increasing the quantity of fibre in your diet may relieve irritable bowel syndrome, but some people find that it makes their symptoms worse in that, while the additional fibre treats their constipation effectively, it exacerbates bloating and flatulence. Foods that contain plenty of fibre include fruit and vegetables, whole grains and beans. A fibre supplement such as ispaghula husk (psyllium) can be taken, but it may also make bloating worse.

● **Turn off the gas** If bloating and intestinal gas are prominent symptoms, cut down or reduce your intake of gas-producing foods such as beans, cabbages, broccoli and cauliflower. Some raw fruits and vegetables should also be avoided. Frequent consumption of fizzy drinks, chewing gum or drinking through straws can increase the amount of air passing into the intestines, producing gas.

● **Eat and drink regularly** Hurried and irregular meals can contribute to irritable bowel syndrome. Adopt regular mealtimes and allow yourself the time to eat in a relaxed fashion. Your bowel gets into the habit of being 'fed' at consistent intervals, so try to eat at roughly the same time each day. Eating small, frequent meals tends to help those for whom diarrhoea is a troublesome symptom, while fewer, larger, fibre-rich meals may be of benefit to people whose main symptom is constipation.

It is a sensible idea to increase the amount you drink because consuming more fluid, especially water, helps to relieve constipation. But be aware that alcoholic drinks or tea, coffee and other beverages containing caffeine may worsen diarrhoea.

● **Take more exercise** Irritable bowel syndrome is a complicated condition in which both physiological and psychological factors play a role. Most doctors recommend taking more exercise – not only will this help to counteract stress and depression, but it also encourages regular intestinal movements and keeps your bowels running smoothly.

BEST HYGIENE PRACTICE

If you or someone else in the family has diarrhoea and/or vomiting, you must take strict hygiene measures to prevent the spread of infection. This includes washing hands thoroughly after using the toilet, changing nappies or cleaning up after the affected person and before preparing food or drink. Disinfect all surfaces and items that have come into contact with the person or their body fluids. Someone who is recovering from a gastrointestinal bug should stay away from work or school for 48 hours after the symptoms have cleared, to avoid spreading the infection.

● **Manage stress** If you suffer from stress, try to learn to manage it. Although stress and tension don't cause irritable bowel syndrome, they can worsen the symptoms. Get plenty of fresh air – in a calming countryside setting, if possible – and make some time to relax every day.

● **Try probiotics** A probiotic supplement can be helpful for the relief of abdominal pain and bloating. 'Friendly' bacteria found naturally in your gut may be disturbed in irritable bowel syndrome, and some studies suggest that foods such as yoghurt containing live probiotic organisms, or probiotic supplements, help to restore your bowel to health.

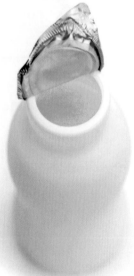

Common culprits include alcohol, tea, coffee, chocolate, dairy products and sugar-free sweeteners such as sorbitol

URINARY AND VAGINAL INFECTIONS

Varying from an irritating minor annoyance to a more serious long-term problem, urinary-tract and vaginal infections are among the most common ailments affecting women. There is plenty you can do to complement any treatment prescribed by your doctor, ensure a rapid recovery and prevent a recurrence.

● **See your doctor** If you suspect a urinary-tract infection, see your doctor. Untreated infections can spread further up the urinary tract to the kidneys, leading to a more serious problem. If an infection is confirmed, you'll probably be given antibiotics, which usually produce rapid and effective relief.

● **Flush out the problem** Increasing your fluid intake dilutes urine and helps to flush out bacteria. Aim to drink six to eight glasses of fluid a day.

● **Urinate after sex** In women especially, bacteria may enter the urethra during sex. Passing urine immediately afterwards helps to flush them out. Some women find that using a diaphragm or spermicidal gel promotes infection. If so, it may help to change your method of contraception. Unlubricated condoms or those impregnated with spermicide can also cause problems – use the lubricated type without spermicide.

● **Be careful what you drink** Avoid drinking alcohol, fruit juices (other than cranberry juice), coffee, tea and other caffeine-containing drinks, which can further irritate the bladder and increase frequency or urgency of urination.

● **Urinate frequently** Don't put it off because you know it might hurt – go as soon as you feel the urge because bacteria are more likely to grow if urine sits in the bladder for too long. If it's very painful, passing urine while sitting in a warm bath can lessen the burning sensation.

● **Wear loose clothes** Keeping the air circulating helps to counter infection, which thrives in moist, sweaty conditions. Avoid nylon underwear and tight jeans.

● **Wipe from front to back** To avoid introducing germs from the intestines into the urethra, women should always wipe from front to back after a bowel movement, or wipe each area separately.

Avoid drinking alcohol, fruit juices (other than cranberry juice), coffee, tea and other caffeine-containing drinks

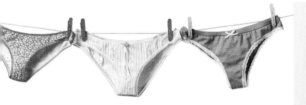

● **Choose cotton underwear**
Underwear made of cotton rather than synthetic fabrics such as nylon reduces sweating and allows the genital region to 'breathe', so that it stays drier, which helps to counteract yeast infections. If you are prone to such infections, avoid wearing tights or close-fitting jeans.

● **Don't lounge around in a wet swimsuit** After a swimming session, dry yourself thoroughly and put on clean, dry underclothes as soon as possible.

● **Treat yeast infection with an antifungal medication** The most common yeast infection, known as thrush or candidiasis, which causes a thick white vaginal discharge, can be effectively treated with an over-the-counter antifungal medication.

If you're not sure you have thrush, or if symptoms are slightly different from those you've had before, or if you have had a recent new sexual partner or are pregnant, consult your doctor.

● **Avoid products containing chemicals and perfumes** Anything that potentially irritates the delicate skin and membranes of the vulva and vagina can encourage infections to take hold, so avoid talc, deodorant sprays, bubble baths and coloured or scented toilet paper.

Choose plain, unperfumed soap or select a pH-balanced wash specially formulated for the genital area. A flannel soaked in cool water laid over the affected area can provide temporary relief of external itching.

did you know?

A 'silent' disease that can cause infertility Chlamydia is one of the most common sexually transmitted infections in the UK – but most people who have chlamydia don't notice any symptoms, and so don't know they have it. Symptoms could include painful urination, unusual discharge from the vagina, penis or rectum or, in women, bleeding between periods or after sex.

Chlamydia is easily treated with antibiotics, but, if left untreated, the infection can sometimes spread to other parts of your body and lead to serious long-term health problems such as pelvic inflammatory disease and infertility. If you think you may have chlamydia, or would like to be screened for the disease, you can get a free confidential test at a sexual health clinic or a GP surgery.

● **Use supplements to counteract thrush** Strengthening your immune system with vitamin C and echinacea will help your body to fight an acute yeast infection. The herb echinacea seems to stimulate white blood cells to destroy the yeast, and vitamin C may inhibit yeast growth. Probiotics – available as bioyoghurts as well as in the form of oral supplements and a topically applied cream – will boost your body's supply of 'friendly' bacteria.

great idea!

Drink cranberry juice Numerous studies have shown that cranberry juice may both prevent urinary-tract infections and relieve symptoms. Cranberries contain substances that discourage bacteria from sticking to the bladder wall. Including cranberries or cranberry juice (a 300ml/½ pint glass twice a day) in your regular diet can help to keep infections at bay. You can also buy supplements – take 400mg twice daily. But if you take the anticoagulant warfarin, check with your doctor first; cranberries may interact dangerously with this drug.

LOWER YOUR CHOLESTEROL

About 70 per cent of adults in the UK have high cholesterol, increasing their risk of heart disease and stroke. Eating a healthy diet and regular exercise can help to lower the level of cholesterol in your blood. Adopting healthy habits will also help to prevent your cholesterol from becoming high in the first place.

● **Choose wholemeal sandwiches** Cutting back on simple carbohydrates such as white bread and white rice and eating more complex carbohydrates, including wholemeal bread, can increase HDL levels slightly and significantly lower triglycerides, another type of blood fat that contributes to heart disease.

● **Have six or more small meals a day** A large study of British adults found that people who ate six or more small meals daily had significantly lower cholesterol than those who ate twice a day, even though the 'grazers' got more calories and fat. In fact, the differences in cholesterol levels were large enough to reduce the grazers' risk of heart disease by 10 to 20 per cent.

● **Eat foods enhanced with plant sterols and stanols** Studies suggest that eating products enhanced with plant sterols and stanols – naturally occurring substances similar to cholesterol in terms of their chemical structure – may help to reduce levels of harmful LDL cholesterol. Consuming around 2g of plant sterols/stanols can lower LDL levels by 10 to 15 per cent, although the amount varies from one person to another. So seek out sterol-enhanced margarines, yoghurts and other milk products and eat some every day. Names to look out for include Flora Proactiv, Benecol and Danacol.

● **Eat oily fish** Oily fish such as mackerel, herring, tuna and salmon provide the richest source of omega-3 essential fatty acids, which help to reduce the level of triglyceride fats in your blood (high triglyceride levels lead to a greater risk of cardiovascular disease).

> **did you know?**
>
> **What it means to have high cholesterol** If you have a high level of cholesterol in your blood, your body is producing too much 'bad' low-density lipoprotein (LDL) and too little 'good' high-density lipoprotein (HDL). 'Bad' LDL carries cholesterol into your arteries, contributing to artery-clogging plaque, while 'good' HDL carries cholesterol away to the liver and out of the body. The biggest dietary cause of high cholesterol is eating too much saturated fat. By choosing the right foods and taking good care of yourself, you can do a great deal to reduce your risk of heart disease and stroke.

● **Drink more orange juice** Some studies suggest that drinking 2 glasses of orange juice a day helps to cut total cholesterol, and a Canadian study found that drinking 3 glasses a day for four weeks raised healthy HDL levels by 21 per cent and improved the ratio of good to bad cholesterol by 16 per cent.

● **Whip up some guacamole** Several studies find that eating one avocado a day as part of a healthy diet can lower your LDL cholesterol by as much as 17 per cent while raising your HDL.

● **Drink a few glasses of cranberry juice** Cranberries are rich sources of anthocyanins, proanthocyanidins and flavonols, plant chemicals that prevent LDL cholesterol from oxidizing, a process that makes it more likely to stick to artery walls. These chemicals also keep red blood cells from getting too sticky. Not only do they decrease LDL cholesterol levels, but, according to one American study, three glasses of cranberry juice a day can raise HDL cholesterol levels by up to 10 per cent.

● **Eat a grapefruit every other day** Grapefruits are particularly high in pectin, a soluble fibre that can help to reduce cholesterol levels. Grapefruits interfere with the absorption and processing in the liver of several medicines, however, so check with your doctor first. Other good sources of pectin include apples and berries.

● **Have oatmeal for breakfast** Rich in a soluble fibre called beta glucan, oatmeal can reduce your LDL by 12 to 24 per cent if you eat a bowl of oats every day, combined with other foods rich in soluble fibre such as beans and pulses. Choose old-fashioned oats rather than instant.

try it... **A slow cooker** Slow cookers are perfect for making bean-based soups and stews high in cholesterol-lowering soluble fibre. They are also ideal for simmering lean cuts of meat, which are healthier due to their low fat content, but tend to be tougher than fattier cuts unless cooked slowly.

● **Pour soya milk over your cereal** A Spanish study of 40 men and women found that those who drank around 2 cups of soya milk a day for three months reduced their LDL cholesterol levels, while at the same time increasing their HDL levels. Make sure that you buy soya milk fortified with calcium.

● **Have a small glass of wine – or purple grape juice** A daily glass of wine or beer a day can boost levels of HDL cholesterol. Opt for red wine as it is three to ten times higher in plant compounds called flavonoids, believed to be responsible for much of wine's beneficial effects on cholesterol. If you don't like red wine, try purple grape juice, which is rich in cholesterol-lowering flavonoids.

● **Sip black tea every 4 hours** Scientists found that drinking 5 cups a day of black tea for three weeks reduced cholesterol levels in people with mildly high levels.

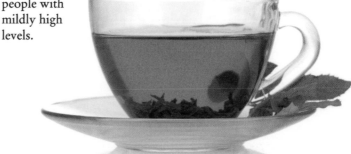

MONITOR YOUR BLOOD PRESSURE

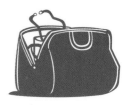

You can't see it, you can't feel it and, if you don't get it checked, you may not even know you have it. That makes high blood pressure a quiet killer, which slowly damages your blood vessels, heart and eyes while increasing your risk of serious diseases – but there are many things you can do to counteract it.

● **Stop smoking** The nicotine in tobacco constricts blood vessels and raises blood pressure in the short term.

● **Watch a yoga DVD** The stress-reducing and blood-pressure-lowering benefits of yoga are well documented. A DVD is a great way to introduce yourself to yoga in the privacy of your own home, with just a minimal investment.

● **Pay extra attention to diet** Follow a diet high in fruit and vegetables and low in high-salt, high-fat and high-cholesterol foods. One of the quickest ways to lower your blood pressure is to reduce your salt intake. Combine this with eating your five portions of fruit and vegetables a day and reducing your fat intake, and you're well on the way to getting your blood pressure down.

● **Snack on roasted soya nuts** Studies show that people with high blood pressure can lower their systolic readings by an average of 10 points by eating 30g (1oz) of soya nuts (roasted soya beans) a day for two weeks. Soya nuts are available at some supermarkets and health-food shops. Buy the unsalted variety.

● **Eat avocados** Avocados have more blood-pressure-lowering potassium than any other fruit or vegetable. We should get about 3,500mg a day of potassium, but one in three women in the UK gets just half this amount.

● **Flavour food with lots of pepper** Pepper is a strong, dominant flavour that can help you to reduce your taste for salt. Without salt, meals may seem bland for a couple of days, but your taste buds can easily be retrained. Add more pepper and, if that doesn't appeal, try garlic, lemon, ginger, basil or other spicy flavours you enjoy. After a week, some favourite foods will taste oversalted and your blood pressure will be singing your praises.

● **Measure your blood pressure at home** A study in the *Journal of the American Medical Association* found that home blood-pressure testing can provide a better overall picture of blood-pressure levels than readings in a doctor's surgery. Another study found that people who monitored their blood pressure at home had lower overall blood pressure than those who had their pressure taken only at the doctor's surgery.

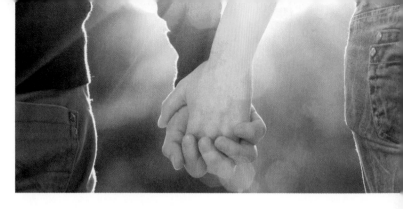

● **Find (and eliminate) one hidden source of salt a day** For instance, did you know that many breakfast cereals contain salt? Who needs salt in their cereal? Find a brand that's salt-free.

● **Eat a handful of dried apricots every afternoon** Apricots are another excellent source of potassium. Plus they have lots of fibre, iron and beta carotene. The drying process actually increases the concentration of these nutrients, which are all good for your circulatory system. And as a snack, dried apricots are low in calories: roughly eight total just 100kcal. Choose an unsulphured brand.

● **Sprinkle linseeds on your yoghurt** Linseeds are rich in many nutrients and in fibre. Sprinkle 2 tablespoons on your yoghurt in the morning and mix 2 tablespoons into your soup, spaghetti sauce or other food later in the day. One small study found that adding 4 tablespoons of the seeds to the daily diet significantly lowered systolic blood pressure in postmenopausal women with a history of heart disease.

● **Sleep with earplugs** Studies suggest that being exposed to noise while you're sleeping may increase your blood pressure as well as your heart rate, so block out any noise.

● **Get out every day for a walk** If you're overweight, make that two walks. Losing just a few pounds will make an enormous difference to your blood-pressure readings.

● **Take daily supplements** Supplements of garlic, fish oil, calcium, CoQ10 all have blood-pressure-lowering effects. Check with your GP first about whether a supplement is right for you.

● **Hold hands with your partner** Holding hands with a partner for 10 minutes (plus a brief hug) is all it took in one study to keep blood pressure steady during a stressful incident.

● **Think about your sleep** Do you wake up tired? Does your partner say that you snore a lot? Talk to your doctor. You may have sleep apnoea. Studies find that half the people who have the condition, in which you stop breathing dozens or hundreds of times during the night, also have high blood pressure.

● **Drink tea instead of coffee** An Australian study found that each one cup increase in daily tea consumption decreased systolic blood pressure (the top number) by 2 points and diastolic pressure (the bottom number) by 1 point. But the benefits ended after 4 cups.

great idea!

Turn to dark chocolate Unlike milk chocolate, dark chocolate is rich in flavonoids, which keep your arteries flexible, preventing the increases in pressure that come with stiffer blood vessels. That's thought to be one reason for the healthy blood-pressure readings of a tribe of indigenous Panamanians who eat a high-salt diet but also consume massive amounts of cocoa. A study in the *Journal of the American Medical Association* found that 85g of dark chocolate a day helped to lower blood pressure in older people with isolated systolic hypertension (when only the upper number of a pressure reading is high).

LIVING WITH **DIABETES**

Whether you have Type 1 or Type 2 diabetes, it is crucial to stick to your care plan, follow a healthy lifestyle and go for regular check-ups to ensure that your condition remains under control. Uncontrolled diabetes can lead to many health problems, including narrowing and furring of the large arteries, as well as foot problems (caused by poor blood circulation), kidney failure, eye problems and gum disease.

● **Eat the Mediterranean way** A Mediterranean diet can help to delay the need for blood glucose-lowering medication, according to a study of 215 overweight people newly diagnosed with Type 2 diabetes.

The study compared the standard low-fat, calorie-restricted diet usually recommended by the American Diabetic Association for people with Type 2 diabetes with a Mediterranean diet containing a high proportion of vegetables, fruit, grains, pulses and nuts with some cheese or yoghurt, fish, poultry and eggs. The overall proportion of calories derived from carbohydrates in such a diet is relatively low (less than 50 per cent) and its fats are mostly monounsaturated, mainly olive oil.

After four years, just 44 per cent of people on the Mediterranean diet needed blood-sugar-lowering medication compared with 70 per cent on the low-fat diet. Those eating the Mediterranean way also lost more weight and had lower levels of blood fats and blood pressure.

● **Be 'hypo' aware** A hypoglycaemic incident – colloquially known as a 'hypo' – occurs if your blood-glucose level drops to less than 4.0mmol/l. Hypos can happen if you are taking insulin or tablets for diabetes. They may result from taking too much insulin or other diabetes medication, missing or delaying a meal, not eating enough carbohydrates, taking more exercise than usual, hot weather, having too much alcohol or drinking alcohol without food.

Immediate action is needed to deal with hypoglycaemia (see page 119).

● **Lose weight slowly** If you're overweight, losing just 10 per cent of your body weight can improve your insulin sensitivity and glucose tolerance as well as reducing your blood pressure and cholesterol levels.

The best way to shed weight is to make small, healthy changes to what you eat and increase your activity levels. Diabetes UK advises filling half your plate with vegetables or salad, a third with starchy foods and most of the rest with low-fat protein such as lean meat, fish, chicken, lentils or beans.

Aim for a modest weight loss of 0.5–1kg (1–2lb) a week.

Insulin enables blood glucose to enter body cells to be used as fuel

● **Include carbohydrates in every meal** Try to include starchy carbohydrate foods, such as bread, pasta, rice, noodles, cereals and potatoes, in every meal. This will help to stabilize your blood-glucose levels throughout the day. Starchy carbohydrates that contain higher levels of fibre, such as whole-grain products, are digested more slowly, helping to keep your glucose levels steady.

● **Match meals with medication** Too little food in relation to medication – especially insulin – can result in hypoglycaemia, while too much can lead to high blood glucose (hyperglycaemia). Your health-care team will advise you on how to strike a balance. It's best to match your insulin dose to food intake, rather than vice versa.

● **Create a routine that works for you** To control your diabetes effectively, you need to establish a schedule for taking medication when your body needs it. This is determined by your intake of food and how much energy you expend. Initially you will have to monitor your blood-glucose levels several times a day and discuss the results with members of your health-care team. The team will help you to create a medication schedule based on your lifestyle.

● **Ease up on alcohol** Your liver normally releases glucose that has been stored as glycogen to offset falling blood-glucose levels, but if it's processing alcohol it may not work as effectively. If you're on insulin or some oral medications, even a small amount of alcohol can cause hypoglycaemia shortly after drinking and for up to 16 hours afterwards. It's generally safe to have a little alcohol as long as you stick to the following guidelines:

UNDERSTANDING DIABETES

Diabetes results in high levels of glucose (sugar) in the blood. It occurs when the pancreas stops making the hormone insulin, or does not make enough insulin, or the insulin it produces does not work as well as it should (insulin resistance). Insulin is a chemical messenger in the blood that enables blood glucose to enter body cells to be used as fuel. If the amount or action of the insulin is inadequate, glucose levels in the blood become too high. Most people with diabetes have to take lifelong medication – tablets, injections or both – to help to control blood glucose, blood pressure and cholesterol.

• **Type 1** occurs when the body's immune system destroys the insulin-producing cells in the pancreas. It usually appears during childhood. Treatment involves daily insulin injections that must continue for life.
• **Type 2** tends to appear after the age of 40, although younger people, including children and teenagers, can develop it too, and it's often linked to being overweight. It occurs when the pancreatic cells don't produce enough insulin or the body develops insulin resistance. Treatments include weight loss for those who are overweight, a healthy diet, regular activity and medication and/or insulin.

• Never drink if your blood glucose is low or your stomach is empty.
• Eat a low-fat snack with your drink.
• Don't exceed 2 units (women) or 3 units (men) a day.
• Check your blood glucose before drinking and before going to bed.
• Always wear medical ID. To people unfamiliar with diabetes, the symptoms of a hypo can be similar to drunkenness.
• If you're watching your weight, choose lower-calorie drinks such as dry white wine. And don't forget to count alcohol in your daily carbohydrate or calorie allowance.

● **Be more active** Being active is vital for your health, regardless of your circumstances, and especially if you have diabetes. Pick activities you enjoy and get moving – you'll feel much better for it. Becoming more active will help to improve your insulin sensitivity (which means that you'll need a lower dosage of insulin or other medication), lower your blood glucose, control your weight, lower your blood pressure and levels of harmful blood fats, and help to shift excess abdominal fat.

● **Be prepared** Always carry a starchy snack, such as an energy bar or banana, as well as a fast-acting carbohydrate source, such as glucose tablets or gel, in case you have a hypo while you are exercising. Make sure you drink plenty of fluids before, during and after exercise, and never drink alcohol before exercising, as it increases the risk of hypoglycaemia.

● **Get started** Choose light to moderate activities to begin with. Options include brisk walking (outside or on a treadmill), swimming or aqua aerobics, cycling (outside or on a stationary exercise bike), dancing, yoga, gardening, golf and racquet sports such as badminton or tennis. Water-based exercises put less strain on the joints.

● **Set goals** Decide which activities you want to do and for how long, then work out how to achieve this. Start slowly – for example, three 5–10 minute walks a week – and build up gradually to 30 minutes most days. Keep a record of what you do, along with any changes in your blood glucose, blood pressure and weight.

● **Ring the changes** Avoid boredom by varying your activities. Pick something you enjoy – dancing may be more appealing than jogging. Or how about something you enjoyed at school, such as basketball, hockey, netball or skipping?

● **Adopt a NEAT lifestyle** Being more active generally – what experts call non-exercise activity thermogenesis or NEAT – can burn 350kcal a day, equivalent to about a sixth of a woman's recommended daily calorie intake and about a seventh of a man's. Do all you can to exercise when moving from one place to another. Take the stairs instead of the lift, walk to the shops instead of driving, cycle to work.

● **Stay safe** Always carry or wear some medical ID. Make sure your exercise companion, trainer or fitness centre staff are aware that you have diabetes and know what to do if you have a hypo.

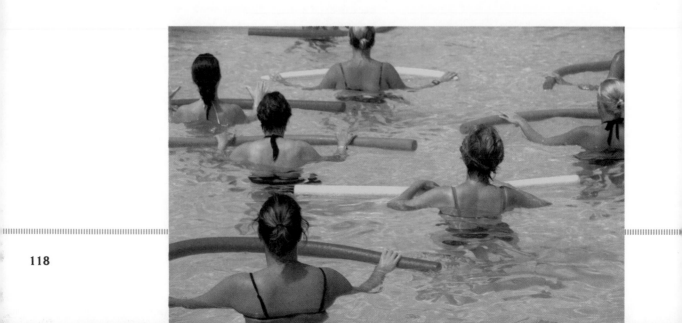

MANAGING **HYPOGLYCAEMIA**

Be aware of the key signs of hypoglycaemia – a 'hypo' – and make sure your friends, family and colleagues are also aware. Immediate action, by you or someone else, is needed, and treatment depends on severity.

• **Mild hypoglycaemia** In the case of a mild hypo, you are aware of the symptoms and able to act on them yourself.
• Stop and take a rapidly absorbed carbohydrate, such as a sugary drink (not a diet drink) or fruit juice; glucose, in the form of tablets or gel; or a couple of teaspoons of sugar, honey or jam.
• Repeat if there is no improvement in 5–10 minutes.
• Follow this up by eating a more slow-release or starchy carbohydrate snack such as a sandwich, piece of fruit, bowl of cereal, biscuit and milk, or a meal if you're due one.

• **Moderate hypoglycaemia** In a moderately severe hypo, you may become confused, in which case someone else must take the initial action needed to restore your blood glucose levels.
• The helper should squirt or rub a glucose gel or something sweet, but not solid, such as syrup, jam or honey, into the inside of your cheeks.
• The outside of your cheeks should be gently massaged to aid absorption.
• Once you're able to, have a sugary drink, followed by a starchy snack.

• **Severe hypoglycaemia** Severe hypos result in loss of consciousness and, possibly, seizures. If someone with diabetes experiences a severe hypo, summon medical help urgently.
• Do not give the person concerned anything by mouth, but, if you can do so, give a glucagon injection. Glucagon is a hormone that triggers the liver to release stored glucose. It takes around 15 minutes to restore consciousness in someone having a hypo.
• If this is not possible or the person fails to regain consciousness, call an ambulance without delay.
• Once the person has regained full consciousness following a glucagon injection and can swallow again, offer a sugary drink and a starchy snack as described above.

Hypo symptoms

the person with diabetes may notice

hunger • trembling or shakiness • sweating • anxiety or irritability • fatigue • palpitations • tingling lips • headache • blurred vision

other people may notice

pallor • glazed eyes • slurred words/inability to speak • lack of coordination • mood changes • confusion • irrational behaviour

● **Aim for more peaceful nights**
Check your blood-glucose level before you go to bed – if it's too high or too low, it can interfere with sleep.

Keep a high-carbohydrate snack, such as a banana or cereal bar, by your bed to eat if you wake in the night, along with some water. If you have experienced night-time hypos, set your alarm for 3am every night for a week and check your blood-glucose level when you wake up. If it's below 4.0mmol/l, have a snack. If your blood glucose is often low in the early hours of the morning, you may need to adjust your insulin regime or eating plan. See your doctor.

Be more active and go for regular check-ups

TAKING CARE OF
YOUR HEART

There are many different types of heart disease, ranging in severity from mild to life-threatening. Medical science has transformed the treatment of heart conditions in the past 50 years and most people now survive a major incident such as a heart attack, but a full recovery also depends on making important lifestyle changes that encourage the heart to heal.

● **Help yourself** A global study called Interheart has found that 90 per cent of first heart attacks can be attributed to nine controllable major risk factors: smoking, high blood cholesterol, high blood pressure, diabetes, obesity, stress, lack of daily fruit and vegetables, excess alcohol intake, and lack of daily exercise. If any affect you, you must tackle them as part of your recovery:
• stop smoking
• adopt a healthy diet
• lose weight
• take daily exercise
• control stress
• moderate your alcohol intake

● **Brush your teeth** If you don't brush your teeth, your mouth can become infected with bacteria, which can cause inflammation, Inflammation in the body, (including gum disease) is a significant risk factor for heart disease. Dentists recommend brushing twice a day.

● **Use low-fat cooking techniques** These include grilling or roasting, stir-frying, steaming and cooking without oil, such as in a griddle pan or in a parcel of greaseproof paper.

● **Keep taking the pills** If you have heart disease, drugs are likely to be part of your recovery programme. Drugs treat heart disease in different ways: they may target the heart directly, by affecting the way it works, or indirectly, by lowering blood pressure or cholesterol.
Aspirin reduces the stickiness of blood cells called platelets, cutting the risk of clotting or a blocked coronary artery.
Beta-blockers block the effects of stress hormones, which make your heart beat faster. They cut the risk of a heart attack by preventing angina attacks, reducing high blood pressure and improving heart function. They can make an abnormal heart rhythm regular.
Calcium-channel blockers help to dilate constricted blood vessels improving angina, high blood pressure and heart function.
Diuretics remove excess water from the body and are used to treat high blood pressure and heart failure.
Nitrates dilate the coronary arteries to improve blood flow to the heart muscle and are used to relieve angina.
Statins reduce the risk of having a heart attack by reducing the amount of cholesterol in the blood.

● **Follow a heart-healthy diet** Aim to restrict your intake of saturated fat, replacing it with unsaturated fat. Eat two to three portions of fish a week, especially oily fish. Eat at least five portions of fruit and vegetables every day, and select different colours for the healthiest choice. Keep your intake of milk, cheese, butter and red meat to a minimum, and avoid foods such as pastry, biscuits and cakes. Use low-fat dairy products where possible. Include whole-grain bread, pasta or rice with every meal, along with a low-fat source of protein such as chicken breast.

● **Cut down on salt** Common salt (sodium chloride) raises your blood pressure, which puts extra strain on your heart. To aid your recovery from heart disease, you must cut back on salt; you should eat no more than 6g of salt (2.4g of sodium) a day. Your taste buds quickly adjust to eating less.
• Sprinkle less salt or preferably none on your food. In cooking, use lemon juice, vinegar, spices and pepper as alternative flavourings.
• Buy low-sodium salt, which contains potassium. Sea salt, rock salt and natural salt are high in sodium.
• Avoid processed foods, tomato ketchup, stock cubes or other manufactured stock, sausages, bacon and other cured meats, all of which contain high levels of salt.
• Find low-salt varieties of crisps, tinned soups and even breakfast cereals.

● **Reduce the strain** Being overweight is bad for health in general, and your heart in particular. If you are one of the many overweight people with heart disease, you probably know that losing weight will give a huge boost to your chances of a lasting recovery. The most serious problem is abdominal fat.

FOODS FOR A HEALTHY HEART:
THE TOP TEN

• **Oats** contain a high proportion of soluble fibre, which reduces 'bad' LDL cholesterol.

• **Yoghurts and spreads** containing plant sterols (similar to 'good' HDL cholesterol) can reduce blood levels of LDL cholesterol by up to 10 per cent.

• **Olive oil** is a potent mix of antioxidants that reduce LDL cholesterol while leaving your HDL cholesterol untouched.

• **Salmon and fresh tuna** contain high levels of omega-3 fatty acids. Aim to eat three portions of oily fish a week.

• **Tomatoes and tomato paste** are packed with vitamins and the antioxidant lycopene, which benefits the heart.

• **Walnuts and almonds** are rich in essential fatty acids that help to keep your blood vessels healthy by lowering cholesterol levels.

• **Apples** contain quercetin, an anti-inflammatory chemical that can help to prevent blood clots.

• **Onions and garlic** help to cut blood cholesterol, as well as improving circulation and discouraging blood clotting.

• **Red wine** has been shown to clean up the walls of the arteries. But be careful not to exceed healthy guidelines.

• **Dark chocolate** is rich in flavonoids that keep cholesterol from gathering in blood vessels. It also slightly lowers blood pressure. Eat no more than 45g (1.5oz) daily.

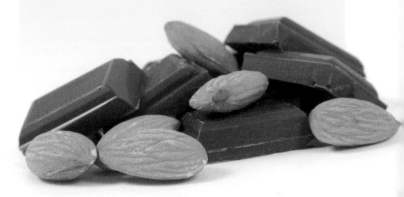

TOP STRATEGIES FOR
GIVING UP SMOKING

Smoking causes one in five deaths from heart disease. Compared with non-smokers, smokers have double the risk of having a heart attack and increase their risk of dying from heart disease by 60 per cent (85 per cent in heavy smokers).

• **Go 'cold turkey'** Choose a day on which you'll have your last cigarette. You'll give yourself the best chance if you avoid highly social or stressful days such as Christmas or a time of demanding commitments. If you're a woman, don't stop just before a period.

• **Try hypnotherapy** There's much anecdotal evidence that a few sessions with a hypnotherapist can change the way you think about smoking and make it easier to break the habit.

• **Try nicotine replacement therapy** Whether you use gum, patch, inhaler, lozenge or pill, it's well documented that taking nicotine without the tar and carbon monoxide in tobacco is a successful way of breaking the smoking habit – especially if you are also using another method of quitting.

• **Ask your doctor to prescribe a stop-smoking drug** These drugs, including varenicline and bupropion, help to suppress the desire to smoke.

• **Go online to www.smokefree.nhs.uk** Order a QuitKit, which includes a 'quit plan' and an addiction test. You can also sign up for emails, texts and phone support. You can chat online or arrange face-to-face support and advice from a trained NHS adviser.

• **Contact the NHS Smoking Helpline** Talk through cravings and get advice on strategies for stopping and encouragement when you need it.

● **Be kind to your heart** Start exercise slowly with a warm-up and slow down gradually ('warm down') before the end of the session. The ideal level of exercise is where you get warm and slightly out of breath but are still able to talk.

● **Strengthen your heart** Aerobic exercise involves working your large muscles hard so that they require more than the usual amount of oxygen. This will force the heart muscle to work harder, helping it to become stronger. If you have heart disease, take your time building up aerobic strength, starting gradually and initially working out only under the supervision of a physiotherapist or other qualified practitioner. Among its many benefits, exercise can:

• Lower blood pressure, reducing the strain on the heart and increasing 'good' HDL cholesterol that transports fat away from the arteries and back to the liver for processing.

• Improve circulation, which prevents the formation of blood clots that can lead to a heart attack.

• Help you to control your weight; thereby reducing the extra load of fat you are carrying and the workload that your heart has to undertake.

• Strengthen and enlarge heart muscle so it can pump more blood around the body and sustain its maximum level with less strain. The resting heart rate of those who exercise is slower because less effort is needed to pump blood.

● **Know your target heart rate** Before you start exercising, check with your GP or cardiologist. Your doctor may organize a stress test, which involves having an ECG test while on a running machine or exercise bike to find out how much activity is safe for you. Discuss what your target heart rate should be. A healthy person's target heart rate is 60–85 per cent of their maximum heart rate (220 minus their age). If you are taking drugs that slow your heart rate, such as beta-blockers or calcium-channel blockers, you may not reach your target despite intense exercise.

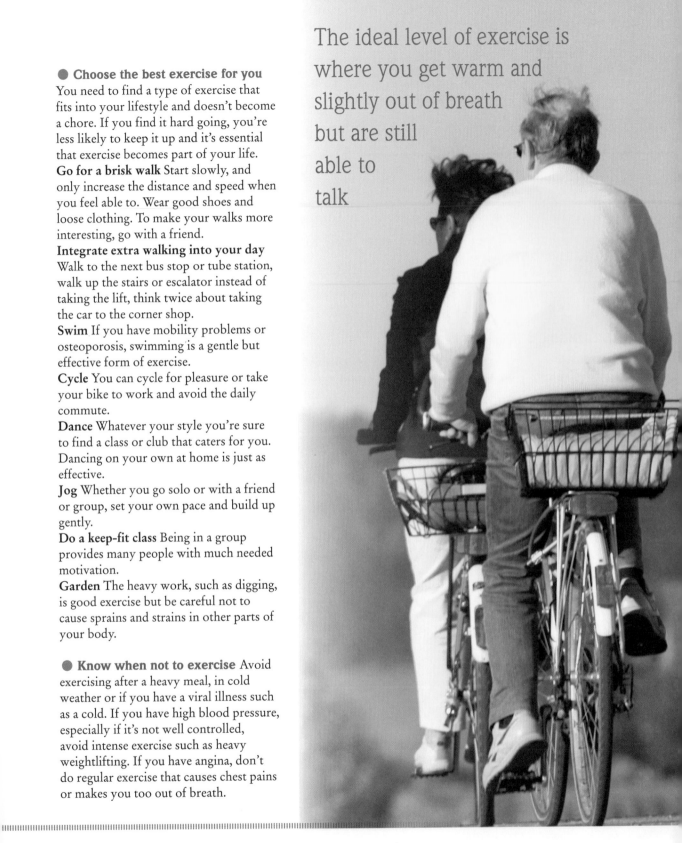

● **Choose the best exercise for you**
You need to find a type of exercise that fits into your lifestyle and doesn't become a chore. If you find it hard going, you're less likely to keep it up and it's essential that exercise becomes part of your life.

Go for a brisk walk Start slowly, and only increase the distance and speed when you feel able to. Wear good shoes and loose clothing. To make your walks more interesting, go with a friend.

Integrate extra walking into your day Walk to the next bus stop or tube station, walk up the stairs or escalator instead of taking the lift, think twice about taking the car to the corner shop.

Swim If you have mobility problems or osteoporosis, swimming is a gentle but effective form of exercise.

Cycle You can cycle for pleasure or take your bike to work and avoid the daily commute.

Dance Whatever your style you're sure to find a class or club that caters for you. Dancing on your own at home is just as effective.

Jog Whether you go solo or with a friend or group, set your own pace and build up gently.

Do a keep-fit class Being in a group provides many people with much needed motivation.

Garden The heavy work, such as digging, is good exercise but be careful not to cause sprains and strains in other parts of your body.

● **Know when not to exercise** Avoid exercising after a heavy meal, in cold weather or if you have a viral illness such as a cold. If you have high blood pressure, especially if it's not well controlled, avoid intense exercise such as heavy weightlifting. If you have angina, don't do regular exercise that causes chest pains or makes you too out of breath.

The ideal level of exercise is where you get warm and slightly out of breath but are still able to talk

RECOVERING FROM A STROKE

A stroke can occur at any age, but it is most likely from middle age onwards. Once diagnosed, stroke patients are likely to be cared for by a specialist multi-disciplinary medical team and given highly effective drug treatments. Although strokes may lead to permanent disability, many people suffer only temporary symptoms and make an excellent recovery.

● **Focus on your muscles** More than a third of stroke patients suffer spasticity, meaning tight or stiff muscles. Moving your limbs can be hard as well as painful, and simple daily activities become time-consuming for you and your carers. Talk to your health-care team about effective treatments for spasticity including drugs, physiotherapy and occupational therapy.

● **Do more each day** Stand for longer, walk a bit farther, climb the stairs more than once a day.

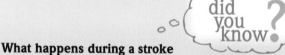

What happens during a stroke
Four out of five strokes occur when blood flow to the brain is blocked by a blood clot. People who experience clots may have chronic health problems that affect the normal flow of blood, such as heart disease or hardening of the arteries (atherosclerosis). Other (haemorrhagic) strokes occur as a result of bleeding into or around the brain – these are often more severe than strokes caused by a clot. A stroke may cause only temporary symptoms such as facial palsy that disappears within hours. This is known as a TIA (transient ischaemic attack, or 'mini-stroke').

● **Don't neglect the weaker side** Try not to do everything with the stronger side of your body. For example, attempt activities that require you to move or put weight on your weaker leg.

● **Don't overdo it** Becoming exhausted will set you back rather than push you forward.

● **Seek stimulation** Mental and physical stimulation are vital for rediscovering yourself after your period in hospital. Try to arrange regular challenges for your body and mind – for example, by setting goals for your physical exercise programme or mental workouts such as puzzles.

● **Listen to your favourite music** You can get better more quickly by listening to your favourite music CD, according to Finnish researchers. The study, reported in the journal *Brain*, showed that stroke patients who listened to their favourite music in the early days of recovery were better at remembering language later on than those who did nothing or just listened to audio books. They had better cognitive recovery and were less likely to develop depression.

● **Control chronic health problems**
Once you have had a stroke, there are several long-term conditions that you need to focus on to reduce your risk of having a second stroke.

High blood pressure This is perhaps the most important. If your doctor prescribes medication for high blood pressure, make sure you take it and go for regular blood-pressure checks.

High cholesterol levels Ask your doctor if you should be prescribed a statin to reduce levels of 'bad' LDL cholesterol.

Abnormal blood-glucose levels
Aim to keep your blood-glucose levels as normal as possible.

Abnormal heart rhythms Unless you had a haemorrhagic stroke (a stroke resulting from a bleed), your doctor will probably prescribe a blood-thinning drug such as aspirin or warfarin to reduce the chances of a blood clot.

● **Don't despair** If you can't do everything you used to be able to do, there will be many things you can still enjoy and new possibilities to explore. If you are feeling sad, consider treatment, whether this involves seeing a therapist or clinical psychologist, or taking a course of antidepressant medication.

● **Get the family involved** During your stay in hospital, surround yourself with photographs of your family and friends, and ask your visitors to bring in souvenirs and keepsakes – objects that will remind you why it's worth striving to return to normality.

Mental and physical stimulation make a vital contribution to recovery

● **Get moving** A stroke may have affected your mobility, but the sooner you get out of your hospital bed and start walking around the better your chances of making a good recovery. While you are still in hospital and have begun to walk, try to do some gentle aerobic exercise under the guidance of a physiotherapist.

● **Try not to push people away** Even if you have difficulty communicating, spending time with your family and wider social circle is healthy.

MEDICATIONS YOU MAY NEED

The three most common types of medication that are prescribed for stroke patients are statins, blood-pressure drugs and warfarin.

• **Statins** These drugs work by controlling the level of cholesterol in the blood, which is a major risk factor in the build-up of plaque in the blood vessels and thus a clot. By taking a statin, in combination with other medication, you are also likely to suffer less extensive brain damage if you do have a stroke.

• **Blood-pressure medication** Lowering your blood pressure will help to prevent further strokes no matter what sort of stroke you've had. Several different types of blood pressure medication are prescribed, depending on your symptoms and how well you tolerate them. They are most effective if you also make lifestyle changes such as reducing your alcohol consumption, increasing your activity and exercise levels and eating a healthier diet.

• **Warfarin** If you've had a stroke caused by a blood clot and have an abnormal heart rhythm, you are likely to be prescribed warfarin because it substantially reduces the risk of a subsequent stroke.

DEALING WITH **CANCER**

Positive thinking will not make your cancer disappear, but it can help you to take control of your situation and get through the sometimes gruelling recovery process. The better you feel physically and psychologically, the better you'll be able to deal with the bumpy road ahead and develop ways of coping that are right for you.

● **Cut down on drinking** The Million Women Study has established that there is a link between alcohol consumption and some cancers, including cancer of the breast, liver and bowel. A recent study of 365 women who had had breast cancer showed that those who consumed more than six alcoholic drinks a week had a 90 per cent greater risk of developing a second breast tumour.

● **Ditch tobacco** If you make just one resolution after a cancer diagnosis, it should be to give up smoking. Smoking is not just a cause of cancer; studies also suggest that cancer patients are more likely to survive if they do not smoke. Smoking may also make some treatments less effective.

● **Look at your lifestyle** Some people with cancer describe the illness as a wake-up call that gives them an opportunity to rethink their priorities. Faced with a life-threatening condition, they find themselves reassessing all aspects of their lives – work, relationships, diet, leisure.

Reassess every aspect of your life – work, relationships, diet, leisure

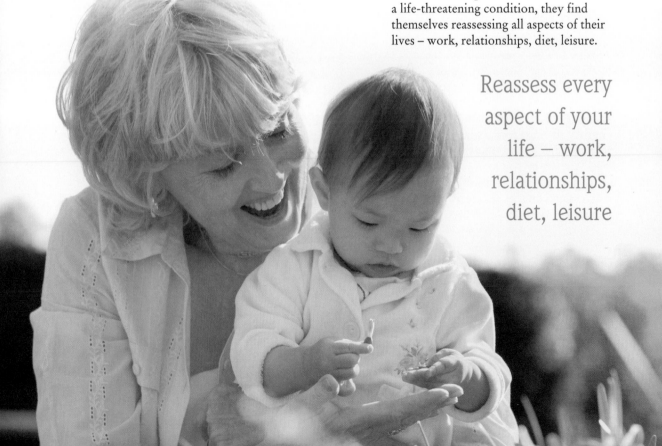

● **Go for a spray-on tan** Spray-on tans are available in most cosmetics departments and tanning salons and, unlike sunbeds, there's no evidence that they increase your risk of skin cancer.

● **Ask your partner to feed you grapes** Grapes are a wonderful source of resveratrol, the cancer-protecting compound that is also found in wine. Plus, the closeness engendered by such an activity as being fed by your loved one will strengthen your immune system.

● **Have a beer** Beer protects against the bacterium Helicobacter pylori, known to cause ulcers and possibly linked to stomach cancer. But don't overdo it. More than one or two alcoholic drinks a day may increase your risk of mouth, oesophageal, liver and breast cancer.

● **Take a multivitamin and multimineral** Many studies suggest that getting optimum levels of vitamins and minerals can boost your immune system and help to prevent a variety of cancers. If you're not eating a balanced, healthy diet, a daily supplement could help.

● **Take a calcium supplement with vitamin D** A US study suggests that calcium supplements reduce colon polyps (a risk factor for colon cancer) in susceptible people. Make sure, if you can, that all the dairy products in your diet are fat-free.

● **Take up the tea habit** The healing powers of green tea have long been valued in Asia. Now new research reveals that it protects against various cancers as well as heart disease. Some scientists believe that a chemical in green tea called EGCG could be one of the most powerful anti-cancer compounds ever discovered.

 great idea!

Add garlic to (almost) everything you eat Garlic contains sulphur compounds that stimulates the immune system's natural defences against cancer, and may have the potential to reduce tumour growth. For a perfectly healthy pasta dish, sauté two cloves of crushed garlic in 2 tablespoons of olive oil, then mix in a can of chopped tomatoes. Stir gently until heated and serve over wholemeal pasta. The lycopene in the tomatoes protects against prostate, colon and bladder cancers; the olive oil helps your body to absorb the lycopene; the fibre-filled pasta reduces your risk of colon cancer.

● **Get sunlight on your skin each day** Getting too little vitamin D, the sunshine vitamin, increases the risk of various cancers, including cancer of the breast, colon, prostate, ovarian and stomach, as well as other serious diseases such as osteoporosis, diabetes, multiple sclerosis and hypertension.

UVB rays in natural and artificial sunlight are the best source of vitamin D. About 15 minutes of exposure a day is enough to meet your needs.

● **Get out more** Exercise can help with the side effects of treatment, such as fatigue, pain and nausea, and can also improve your mood. What you can do will depend on the type of cancer, your treatment, stamina, strength and fitness. Build up gradually to more strenuous exercise as you feel stronger.

● **Eat to beat cancer** If you already eat healthily, you will be starting your cancer journey in good shape. If not, now is the time to change your diet for the better, so that you feel stronger and more energetic.

According to Cancer Research UK, a good diet can help your body to cope with the side effects of cancer treatments, to recover and heal faster, and to fight off infections.

CANCER TREATMENTS

Cancer treatments are widely thought to be almost as challenging as the illness itself. This is much less true today than it was in the past. The three main therapies – surgery, radiotherapy and chemotherapy – are constantly being refined to increase their effectiveness and reduce side effects, but you will need support from others during and after treatment.

● **Make an informed choice** In the past, doctors used to make all the clinical decisions for their patients, but times have changed. If two or more treatments are likely to be equally successful – for example, radiotherapy or surgery for prostate cancer – your doctor may ask which you would prefer. To help you to make up your mind, find out as much as you can from your doctor or specialist nurse, including side effects, possible complications and ease of treatment.

● **Consider body image** Cancer surgery can save your life, but it may also change your body and, with it, the way you see yourself.

The difference may be obvious – for example, the amputation of a limb – or seen only by those closest to you, such as a mastectomy or the removal of a testicle. It may also be totally invisible as in a hysterectomy or the removal of a kidney.

In all such cases, the psychological effects can be profound. Ask in advance about the opportunities for talking to experts who could help you to come to terms with your altered body.

● **Find out about chemotherapy** Chemotherapy uses powerful drugs to destroy cancer cells by interfering with the cell-division process.

Many people experience an array of side-effects from chemotherapy, which vary according to the type of drug, and you should ask your doctor about any specific problems you experience. Knowing what to expect can make you less fearful. Different people react differently to chemotherapy, and each person has an individual threshold for certain symptoms, such as pain.

● **Combat sickness** Modern anti-emetic drugs are usually effective against sickness or nausea caused by chemotherapy.

● **Learn about radiotherapy** For many forms of cancer, it is likely that you will be offered radiotherapy – the use of radiation to destroy cancer cells. The type of radiotherapy you are offered will depend on the type and site of your cancer, what other forms of treatment you are having and your general health.

If two or more therapies are likely to be equally successful, your doctor may ask which treatment you would prefer

● **Lessen the side effects** Common side effects of radiotherapy are fatigue, poor appetite and sore skin. If you have other troubling side effects, including depression, seek medical advice.

Pace yourself If the hospital where you are being treated is a far from home, travelling there and back may be tiring. Try to stay with someone who lives nearer or ask friends to give you a lift. Allow yourself time to rest but do some gentle exercise, such as a short daily walk.

Eat little and often Eat healthily and drink plenty of liquids while your body is under assault from radiotherapy. The hospital dietitian may be able to help.

Have a nice bath Bathe or shower in warm water rather than hot. Use unperfumed soap and pat the treated area rather than rubbing with a towel.

Avoid using creams Do not use any creams on sore areas unless recommended by your health-care team.

Choose clothes with care Try to wear soft, loose clothes that don't chafe.

Cover the treated area This will provide protection from sun and wind.

● **Reduce nausea** Research suggests that acupuncture, hypnotherapy and relaxation can reduce nausea. Travel sickness wristbands can also be helpful. Don't have a meal just before treatment or prepare or eat food when you are feeling sick. Avoid hot, fried or spicy food. Have several small meals throughout the day and plenty of soft drinks. Many people find mint or ginger tea or pastilles effective against nausea.

● **Get plenty of rest** You may feel exhausted during chemotherapy. Get plenty of rest but don't be afraid of gentle exercise such as walking or yoga. If your energy levels suddenly plummet, tell your doctor – you might have become anaemic.

Preventing infection
Chemotherapy can lower your resistance and make you more prone to infection. Your doctor may give you antibiotics to protect you. If possible, avoid large crowds, public transport, swimming pools and people with infectious illnesses. There are other precautions you can take.
• Clean your teeth thoroughly but gently morning, evening and after meals with a soft brush; floss daily.
• Use a mouthwash three times a day.
• Wash your hands thoroughly before eating, after using the toilet and if you've been in contact with other people or animals.
• Shower every day.
• Make sure friends and family always wash their hands before seeing you.
• Have your room cleaned every day.
• Eat only freshly prepared and well-cooked meals.
• Wash and peel all fruit and avoid eating salads.
• Do not eat fresh cream or soft cheese or raw or lightly cooked eggs, or dishes or sauces containing them, such as homemade mayonnaise.

● **Keep up appearances** Losing your hair, eyebrows and eyelashes can feel like the final straw on top of the diagnosis, but the lost hair usually grows back within six months. It isn't vain to worry that chemotherapy will change the way you look, and you shouldn't be afraid to discuss your anxieties with medical staff.

● **Wear a cold cap** Not all chemotherapy drugs make your hair fall out and, even if you are on one that does, you can ask about wearing a cold cap. This reduces the blood flow in the scalp by lowering the temperature, so less of the drug reaches the hair follicles on your head. Cold caps are only suitable for some chemotherapy drugs and some cancer types and, even then, they don't work for everybody.

15 great ways to boost your sex life

Regular sex increases immunity from viruses, relieves stress and triggers the release of chemicals that improve mood and ease pain. So, if your sex life is not what it was, giving it renewed impetus will benefit your health as well as increasing your pleasure.

1 HAVE SEX TONIGHT

Having intercourse regularly helps to keep your sex drive in high gear by increasing the production of testosterone, the hormone mainly responsible for libido in both men and woman.

2 WEAR SENSUOUS UNDERWEAR & LINGERIE

The feel of soft silk and other sensuous fabrics against your skin will help to stimulate those sensitive nerve endings and put you in the mood for sex.

3 MAKE PESTO AND SERVE IT WITH PASTA

Pesto contains pine nuts, a great source of arginine. This is the precursor for nitric oxide, a main ingredient in drugs such as Viagra. Arginine helps to open blood vessels so that blood flow improves.

4 TOUCH OR KISS YOUR PARTNER OFTEN

Every time you pass your partner, reach out to touch or kiss him or her. Don't allow these moments to go beyond a kiss or hug. Simply increasing the amount of physical contact you have with your partner will help with desire.

5 GET PLENTY OF ZINC

Sprinkle 1 tablespoon of wheatgerm on every pot of yoghurt and bowl of cereal that you eat. Wheatgerm is rich in zinc, which is important to the production of that all-important hormone, testosterone. You can also get your fill of zinc from beef, eggs and seafood – especially oysters.

6 READ A 'BODICE RIPPER' WITH YOUR PARTNER

The two of you can play-act the parts of the ravishing heroine and her handsome, yet dangerous lover.

7 KEEP YOUR EYES OPEN

Open your eyes when you kiss and when you're having sex. Looking into your partner's eyes during such times sends a wonderful message of trust and honesty.

8 SAY EXACTLY WHAT'S ON YOUR MIND – SEXUALLY

If watching your partner pull out the tree stump in the garden makes you go weak at the knees, tell him. Simply expressing in words how everyday things make you feel will add extra depth to the intimacy between the two of you.

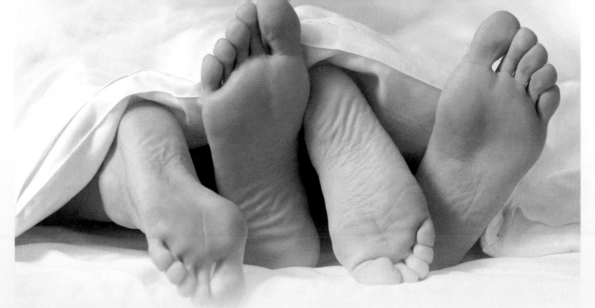

9 TALK TO EACH OTHER ABOUT WHAT MATTERS

Turn the timer on for 15 minutes and talk to him (or her) about anything other than children, money problems or work issues. Talk about the dream you had last night, an article you read, the great presentation you made, the hopes you have for the future. When the timer goes off, it's your partner's turn to have a say.

10 CREATE YOUR OWN INTIMATE RITUALS

What about waking your partner up with a steaming cup of coffee instead of the alarm every morning? What about having a hot bath ready in the evening? How about a meal out every Tuesday – or massaging your partner's feet while you watch a DVD together? The key is consistency. These are not things you do just once, but over and over again.

11 GET A MASSAGE

Having a professional massage can make you feel at your physical peak. Alternatives include a pedicure or a facial – whatever makes you feel better about yourself. If you take care of your own body, you're much more likely to enjoy it. Another good way to take care of yourself is to exercise regularly.

12 GO AWAY FOR A COUPLE OF DAYS – BY YOURSELF

While you're staying at your solitary retreat, make a list of all the things you love and like about your partner. Close your eyes and picture yourself making love. Call him or her and have an erotic phone conversation. By the time you get home, you'll be greedy for each other.

13 TOUCH WITHOUT USING HANDS

Spend an hour touching every part of your partner's body – without using your hands. Use other parts of your body instead. Conversely, caress one another, with your hands touching every part of the body except the genital zones.

14 SHOW RESPECT

Tell your partner two things you love about him or her every day. Love, affection and mutual respect are the bases for a steamy sex life.

15 DO SOMETHING PHYSICAL TOGETHER

Skiing, a long country walk, a stroll along a beach, canoeing – whatever you prefer. Such activities create a sense of physical vitality that readily translates into intimacy.

BEST WAYS TO LOOK AFTER YOUR EYES

Most of us take our eyesight for granted, but imagine if you couldn't gaze at your family or even navigate your way safely round the kitchen. There is much you can do to look after your eyes. For example, a well-balanced diet can protect against age-related macular degeneration, the leading cause of blindness in older people.

● **Switch to 'low' salt** Studies find that a high-salt diet increases the risk of certain types of cataracts, so stay away from the salty stuff. And don't forget the high salt content in many processed foods. Check labels for 'no-salt', 'no-sodium', 'low-salt' or 'low-sodium' tags when buying tinned and other prepared foods.

great idea!

The power of essential oils Dab essential oil of jasmine, peppermint or vanilla on your arm and sniff. Jasmine increases the beta waves in the frontal lobes of your brain, promoting wakefulness and enabling you to focus better and see things more acutely, says scent researcher Dr Alan R. Hirsch, of the US Smell and Taste Treatment Research Foundation. All three scents stimulate the limbic system in your brain, which, in turn, stimulates the rods in your eyes, helping you to see in dim light.

● **Wear sunglasses whenever you go out** When researchers examined the relationship between exposure to sunlight and cataracts or age-related macular degeneration in fishermen, they found that those who protected their eyes from the sun's glare and its damaging ultraviolet rays were significantly less likely to develop these conditions than those who went bare-eyed. Wear sunglasses even when it's not sunny outside to protect your eyes from the drying effects of wind.

● **Have spinach or kale twice a week** It could be a spinach quiche, steamed kale or maybe Tuscan spinach – sautéed in some olive oil with garlic and raisins. Studies find that lutein, a nutrient that is abundant in spinach and kale, may prevent age-related macular degeneration and cataracts. Ideally, get your lutein in combination with some form of fat (olive oil works well) for the best absorption.

● **Cook with red onions, not white** Red onions contain far more quercetin, an antioxidant that is thought to protect against cataracts.

● **Turn down the heating** Heat dries out the air and this dries out your eyes. In winter, you might also try adding some humidity with a humidifier or even grouping a few plants together in the room in which you spend the most time.

● **Eat fish twice a week** A study by Harvard researchers evaluated the diets of 32,470 women and found that those who ate the least amount of fish (thus getting the smallest amount of omega-3 fatty acids) had the highest risk of a condition called dry-eye syndrome. If you don't like fish, or are worried about mercury consumption, try fish-oil supplements to get your omega-3s.

● **Sprinkle a handful of blueberries on your breakfast cereal** Blueberries are a rich source of health-preserving antioxidants. A study published in the *Archives of Ophthalmology* found that women and men who ate the greatest quantity of fruit were the least likely to develop age-related macular degeneration.

● **Aim your car vents at your feet, not your face** Dry, air-conditioned air will suck the moisture out of the eyes. Aim the vents in your car away from your eyes, or wear sunglasses as a shield. Dry eyes can be more than an inconvenience; serious dryness can lead to corneal abrasions and even blindness if left untreated.

● **Twice a week, walk away from greasy or sweet snacks** A 2001 study found that people whose diets were high in omega-3 fatty acids and low in omega-6 fatty acids (found in many fat-filled snack foods such as pre-prepared pies, cakes, biscuits and crisps) were much less likely to develop macular degeneration than those whose diets were high in omega-6 fatty acids and low in omega-3 fatty acids.

● **Wear goggles** When doing carpentry or gardening, always wear goggles. Debris in the eye can lead to corneal abrasions, which can ultimately damage vision. Also use protective goggles when swimming to protect your eyes from chlorine.

● **Have sweet potatoes for dinner tonight** Rich in vitamin A, sweet potatoes can help to improve your night vision.

● **Wear a wide-brimmed hat along with your sunglasses** A wide-brimmed hat will block about half of the ultraviolet (UV) radiation, as well as reducing the UV radiation that may enter your eyes from above or around the glasses.

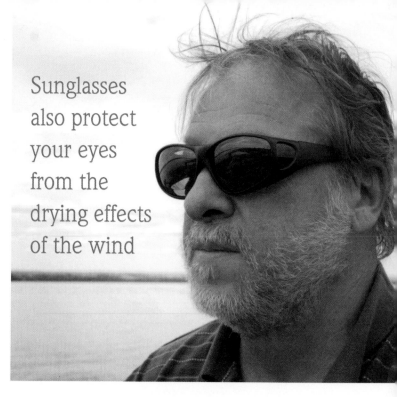

Sunglasses also protect your eyes from the drying effects of the wind

● **Roast some fresh beetroot as a side dish** Beetroots get their deep red colour from phytochemicals called anthocyanins, powerful antioxidants that protect the smaller blood vessels in your body, including those in your eyes.

● **Prevent eye strain** While you are working or reading, set your alarm to beep every 30 minutes. When it goes off, look up and away from your computer or look to some distant point for 30 seconds. This helps to prevent eye fatigue and eye strain.

● **Check your blood pressure every month** You can do this yourself with a home blood pressure kit, at your GP's surgery or at some pharmacies. Two leading causes of blindness are high blood pressure and diabetes, both of which damage blood vessels.

● **Replace your mascara every three months** Eye make-up is a great repository for bacteria, which can be transferred to your eyes and cause infections.

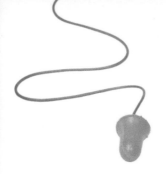
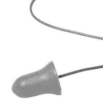

PRESERVE
YOUR HEARING

Nearly 9 million people in the UK are deaf or hard of hearing. Although more than 70 per cent of these are over the age of 60, plenty of younger people have hearing problems too. Unfortunately, once you lose your hearing, you can't get it back without help from hearing aids, so it's worth trying to preserve what you've got.

● **Go for a regular walk in the woods** Not only will the experience of silence help you to focus better on sounds, but also physically fit people tend to have better hearing than those who are unfit. The reason? Aerobic exercise brings more oxygen into your system and improves blood flow to your ears.

● **Carry earplugs** Keep a pair of earplugs in your bag, in your car, in the garage with the gardening tools and by the lawnmower. If you find yourself unable to avoid loud noise, you'll always be prepared to protect your hearing.

● **Eat guacamole as a snack or starter** Guacamole is rich in magnesium. Low levels of magnesium may increase the risk of noise-induced hearing loss.

● **Hang on to your teeth** For optimum dental health, brush your teeth at least twice a day and floss after every meal. The more of your own teeth you retain in old age, the better your hearing.

● **Serve whole-grain bread and split-pea soup** Whole grains and pulses are great sources of B vitamins, which protect the neurons and blood vessels connected to the cochlea, the tiny bone found in your inner ear.

● **Get wax cleared** Clearing the wax from your ears is often all that's needed to improve your hearing, but don't try it yourself. Ask at your GP surgery about ear syringeing.

did you know?

How loud is too loud?
Exposure of just 1 minute to sounds of 110 decibels or higher can damage hearing. No more than 15 minutes of unprotected exposure is recommended for noises of 100 decibels, or several hours' exposure to noises of 90 decibels or higher. Here are the decibel levels of some common noises:

- 140 decibels: rock concerts, fireworks
- 110 decibels: chainsaw
- 100 decibels: woodworking equipment
- 90 decibels: lawnmower, motorcycle
- 80 decibels: city traffic noise
- 60 decibels: normal conversation
- 40 decibels: refrigerator humming
- 20 decibels: whispered voice
- 0 decibels: threshold of normal hearing

SHARPEN YOUR SENSES OF **SMELL AND TASTE**

Your senses of smell and taste naturally decline as you age. Often the change is so gradual that you barely notice it. But studies find that people with an impaired ability to smell and taste tend to follow less healthy diets. It also puts you in danger: your sense of smell serves as an early-warning system for things such as gas leaks.

● **Add spices to your food** Even if your senses of smell and taste are a little jaded, you should still retain full function in your 'irritant' nerve, the nerve that makes you cry when you cut an onion. So use spices such as hot chilli powder to liven up your food.

● **Indulge in a dozen oysters** Among their other benefits, oysters are one of the highest food sources of zinc, and zinc deficiencies contribute to a loss of the senses of smell and taste.

● **Eat only when you are hungry** Our sense of smell (and thus taste) is strongest when we're hungriest.

try it... **Sniff therapy** It's possible to train your nose (and brain) to notice smells better. Start by sniffing something with a strong odour for 2 minutes a few times a day. Do this for three or four months and you should notice your sense of smell getting stronger – at least for that item.

● **Serve food that looks like itself** Forget fancy presentation. If you're serving fish, keep it looking like a fish. Your sense of taste is stronger if your brain can connect what you're eating with how it looks.

● **Chew thoroughly and slowly** This releases more flavour and extends the time that the food lingers in your mouth so that it spends more time in contact with your taste buds. Even before you start chewing, stir your food around – this aerates the molecules in the food, releasing more of their scent.

● **Humidify the air in the winter** Our sense of smell is strongest in the summer and spring, most likely because of the higher moisture content in the air.

● **Go for a brisk 10 minute walk or run** Our sense of smell is higher after exercise. Researchers think it may be related to additional moisture in the nose.

● **Drink a glass of water every hour or so** Dry mouth – whether due to medication or simply dehydration – can adversely affect your sense of taste.

STAY MOBILE
WITH ARTHRITIS

Arthritis describes more than 200 different joint disorders, which have the following symptoms in common: pain, stiffness, restricted mobility, inflammation and swelling. The two main types are osteoarthritis and rheumatoid arthritis. To ease the problems of living with arthritis, you can make all sorts of subtle changes at home and at work.

● **Stay active** With all musculoskeletal problems, it's important to keep moving. This may not be possible initially if your pain is severe, but don't put your feet up for too long. Resume everyday activities such as walking to the shops, going to work and light gardening as soon as possible.

● **Wash dishes by hand** The combination of warm, running water and light exercise, requiring complex movement of the wrist and hand, is an effective and low-cost way of rehabilitating the hand and wrist after injury or surgery. It will also keep your wrists and hands flexible with good blood circulation if you have arthritis or other painful problems.

● **Squeeze a ball** Keep a small rubber ball on your desk and in your car. Every time you get up for a screen break (at work) or stop at a red light (when you're in the car), squeeze the ball 20 times in each hand. This helps to strengthen your hands and improves flexibility.

● **Exercise your wrists** Enhance the range of motion in your wrist with this exercise. Slowly bend your wrist backwards and forwards, holding for a 5-second count in each position. Do three sets – ten times for each hand – twice a day.

● **Follow an anti-inflammatory diet** Eating too many fatty and sugary foods worsens the pain, swelling and redness that characterize inflammation. You can counter inflammation by eating plenty of fresh fruit and vegetables and a good intake of omega-3 fatty acids, found in fish and fish oils and foods such as walnuts, hempseed and flaxseed.

● **Switch to spicy foods** Try changing your diet when your arthritis flares up. Spices such as cayenne pepper, ginger and turmeric contain compounds that reduce swelling and block a brain chemical that transmits pain signals.

● **Let stronger parts take the strain** Ease strain on smaller, weaker joints by using larger parts of your body to carry heavy items. For example, carry shopping bags using your forearms or the palms of your hands, rather than your fingers.

● **Sip a cup of green tea every day**
Polyphenols called catechins in green tea can significantly reduce cartilage damage.

● **Use a wrist pad with care** Resting your wrists on a wrist pad when typing can compress soft tissues – such as tendons, nerves and blood vessels – in your forearms, reducing blood flow to your wrists and fingers. This, in turn, can increase pressure in the carpal tunnel located inside your wrists and ultimately lead to nerve damage. Instead, use the pad only for support during typing breaks.

● **Select the right shoes** For everyday wear, choose well-cushioned lace-up or bar shoes with good arch support. Avoid raised heels – or choose heels no higher than 2.5cm (1in).

● **Adopt a good sleeping position**
If you're waking up sore and aching every morning, think about how you're sleeping. Lying flat on your back forces your spine into an unnatural position, which can strain muscles, joints and nerves. Your spine isn't meant to be straight. It has three natural curves: one in your lower back, one in the middle of your back, and one near your neck. You may benefit from this advice:
• Lie on your side in the foetal position with your knees bent and a pillow tucked between your legs. This will take the most stress off your back.
• If you must sleep on your back, prop a big, fluffy pillow under your knees to reduce the pressure on the sciatic nerve in your lower back.
• Use a small pillow or a rolled-up towel under your neck as long as it doesn't push your chin too far forward.
• Don't sleep on your stomach. Sleeping face down can exaggerate the arch at the base of your spine and cause strain.

With all musculoskeletal problems, it's important to keep moving

● **Consider joint-replacement surgery** Surgery such as a hip-joint replacement can help to alleviate pain and improve movement – depending on the severity of your arthritis and the strength of the surrounding muscles. You may want to consider surgery in the following circumstances.
• Arthritis is interrupting your sleep.
• Lack of mobility makes everyday activities difficult – for example, going up stairs, going to the toilet or working.
• Your symptoms mean that you put off doing activities you enjoy such as visiting friends or taking a holiday.
• Your medication is ineffective.

did you know?

Supplements can help
• **Ginger** US researchers found that taking ginger extract twice daily reduced knee pain significantly in patients with osteoarthritis, as well as improving knee movement. Ginger has some anti-inflammatory effects, like ibuprofen.
• **Fish oils, including cod-liver oil** A British study found that 86 per cent of people with arthritis who took cod liver oil had far fewer enzymes that cause cartilage damage compared to those who took a placebo. Plus, they had far fewer pain-causing enzymes.
• **Glucosamine** It doesn't fight pain immediately in the way that drugs such as ibuprofen do. But, over time, glucosamine becomes an effective pain reliever and anti-inflammatory. More importantly, it can actually help to repair damaged cartilage. You can use a drug such as ibuprofen for prompt pain relief, but start taking glucosamine at the same time. After about a month, you should be getting enough pain relief from the glucosamine to allow you to stop the ibuprofen.

SOLVE BACK PROBLEMS

Four out of five people experience chronic back pain at some time in their lives and it is a major cause of mobility problems – and of lost working days. Learning how to protect and strengthen your back will help you recover and safeguard against future back pain.

● **Pace yourself** Too much activity can be as detrimental as too little to a bad back, so learn to pace yourself and don't do too much too soon, especially when the pain starts to subside.

Keep on working Research shows that people who continue to work during a bout of back pain recover more quickly.

Balance it Both low and high extremes of physical activity are linked to an increased risk of chronic low back pain. Maintain a balance and don't overdo or underdo it.

Relax, relax Feeling tense may cause muscle spasms, which can exacerbate pain and stiffness; and worry about whether you're going to get better can add to stress.

● **Avoid prolonged bed rest** Resting in bed for longer than three days can delay healing – while immobile, the unused back muscles become stiff and weak and other muscles take over, throwing the spine out of balance. People who stay active when suffering back problems tend to have better function and less pain.

● **Bend your knees** Always bend your knees, not your back, when picking up something heavy from the ground. Also, keep the weight you're carrying close to your body, as if carrying a baby.

● **Keep mobile** When you have a back problem it is essential to keep mobile. The sooner you put into place measures to protect your back, the faster you're likely to get better.

● **Rule out an underlying cause** Consult your doctor before embarking on a self-help programme. Your doctor will also be able to provide you with effective pain-relieving medication – a key component of your recovery.

● **Take breaks while driving** During long drives, take a break every 1-2 hours, get out of the car and walk around for 5 minutes, stretching like a cat. Your back will thank you later.

● **Strengthen your muscles** The National Institute for Health and Clinical Excellence (NICE) says that people who have had lower-back pain for longer than three months should be prescribed an exercise programme under professional supervision. The aim is to strengthen the muscles that support the back, improve flexibility and increase stamina. Even if you are not enrolled in a formal course, your goal should be to include a variety of physical activities in your life.
Walking A simple and effective low-impact aerobic activity that should cause minimal pain if your back is strained. Using a pedometer will help you record your progress and provides an incentive. Try to work up to 10,000 steps a day.
Swimming Front crawl or backstroke is better for your back than breaststroke, which can strain the back muscles if you keep your head above water.
Yoga Yoga strengthens back muscles and improves flexibility and balance. American studies suggest that people with low back pain who do yoga have less disability, pain and depression. A

A SUCCESSFUL COMEBACK

Here are some ways to improve your working environment when returning after an absence caused by back problems.

• **Change your hours** Shorter periods of desk work in front of a computer screen are more manageable than long hours.

• **Take 15-minute breaks** Try to take a break every few hours, or even arrange a shorter working day.

• **Adjust your tasks** A temporary change to your work can help to lessen the strain on your back. If your job includes lots of lifting and carrying, ask if you can switch to lighter tasks until you feel better. This will allow your back time to recover.

• **Check your desk** Place your monitor about an arm's length away from your eyes with the top of the screen at eye level. Keep other equipment within easy reach so you don't have to keep stretching or twisting to pick them up. Use a headset if your job involves regular long phone calls.

• **Be chair aware** Make sure your chair is at the right height and angle for your desk/workstation. Adjust your chair so that your forearms are resting comfortably on the desk and your elbows are roughly at right angles.

• **Sit correctly** When sitting, keep your shoulders back. Use a small cushion in the small of your back for lumbar support, if you have low back pain. When sitting, your hips should be slightly higher than your knees so that your upper legs are sloping down. If necessary, rest your feet on a footrest or a pile of books.

• **Break up the day** Get up and move around as often as possible. Make a drink, talk to colleagues in person rather than emailing, do some photocopying or filing – anything that gets you moving.

UK pilot study published in the journal *Complementary Therapies in Clinical Practice* in 2010 found that people with chronic low back pain who practised yoga for 75 minutes a week over three months suffered significantly less discomfort.
Pilates classes Practising Pilates is an effective way to strengthen the muscles of the abdomen and back that support the spinal column.

STRONGER **BONES**

Annually, osteoporosis accounts for about 230,000 fractures in the UK. One in two British women and one in five British men over the age of 50 will break a bone, mainly because of poor bone health. Yet even as an adult there's plenty you can do to protect yourself, from increasing your calcium intake to getting the right exercise.

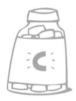

● **Take the right kind of calcium at the right time** Calcium citrate, for instance, is more expensive, but can be absorbed on an empty stomach. Calcium carbonate, the cheapest and most common supplement, is absorbed best with food, particularly acidic foods such as citrus juice or fruit.

● **Drink your milk!** Children who drink plenty of milk (or who get plenty of calcium from other sources) grow up to have less risk of osteoporosis, the disease that causes bones to become thin and brittle.

did you know?

Turn your face to the sun
You should aim for about 15 minutes a day of sun exposure, without sunscreen. That's how much your body needs to make vitamin D, the 'sunshine vitamin' important to bone health. And exposure to sunlight enhances mood because sunlight affects levels of the hormone melatonin. Too little sun can result in a form of depression known as seasonal affective disorder, or SAD. Studies find that women prone to depression are also more likely to have lower bone density.

● **Squat every day** Squats are beneficial for your hips, which are especially prone to fracture. Pretend you're about to sit in a chair, but without a chair behind you. As you 'sit', try to lower yourself enough so that your thighs are parallel or nearly parallel to the floor, but don't let your knees extend beyond your toes. Do 12 to 16 squats nightly before you get into bed.

● **Drink one cup of tea a day** That's all it took in a study of 1,256 women aged 65 to 76 to increase their bone density by 5 per cent. That translates to a 10 to 20 per cent reduction in fracture risk. Another study found that among more than 1,000 Chinese men and women, those who regularly drank tea (usually green tea) had denser bones than those who didn't.

● **Walk for 30 minutes a day** Most women lose 3 to 6 per cent of their bone mass every year during the five years before and after menopause. But women who walked regularly (about 7½ miles a week) took four to seven years longer to lose the same amount of bone as women who didn't walk at all. Brisk walking should enable you to cover 2 miles in 30 minutes. If you walk for 30 minutes just four days a week, you will achieve the target of 7½ miles.

● **Roast a butternut squash**
Butternut squash is high in calcium
(175g/6oz contains about 10 per cent of
your recommended daily amount). Slice
one open, scoop out the seeds, then spray
the top with olive oil and sprinkle with
brown sugar and cinnamon. Roast at
200°C/400°F/gas mark 6 until soft, about
45 to 60 minutes, and scoop out the flesh.

● **Plant a vegetable garden** US
researchers found that gardening was
strongly associated with reducing the
risk of osteoporosis in 3,310 women aged
50 and older. It turns out that pushing
a lawnmower, thrusting a shovel into
the ground, lifting heavy wheelbarrows
filled with mulch, raking, carrying and
pulling weeds are all great weight-bearing
exercises.

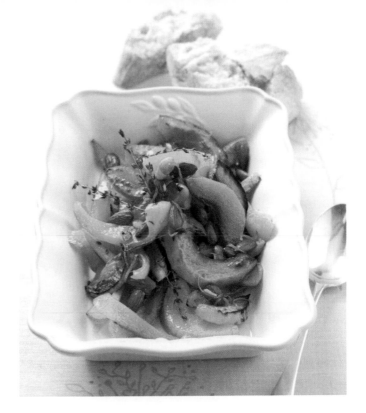

● **Add almonds to everything**
They're packed with bone-strengthening
calcium. Just 25g/1oz of the sweet nuts
provides 60mg of calcium. Try them
toasted and sprinkled over salad or
yoghurt, crushed and mixed into meat or
turkey for meatballs, used in place of pine
nuts for homemade pesto, or as a topping
for ice cream or frozen yoghurt.

● **Have four dried figs for a mid-
afternoon snack** Dried figs are a great
source of calcium. Sprinkle a few diced
figs over your yoghurt and you'll meet
more than half your daily calcium needs
(four dried figs, about 60g/2oz, contain
almost a fifth – 17 per cent – of your
recommended daily amount).

● **Hang room-darkening blinds
in your bedroom** You'll sleep much
better without ambient light, and sleep is
important for bone health. Much of your
bone remodelling, in which old bone is
replaced by new, occurs during sleep.

● **Drink mineral water** Mineral water
contains calcium, and a study published
in *Osteoporosis International* in 2000
found that your body absorbs the mineral
just as well from water as it does from
milk. Try to drink two glasses a day.
Make sure the water is labelled 'mineral
water', not just 'spring water'. If you live
in a hard-water area, rather than a soft-
water area, you will get some calcium
from tap water too.

● **Snack on low-fat yoghurt** Make a
pot of low-fat yoghurt a daily snack. With
210mg of calcium in a small pot (150ml)
of low-fat yoghurt, you're a quarter of the
way to your recommended daily amount.

● **Sign up for a tai chi class** Several
studies have found that tai chi cut the risk
of falling by nearly a half and reduced the
rate of fractures even in people who had
falls. Ideally, you should practise tai chi
for 10 to 15 minutes at a time, once
or twice a week, to gain the benefits.

BEST WAYS TO EASE PAIN

Medical advances and a greater understanding of the benefits of complementary therapies mean that most types of pain can now be eased or controlled. Highly specific medications have been developed in recent years and there are many other effective treatments, ranging from self-help measures to machines that disrupt pain signals. If your pain persists and painkillers don't bring relief, see your doctor for a check-up.

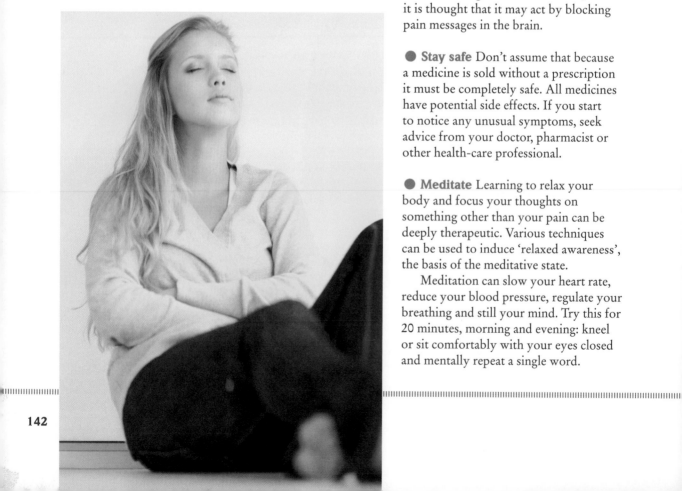

● **Know your painkillers**
Painkillers help with short-term pain, such as headaches, and certain long-term conditions, including some forms of arthritis. In many cases, the relief they bring will enable you to become more active. While mild versions can be bought over the counter, stronger drugs may be available only on prescription from your doctor.

• **Medications** that work by relieving inflammation are known as non-steroidal anti-inflammatory drugs (NSAIDs). Aspirin is often considered as a member of this group.

• **Drugs** that act on specific pain receptors to alter the way your brain perceives pain are known as opioids. They're converted into small quantities of morphine in the body and must be used with caution and for as short a time as possible.

• **Paracetamol** is in a class of its own. How this drug works is unknown, but it is thought that it may act by blocking pain messages in the brain.

● **Stay safe** Don't assume that because a medicine is sold without a prescription it must be completely safe. All medicines have potential side effects. If you start to notice any unusual symptoms, seek advice from your doctor, pharmacist or other health-care professional.

● **Meditate** Learning to relax your body and focus your thoughts on something other than your pain can be deeply therapeutic. Various techniques can be used to induce 'relaxed awareness', the basis of the meditative state.

Meditation can slow your heart rate, reduce your blood pressure, regulate your breathing and still your mind. Try this for 20 minutes, morning and evening: kneel or sit comfortably with your eyes closed and mentally repeat a single word.

● **Change the way you think** How you think about and react to any situation can make it better or worse. This is the basis of cognitive behavioural therapy. If you find yourself thinking, 'This pain is unbearable', you might be advised to adjust the thought to, 'If I breathe deeply, it will pass.' Research shows that if you train your mind to react differently to pain and adopt a positive attitude, you may lessen the effects.

● **Try hypnotherapy** Hypnotherapists help you to focus your attention at the same time as making you feel more relaxed. They then focus on your pain, why you might be feeling it and what you can do about it. The idea is to help you to control your pain yourself by using what you've learnt under your hypnotherapist's guidance. There are also many books and DVDs available from which you can learn the technique of self-hypnosis.

● **Have a good laugh** Being told that you can laugh away your pain might seem like a bad joke, but research increasingly shows that laughter really can be the best medicine. Laughter triggers the production of endorphins, the body's natural painkillers.

● **Flex your neck** This neck exercise is particularly good for relieving pain and stiffness in your neck; it may also help if you get headaches.
• Slowly turn your head to the left as far as you can and hold for 5 seconds. Bring your head back to the centre. Repeat the move to the right. Repeat 5–10 times.
• Keeping your head straight, tilt it over to the right side and hold for 5 seconds (not so far that you touch your shoulder with your ear). Repeat the move to the left. Repeat 5–10 times.

HANDS-ON **THERAPIES**

Pain can be tiring and debilitating, especially if you and your doctors are finding it hard to pinpoint a cause. Hands-on therapies, including acupuncture, massage and reflexology, can sometimes help.

• **Acupuncture** This practice involves inserting needles at specific 'acupoints' around the body and has long been used for pain relief. Research suggests that, as well as triggering 'feel-good' endorphins, acupuncture has a specific effect at the pain site by stimulating the production of adenosine, a natural painkiller.

• **Acupressure and shiatsu** Both therapies work on the same principles as acupuncture but use firm finger pressure instead of needles. For best results, consult a trained practitioner. Many people find them effective for headaches, back pain and pain associated with osteoarthritis.

• **Nerve stimulation** TENS – transcutaneous electrical nerve stimulation – involves applying a mild electrical current via a series of electrodes that you place on your skin at or near the site of the pain. You can get a TENS machine from your doctor or pain clinic, or you can buy or rent one from many pharmacies. TENS It can be effective for low back pain, rheumatoid arthritis, menstrual or labour pain, pain after surgery and headaches.

• **Massage** This is one of the oldest therapies and is offered as part of the pain relief programme in many hospitals and surgeries. Massage is comforting, but it may also have a direct effect on the pain by helping to stimulate endorphins and soothing the nerves that carry pain signals to your brain.

• **Reflexology** Practitioners of reflexology believe that each organ, gland and part of the body is reflected in a corresponding reflex point on the foot. Applying gentle pressure to these points is believed to remove blockages in the flow of energy to organs and tissues in a particular zone, stimulating endorphins and pain relief.

• **Osteopathy and chiropractic** Both of these therapies involve manipulating the spine and other joints and their surrounding soft tissues, to improve nerve function and circulation. Osteopathy and chiropractic have a good track record of relieving pain in a variety of conditions that affect the back, muscles and joints in general, as well as migraine and nerve pain.

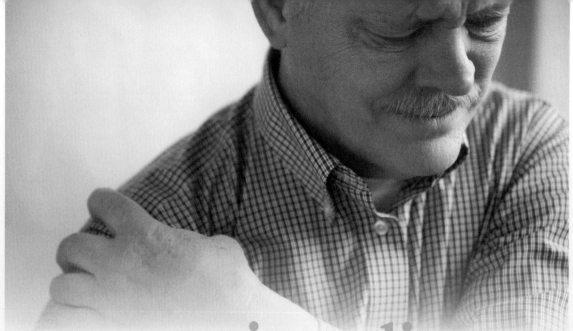

8 great pain-relievers for common conditions

Your first reaction to pain may be to take a pill or seek medical advice but, if the pain persists, a mixture of treatments and lifestyle changes often brings lasting relief.

1 BANISH BACK PAIN

Ranging from a dull ache to a sudden sharp pain, back pain affects four out of five of us at some time. **Painkillers** Paracetamol and ibuprofen are often effective; stronger painkillers such as codeine and dihydrocodeine may be prescribed if pain is severe. **Spinal manipulation and massage** Physiotherapy, osteopathy or chiropractic are helpful for some back problems. **Yoga, Pilates or Alexander technique** may be beneficial in the longer term.

Self-help Having a hot bath or applying a hot-water bottle or heat pack to the affected area can ease muscular pain. In other cases, the application of cold is more effective. Use a specially designed cool pack or a bag of frozen peas wrapped in a towel.

2 EASE TENSION HEADACHE

A tension headache is typified by a dull steady ache that spreads to or from the neck. It can feel as though a band is being pulled tightly around your head. **Painkillers** Paracetamol, aspirin or ibuprofen may work for you. If the headache becomes chronic, consult your doctor who may suggest an antidepressant. **Yoga and Pilates** Both activities will relax muscular tension and improve posture. **Cranial osteopathy** This practice involves gentle manipulation at the base of the skull and top of the neck. **Acupuncture** is another option.

Self-help Take a holiday or at least some time away from work or home pressures and try to relax. Get plenty of sleep and take regular walks. Keep a headache diary to pinpoint triggers.

3 ALLEVIATE NERVE PAIN

Nerve pain is often caused by a trapped, damaged or pinched nerve. Shooting or burning pain and tingling or numbness are among the symptoms. Always talk to your doctor about this type of pain. **Drug treatments** You may be prescribed antidepressants, anti-epileptics or opioids, depending on the type of pain. **Acupuncture and relaxation training** may also be recommended.

Self-help High blood-sugar levels have been linked with nerve pain in people with diabetes, so keep an eye on these. There is some evidence that taking B vitamins can help, especially if the nerve pain is linked to a medical condition such as diabetes.

4 RELIEVE FIBROMYALGIA

Fibromyalgia causes widespread pain across the body that last for three months or more. The cause is unknown. **Painkillers** If paracetamol and ibuprofen are not effective, a stronger drug such as codeine may be recommended. **Physiotherapy** Exercise advice from a physiotherapist may help you to become more active. **Chiropractic and osteopathy** are also worth considering.

Self-help Take regular exercise, such as walking, swimming or yoga. Make time to relax.

5 OVERCOME MENSTRUAL PAIN

This involves pain or cramps in the lower abdomen just before or during a period. **Painkillers** If over-the-counter drugs do not give relief, a stronger medication, such as co-codamol (codeine with paracetamol), may be prescribed. **Hormones** If you are not trying to get pregnant, you could try the combined contraceptive pill. **TENS** Use of this device (see page 143) can sometimes relieve symptoms. **Acupuncture, acupressure, spinal manipulation and herbal remedies** are among the other options.

Self-help Try activities such as swimming, cycling or walking. Self-massage can also be comforting; use light circular movements around your lower abdomen.

6 COPE WITH CYSTITIS

Cystitis is a urinary-tract infection affecting the bladder that can cause abdominal pain and discomfort when passing urine. Your doctor may prescribe antibiotics. **Painkillers** Paracetamol and ibuprofen can help. **Potassium citrate or sodium citrate** will make the urine less acidic and therefore less painful to pass.

Self-help Drinking plenty of water helps to flush out the bacteria. Warmth from a hot-water bottle can be soothing.

7 CONTROL IRRITABLE BOWEL SYNDROME

An intermittent cramp-like abdominal pain. **Anti-spasmodic drugs** help to ease pain and bloating. **'Gut-directed' hypnotherapy** teaches you how to control gut activity. **Acupuncture** may also be effective.

Self-help Cut out wheat fibre and increase the bulk in your diet by eating more pulses, fruit and vegetables, which provide soluble fibre. To help you to pinpoint problem foods, keep a food diary where you can record what you eat each day.

8 HELP TO HEAL A PEPTIC ULCER

An open sore develops in the stomach lining (a gastric ulcer) or the small intestine (a duodenal ulcer). A type of bacteria, *Helicobacter pylori* (*H. pylori*), is thought to be the main cause. The main symptom is a recurrent gnawing pain in the centre of the abdomen. **Antibiotics** If *H. pylori* is causing your ulcer, tackling the infection can allow the ulcer to heal. **Proton pump inhibitors** A course of drugs that reduce the amount of acid made by your stomach often provides effective relief in the long term.

Self-help Avoid spicy foods and alcohol, which can trigger or worsen symptoms. Aloe vera juice (available in health-food shops) may help to quell inflammation and reduce stomach-acid secretion. Cut back on coffee and tea, which can increase production of stomach acid. Drink herbal teas such as camomile or fennel instead.

ACCIDENTS & INJURIES

Accidents can occur at any time and anywhere – an inadvertent trip, a fall, a burn, a cut or, more seriously, a road accident. Some can result in injuries such as fractures, sprains, strained muscles or tendons, cuts and bruises. Although these can be painful and temporarily disabling, most people make a full recovery.

● **Do a first-aid course** Giving first aid to a casualty in an emergency can turn a potentially permanent injury into a temporary one, as well as ensuring a rapid recovery rather than a prolonged period of disability. Dealing with minor injuries such as burns and cuts or stings in the correct way can avoid complications and help to make healing quicker and more straightforward.

● **Keep cool** For the first 72 hours after a sprain or muscle strain, you should avoid hot baths, saunas and heat packs. Also avoid massage and alcohol because they can increase bleeding and swelling, and delay healing.

● **Prevent recurrence** Exercises that improve strength, balance and core strength – for example, Alexander technique, Pilates and tai chi – can help to prevent a repeat injury.

● **Try a wobble board** Readily available on the internet, wobble boards can promote fast recovery from injuries, such as a sprained ankle, or a hip replacement. Trying to balance – first with both legs, then alternately on each leg – strengthens the muscles that maintain balance and posture, and support the joints. Before using a wobble board, consult your physiotherapist.

● **Improve core strength** The core muscles of the abdomen stabilize and protect the spine. Strengthening the core can speed recovery from a back injury and help you to avoid further injuries. Contract the abdominal muscles below your navel, without moving the 'six pack' muscles above, and hold – building up over time to a count of ten. Repeat three times, as often as possible.

Treat injuries correctly to avoid complications and speed healing

did you know?

Breaks, sprains and strains
In the aftermath of an accident, fall or injury, it may be hard to know whether the casualty has suffered a broken bone (fracture), a joint injury (sprain) or a muscle injury (strain). In fact, healthy bones are extremely strong and are usually able to withstand strong forces, so most fractures are sustained only as a result of a bad fall or another type of impact, such as a car crash.

The most common types of sprain occur in the ankle, knee, wrist and thumb, while the most common strains affect muscles in the thighs, calf and lower back.

● Learn the PRICE procedure

If you or someone else suffers a sprain or strain, you can aid recovery by implementing the PRICE (Protection, Rest, Ice, Compression, Elevation) procedure as soon as possible.

• **Protect** the area from further strain or damage.

• **Rest** the injured joint or muscle for the first 48–72 hours.

• **Ice** the injury for the first 48–72 hours. Wrap crushed ice or a packet of frozen vegetables in a damp towel and place on the injured area for 15–20 minutes every 2 to 3 hours. Never place ice directly on the skin as this could cause a cold burn.

• **Compress** or bandage the injured area to limit swelling and movement (crêpe, elastic or tubular bandages are ideal), but remember to remove the bandage before you go to bed. It should be snug but not too tight, or you risk restricting the circulation of blood.

• **Elevate** the injured area, supported by a pillow if possible.

● Take measures against shock

If you are present at a serious accident, the top priority is to call an ambulance. Then take these simple steps to protect any injured person from medical shock – a potentially life-threatening drop in blood pressure:

• Treat any obvious injuries, such as bleeding, if you have first-aid training and know what to do.

• If you are certain there is no back injury, lay the casualty down, keeping the head low and supporting the legs above the level of the heart.

• If possible, cover the casualty to keep him or her warm. Offer reassurance.

• Loosen tight clothing, straps or belts to reduce constriction.

• Don't let the person eat, drink, smoke or move unnecessarily.

BEST WAYS TO **GET BETTER**

Recovering after a major accident or fall requires patience. Allow yourself time to heal and to get over the physical and emotional effects of the trauma but remember that there is a great deal that you can do to help the healing process.

• **Rest** The body heals itself while you sleep so make sure you get plenty of rest, and ensure that you sleep well, whether that means taking painkillers or learning relaxation techniques.

• **Exercise** A physiotherapist or specialist may prescribe exercises that can speed up repair of the damaged part of the body. You should also exercise the joints and muscles on the non-affected side of the body.

• **A nutritious diet** Your diet should be rich in the foods and nutrients that promote healing.

• **Self-help treatments** These range from relaxation techniques, meditation and self-massage, through herbal teas, flower essences and aromatherapy oils, to consulting relevant therapists and practitioners.

● Recognize a fracture

If you suspect a broken bone, secure and support the injured part and take the casualty to hospital. The signs of a broken bone are:

• severe pain and swelling

• bruising or discoloration around the bone or joint

• inability to bear weight on or move the injured limb/part of the body

• a bend or unusual angle in the limb or part of the body affected

• a grating sensation or sound in the bone or joint

BEFORE & AFTER SURGERY

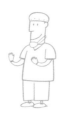

If you need to go into hospital for a surgical operation, preparing yourself physically and mentally can work wonders. And a positive strategy for the days and weeks that follow, while you are in hospital and when you go home, can help to ensure a full and speedy recovery.

● **Guard against infection** Do not be reluctant to challenge staff who don't appear to be cleaning their hands regularly. Handwashing is the most important thing everyone can do – nurses, doctors, hospital visitors – to protect against the spread of hospital-acquired infections such as MRSA and Clostridium difficile. Many wards now have dispensers for alcohol-based hand rubs.

Handwashing protects against infections such as MRSA and Clostridium difficile

● **Accept help graciously** You'll need support at this time, so in the run-up to your operation don't be embarrassed to ask friends and family for help.

● **Get fit for theatre** You can make a real difference to the outcome of your operation if you take steps to get fit in the time remaining before your admission date. For example, if you are a smoker, quitting at least six weeks before has been shown to bring about a significant reduction in health problems resulting from surgery.

● **Lose weight – gradually** Losing excess weight can be one of the most worthwhile contributions you can make to a successful outcome of an operation – especially if it involves weight-bearing joints. Aim for gradual, healthy weight loss (no more than 2lb (1kg) a week).

● **Exercise gently** If your physical condition before your operation does not prevent it, get into the habit of gentle exercise. Aim to resume the exercise programme as part of your recovery.

● **Adjust your attitude** Being relaxed has many benefits, including soothing your nervous system, boosting your immune system, balancing your heart rhythms and promoting healing. In the period before your operation, focus on positive thoughts and your goal of a full and speedy recovery.

● **Get moving** After the operation, you will be encouraged by hospital staff to get active as soon as possible. Moving your legs to get out of bed, sitting, standing up from a chair and walking to the toilet are your first 'mountains to climb'. Wear your slippers whenever you get out of bed to avoid picking up an infection.

● **Pace yourself** When you start exercising, follow the 'do a bit and rest a bit' rule. Listen to your body and stop whenever you feel pain. At this time, the 'no pain, no gain' mantra does not apply. Exercise that causes you excessive pain will slow your recovery.

● **Create an island of calm** Try to stay relaxed during your hospital stay. With busy medical staff and large numbers of visitors coming and going, hospital wards are often far from peaceful. Create your own island of calm with deep-breathing exercises, meditation and, when necessary, by wearing earplugs.

● **Regain your emotional health** If you're feeling in low spirits after your surgery, discuss this with your GP. Once diagnosed, depression can almost always be successfully treated with talking therapies and medication where necessary. Here are some suggestions for how to take care of your emotional wellbeing in the days and weeks after your surgery:
• Try not to panic or feel guilty if you feel depressed following surgery. It's normal.
• Give yourself permission to cry and talk about it. Just being able to express your feelings goes a long way towards helping you feel better.
• Make sure you drink plenty of water. Drinking water is good for you in any case but it will also help to flush out the large amounts of medication pumped into your body in a short period of time, which may be affecting your mood.
• Rest. Having been through surgery, your body needs every available resource to heal what it perceives as 'injuries'.
• Relax. Ask someone to give you a foot massage, hand massage, back rub or a shoulder and neck rub. Do what you can to pamper yourself and allow others to pamper you.

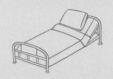

CARING FOR YOURSELF
AFTER AN OPERATION

The recommended self-help recovery measures after an operation depends on the nature of your surgery.

• **Laparoscopic or 'keyhole' surgery** Frequently used for gall-bladder operations as well as hernias and other abdominal surgery, laparoscopy avoids the need for large incisions through muscle and flesh, so recovery is relatively quick. But it still involves cutting soft tissue. It's vital not to engage in vigorous activity, including heavy housework, for four to six weeks, until that tissue has healed.

• **Vaginal and abdominal surgery** Be very careful when lifting for the first six weeks after the operation. If you do have to lift something, brace your tummy and pelvic floor muscles, then raise yourself up using a smooth action without jerking.

• **Shoulder surgery** Make sure that you maintain good posture, and resist slumping forward. This is vital for speedy recovery.

• **Knee surgery** As soon as you're mobile, avoid keeping your knee in one position for any length of time as this can lead to stiffness, pain and swelling. Get up frequently and move around. On long car journeys, stop every hour or so and walk around for 5 minutes before continuing. Similarly, if you're travelling by train or air, get up and walk around at regular intervals.

• **Ankle and wrist surgery** For optimum recovery, do the exercises prescribed by your physiotherapist to ensure that the joints regain their strength and mobility.

• **Foot or toe surgery** Don't walk unaided until your physiotherapist has given you the all-clear. Try to avoid standing for too long as it will cause pain and swelling in your foot.

• **Heart surgery** In many parts of the UK, the NHS provides cardiac rehabilitation in the form of weekly exercise and information sessions. If you've had heart surgery, you'll be invited to participate. The aim is to start you on an exercise programme to get you fit after surgery.

SKIN **INJURIES**

The skin, the body's first line of defence, is the largest organ in the body and, although susceptible to injury, it has amazing powers of regeneration. Prompt action at the time of injury is the key to rapid healing and minimizing the risk of scarring. There are also various follow-up steps that will help the skin to heal more quickly.

● **Treat burns and scalds** A painful burn or scald needs fast, appropriate first-aid treatment. Never be tempted to put ice directly on a heat injury, as this can produce an additional cold burn. It can also cause the victim's body to cool to a level that is dangerous for other organs.
• Cool the burn immediately by running cool water onto the area for at least 10 minutes or until the pain is relieved.
• Carefully remove jewellery, a watch or clothing from around the burn unless it is sticking to the skin.
• Raise the limb to reduce swelling.
• Cover the area of the burn with a clean, non-fluffy, preferably sterile, dressing.
• Avoid using adhesive dressings and be careful not to burst any blisters.
• If the burn is deep or larger than a postage stamp, it is important to seek urgent medical attention.

● **Treat minor sunburn** Take a cool (not cold) shower, then apply pure aloe vera gel, which is instantly cooling. Soak a towel in strong, tepid tea and apply as a compress. Alternatively, aromatherapists suggest a compress dampened by water with a few drops of lavender oil added.

● **Dress a wound with honey** Scientific research shows that some types of honey, particularly manuka honey, contain antimicrobial factors that can kill a range of antibiotic-resistant bacteria, including MRSA.

● **Use cosmetic camouflage** If you are unsure about surgery or other treatments, cosmetic camouflage, which uses make-up to hide scarring and correct colour mismatches, can be effective.

try it… **Scar therapies** While it is not always possible to remove a scar entirely, scar revision treatment can improve the appearance of a scar and ease tightness. Much depends on the type and extent of the scar. Your age and skin type also play a role.

Some scar therapies are carried out by a dermatologist; others require the skills of a surgeon. The options include: laser therapy (suitable for mild scarring); compression therapy, in which pressure is applied to a raised scar; corticosteroid injection; freezing (cryotherapy); and the application of a special silicone sheet. A wide scar can in some cases be minimized by further surgery, perhaps involving a skin graft from another part of the body.

● **Treat cuts and wounds** Knowing how to treat a cut or wound correctly can help to avoid infection and ensure scar-free healing.

• Clean it. Wash the area of the burn under running water. Pat it dry with a sterile dressing or other clean, lint-free material.

• Cover it. Clean the surrounding skin with soapy water. Dry and then cover the cut with a plaster or sterile dressing or use steri-strips to close the edges of the wound. A large or deep cut that cannot be easily closed in this way may need to be stitched in hospital.

• Apply pressure. If bleeding is severe, apply direct pressure to the wound with a clean cloth, pad or even your fingers until a sterile dressing is available. Keep the dressing firmly in place to control bleeding and seek immediate medical attention.

• Elevate the affected area above the heart, if possible, while waiting for help.

● **Protect yourself against the sun** Always seek medical attention for severe (with blistering) or extensive sunburn. Follow these simple guidelines to protect your skin:

• Stay in the shade as much as possible between 11am and 3pm.

• Aim to cover up with T-shirt, hat and sunglasses.

• Never use a sunbed.

• Use sunscreen with an SPF (sun protection factor) of 15 or above.

• Check skin for new abnormalities that don't go away after four to six weeks or existing ones that are getting bigger. See your doctor if you notice such changes.

Sooth inflamed skin by applying calendula gel

BEST **HERBAL SOOTHERS**

Whether your skin damage is caused by a wound, graze, burn or scald, after you have taken essential first-aid measures, certain herbal preparations, essential oils and creams may help your skin to heal speedily and successfully, thereby reducing scarring. Dilute essential oils in a carrier oil before application to the skin. Use up to 12 drops in 6 to 8 teaspoons of a carrier oil such as sweet almond or grapeseed oil. The exception is lavender oil, which can be applied undiluted.

• **Recent wounds or burns** Try aloe vera gel, or lavender, helichrysum, sea buckthorn or carrot root essential oils. An infusion of lady's mantle or St John's wort (especially for burns) can be applied as a cool compress to the affected area. Calendula (marigold) ointment is renowned for its healing properties and can be used for a wide range of minor skin injuries.

• **Scars** Rosehip seed oil is reputed to encourage healing of scars and stretch marks. Alternatively try diluted clary sage oil (not to be used during pregnancy) or neroli oil, or undiluted lavender oil.

• **Sunburn** Sooth inflamed skin by applying witch hazel as a liquid or gel, or calendula or aloe vera gels. Another option is to apply a cool compress soaked in an infusion of dried marigold flowers, or apply neat lavender essential oil or sea buckthorn essential oil diluted in a carrier oil. Contrary to popular belief, the application of yoghurt is not an effective remedy for sunburn.

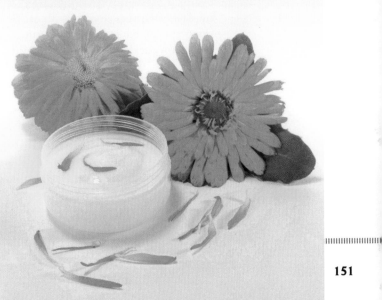

LIVING WITH ECZEMA

The classic signs of eczema are red, itchy patches that scale or weep and crust, most often on the arms and behind the knees. The condition tends to run in families, together with asthma and hay fever, and to occur episodically, flaring up and then subsiding again.

● **Try not to scratch** Eczema can be intensely itchy, but scratching releases chemicals in the skin that actually make the itching worse.

For many people, especially young children, the scratching causes more problems than the eczema, especially if the skin becomes infected. Keep nails well trimmed, and put on a pair of thin cotton gloves at night, when the irritation, and therefore the impulse to scratch, may be at its worst.

● **Use a soothing cream** Choose a simple moisturising cream. Don't use products containing steroids without talking to your doctor first – prolonged use can cause skin thinning and damage, especially on the face.

● **Consider an oral antihistamine** This remedy may help to relieve night-time itching. It may also promote sleep, as drowsiness is a side effect, but don't take these medicines during the day if you intend to drive or to operate potentially dangerous machinery.

● **Minimize house dust** Some people with eczema have a reaction to house-dust mites, so keep your home as dust-free as possible.

● **Avoid stress** Try to keep calm in potentially stressful situations, as stress can provoke a flare-up. It's important to be able to relax and to create a soothing environment at home.

● **Avoid irritating toiletries** Do your best to avoid any soaps, creams, shampoos and detergents that irritate your skin. You may find it helpful to keep a diary of your symptoms and product use. Choose unperfumed products and those designed for people with sensitive skin or allergies, and stick to non-biological washing powder.

● **Choose cotton fabrics** Avoid wearing wool and synthetic fabrics next to the skin: instead, choose cotton or a fabric that is fine and non-scratchy to avoid irritating already sensitive skin.

● **Identify food triggers** For some people, certain foods seem to provoke outbreaks of eczema. The most common culprits are dairy products such as milk and eggs, wheat, fish and foods that contain soya.

Start keeping a food diary and if you are able to pinpoint some potential food triggers, do your best to avoid them.

● **Stay cool** At night, sleep under a cotton sheet rather than a duvet or blankets during hot weather. Try to keep your skin well moisturized, as dry skin exacerbates eczema.

You might find it helpful to use an emollient bath oil or sprinkle bicarbonate or oatmeal into the bathwater to soothe irritated skin.

EASING **PSORIASIS**

Psoriasis causes thick, scaly patches to form on the skin, typically on elbows, knees and scalp. It results from accelerated production of skin cells, leading to thickening and inflammation of the outer layer of skin. The cause is unknown and there is no cure, but there are steps you can take to minimize symptoms and boost skin healing.

● **Seek expert advice** Ask your GP to refer you to a dermatologist, who may prescribe topical medications (drugs applied to the skin, such as salicylic acid) or phototherapy (light therapy).

● **Get some sun** Periods of exposure to sunlight of about 20 minutes three or four times a week can help to keep psoriasis under control. But be careful not to overdo it, as prolonged or intensive sunlight can make psoriasis worse or even trigger a flare-up.

● **Humidify indoor air** Use a humidifier or place bowls of water on hot radiators to avoid dry air sucking more moisture from your skin.

● **Use cling film** Apply an emollient ointment to patches of psoriasis and cover them with cling film overnight. In the morning, wash scales away under a lukewarm shower.

● **Take fish-oil supplements** The omega-3 fatty acids in fish oils reduce inflammation and dampen immune responses thought to underlie skin-thickening in psoriasis. Try 1g to 3g of fish oils daily, but no more, as high doses can interfere with the normal blood-clotting mechanism.

● **Moisturize often** Apply a moisturiser at night, in the morning and every time you wash, while your skin is still damp. You don't need expensive brands; cheaper moisturisers are just as effective.

● **Bathe less** Taking a shower or bath depletes your skin of nourishing oils, so always moisturize afterwards. You may find it acceptable to flannel-wash areas such as armpits, groin and feet daily, and save a full bath or shower for every few days. Avoid long soaks in the bath and keep the water warm rather than hot.

● **Avoid harsh soaps** Try to do without soap altogether, and wash most areas simply with warm water, or use a proprietary wash specially designed for dry skin.

● **Choose fabrics with care** Where possible choose natural fibres such as cotton and silk, which allow your skin to breathe – but avoid wool, which can scratch and irritate. Use non-biological, unperfumed detergents when washing clothes, towels and bedlinen.

There are various ways to minimize symptoms and boost skin healing

BECOMING **A MOTHER**

In the early weeks after childbirth, a mother's wellbeing is closely linked to that of her baby – so pamper yourself. If you've had a vaginal delivery you may be affected by stitches and bruising; if you had a caesarean section, you may have a painful wound. Your emotions will be in turmoil due to hormonal upheaval, and you will be suffering from a lack of sleep.

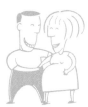

● **Rest when you can** Sleep when your baby sleeps. Put other concerns aside.

● **Interpret sniffles and snorts** Newborn babies often sniffle and snort especially when asleep. This indicates that mucus has accumulated in their nasal passages as a result of lying on their back and is nothing to worry about. More persistent sniffles can be a sign of a cold.

● **Soothe soreness** Stitches, bruising or small tears in or around the vagina are common features of childbirth.
• Keep the vaginal area clean and look out for signs of infection such as redness, swelling or discharge.

• Over-the-counter painkillers may help to reduce discomfort, but if you're breastfeeding ask your GP, health visitor or pharmacist for advice on what medicines are safe for you to take.
• Sit down gently and lie on your side rather than your back. Cushions or a special soft ring-shaped seat on your chair can help to ease pressure while you are sitting down.
• You may feel anxious about passing urine because of the soreness. Try sitting in a warm bath or running a warm shower over the area as you urinate. Drinking lots of water can help to dilute urine so it stings less.

● **Get help** Delegate household tasks and daily chores to your partner, friends, family or other people who offer to help.

● **Stay in touch** Other mothers can be a great source of support when you have a new baby. Arrange get-togethers with women you met at antenatal classes or ask your health visitor to put you in contact with other new mothers.

● **Eat well** Make sure that you have a balanced, nutritious diet. Regular meals are important, especially if you are breastfeeding. Eat plenty of fresh fruit and vegetables to prevent constipation.

> **did you know?**
>
> **Postnatal depression** Most new mothers experience a short period of 'baby blues' a few days after giving birth, which usually passes after 10 to 14 days. Postnatal depression by contrast may develop weeks or months after the birth and last for an indeterminate time. If you think you may have postnatal depression, consult your GP. Left untreated, the condition can adversely affect your relationship with your baby and your partner. Specific treatments may include cognitive behavioural therapy and/or medication as for other types of depression.

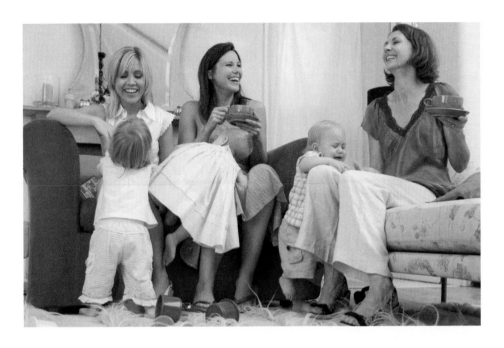
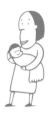

● **Don't neglect your partner** Nurture your relationship by spending time together every day and get a babysitter occasionally so you can go out.

● **Avoid caffeine** Drinking caffeine-containing drinks can increase anxiety and may affect the baby if you are breastfeeding.

● **Lie babies on their back** Placing babies to sleep on their back has greatly reduced the incidence of cot death.

● **Deal with nappy rash** Nappy rash is common. Fast action will prevent it from getting worse.
• Let your baby go without a nappy for as long as possible. Change nappies often.
• Clean your baby's bottom thoroughly using cotton wool and water (not baby wipes) and dry well between changes.
• Use a barrier cream. Preparations containing zinc oxide are good choices.
• A tablespoon of bicarbonate of soda in the bath water helps to soothe soreness.

● **Persevere with breastfeeding**
Although millions of babies every year thrive on bottle-feeding, childcare experts are in no doubt that breast milk provides the best nutrition for a baby. It supplies a perfectly balanced meal at every feed and passes on a degree of resistance to some infections, and its constituents change over the weeks to meet a growing infant's needs. However, breastfeeding does not come easily to many women and gives rise to challenges. It takes practice and perseverence to get it right, so take advantage of every offer of support.
   Even if you are only able to breastfeed for a few days or weeks, you will have given your baby a flying start in life.

● **Look for signs of infection** Proper vomiting – as opposed to bringing up a small amount of milk after feeding (possetting) – can be a sign of an infection. If your baby also has diarrhoea and a temperature, or if the vomiting ejects the stomach contents with force, consult your doctor without delay.

LOOKING AFTER
YOUNG CHILDREN

A healthy, happy childhood depends on a nutritious diet and plenty of sleep, physical activity and loving care. But illness is a normal part of every child's life. Illnesses may come on suddenly and often get better quickly on their own, but you need to be alert for signs of more serious condition. Occasionally a child may develop a more lasting physical or mental health problem such as asthma or attention deficit disorder.

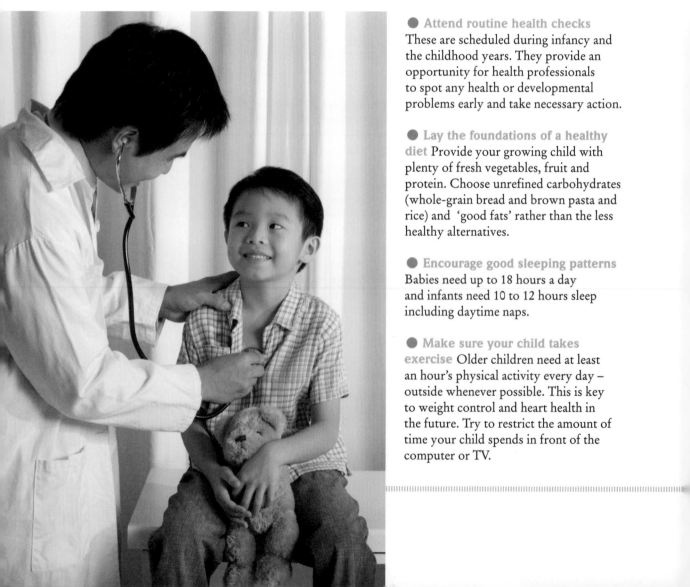

● **Attend routine health checks**
These are scheduled during infancy and the childhood years. They provide an opportunity for health professionals to spot any health or developmental problems early and take necessary action.

● **Lay the foundations of a healthy diet** Provide your growing child with plenty of fresh vegetables, fruit and protein. Choose unrefined carbohydrates (whole-grain bread and brown pasta and rice) and 'good fats' rather than the less healthy alternatives.

● **Encourage good sleeping patterns** Babies need up to 18 hours a day and infants need 10 to 12 hours sleep including daytime naps.

● **Make sure your child takes exercise** Older children need at least an hour's physical activity every day – outside whenever possible. This is key to weight control and heart health in the future. Try to restrict the amount of time your child spends in front of the computer or TV.

● Monitor your child's weight
Childhood obesity is on the increase and with it a greater risk of diabetes, heart disease, cancer, arthritis and many other illnesses. The majority of children can maintain a healthy weight with the right balance of exercise and food intake.

● Stop hiccups Hiccups can be intensely annoying and children tend to get them quite often. One simple thing you can do, which often seems to stop them, is to get your child to put one finger in each ear while you pinch his or her nose, and simultaneously help the child to sip from a glass of water.

● Ease nasal congestion Colds and coughs are very common in young children and will usually get better of their own accord. If mucus is causing your baby or child to have difficulty breathing at night or when feeding, try squeezing some saline (salt) solution (one or two drops) into each nostril before he or she feeds or settles for the night to clear the nostrils. To loosen phlegm when an older child has a cough, sit him or her on your knee, leaning slightly forwards, and pat the child's back.

● Cool a fever A child's normal temperature is between 36.5°C (98°F) and 37.5°C (99.5°F). A temperature above this is considered a fever and is usually a sign of infection. A high temperature can cause convulsions in some children.
• Sponge your child's forehead with lukewarm water.
• Encourage your child to drink plenty of fluids to reduce the risk of dehydration, which can occur as a result of sweating.
• Give children's paracetamol or ibuprofen.
• Dress your child in light clothing and keep the room below 18°C (64°F).

WHEN YOUR **BABY IS ILL**

Knowing how to differentiate between the many variations of normal behaviour and a real cause for concern is one of the hardest things for a new parent to learn. But you should trust your instinct and contact your doctor if you are at all worried.

Call 999 immediately if your baby:
• is not breathing
• is unconscious
• seems breathless, or is breathing much faster than usual
• looks very pale, or the skin is blue or dusky around the lips
• is having a convulsion (fit)
• has cold hands or feet, but also a fever (a temperature above 38°C/100°F)
• feels floppy or limp (perhaps when cuddled)
• has a raised, tense or bulging soft spot (fontanelle) in the centre of the top of the head.

● Be meningitis aware Meningitis (infection of the membranes surrounding the brain) is a frightening possibility for parents dealing with a feverish child. The symptoms are often not easy to recognize and can appear in any order. They may initially resemble those of other more common illnesses including flu. If you suspect that your child may have meningitis, seek an expert opinion without delay. A child with meningitis will usually appear ill and other symptoms may include fever, headache, nausea or vomiting, muscle pain, with cold hands and feet, drowsiness and lethargy, and a rash. A rash that does not fade under pressure is a sign of septicaemia (blood poisoning), and this can be a symptom of meningococcal meningitis. If your feverish child has a rash, press the side of a drinking glass firmly against the skin. If the spots do not fade, seek medical help urgently.

● **Act on anaphylaxis** Some children with a severe food allergy may develop anaphylaxis (severe swelling of the airways and shock) after eating a particular food. This is an emergency – dial 999 or get your child to your nearest A&E department as soon as possible.

● **Support your diabetic child** You don't need to feed a child with diabetes special foods – just provide a healthy, balanced diet. Aim for your child to have a minimum of an hour of brisk exercise every day. But be aware that physical activity causes a fall in blood glucose and it can take trial and error to balance food intake, insulin and exercise.

● **Minimize asthma attacks** If your child has been diagnosed with asthma, learn to spot warning signs of an asthma attack such as sneezing or a runny nose. You may be able to stop an attack by prompt use of appropriate medication.
• Protect your child as well as possible from known allergens.
• Rid your house of dust traps; keep your child's bedroom dust free.
• Keep a diary to identify triggers and situations that set off an attack.
• Keep your child active – swimming and walking are good options.
• Monitor your child's weight. Carrying excess weight can force lungs to work harder.
• Help your child to avoid stress
• Don't overprotect your child. Encourage him or her to join in normal activities as much as possible.

● **Combat eczema** Eczema is a skin rash that is often linked to allergy. It often appears first in babyhood.
• Keep your child's skin well moisturized at all times. Look out for over-the-counter creams and ointments.

• Oral antihistamines can help to relieve troublesome symptoms such as itching.
• Keep your child's skin from coming into contact with potential irritants such as soap.
• Keep your child's bedroom cool – use cotton sheets and a light duvet.
• Keep your child cool.
• Keep fingernails short and put scratch mittens on a baby.
• Try to pinpoint triggers. Keeping a diary can help.

● **Deal with hyperactivity** A child with a hyperactivity disorder may be prescribed medication by the doctor, but there are some non-medical measures you can take to make life easier for your child.
Watch additives Some children with attention deficit hyperactivity disorder (ADHD) may be sensitive to sugar and caffeine. Certain food additives may also exacerbate symptoms. Keep a food diary and discuss patterns with a dietitian.
Structure it A carefully structured environment and a clear understanding of acceptable and unacceptable behaviour can help your child to feel secure.
Work with your child's school Talk to the school about whether they can give extra help in certain subjects or skills.
Get fishy According to some studies, omega-3 supplements can help some children with ADHD, although more research is needed. Always check with a dietitian before making changes to your child's diet.
Talk it through Your GP or your child's psychiatrist may suggest talking therapy to help your child deal with symptoms such as impulsiveness. Family therapy can also help.

● **Get to grips with autism** Having a child with an autistic spectrum disorder can be especially demanding for parents.

Stay on your child's side Recognize your child's difficulties and find ways to structure the environment to minimize challenging behaviour. Praise good behaviour and stay positive.

Get help with behaviour Applied behaviour analysis started before the age of five teaches basic social, educational and daily life skills, which can reduce problem behaviour. Ask your doctor to refer you to a child psychologist.

Be a partner in play Learn about the best ways to communicate with your child. Give your child extra time when playing or doing everyday tasks to enable him or her to think about what to say. Speech therapy may also help.

Get support There are many ways of dealing with autistic spectrum disorders and lots of help available for parents. You may be entitled to benefits to help cover the extra expenses involved.

● **Nurture your child through depression** All children have ups and downs but if your child or teenager is experiencing more persistent low moods, withdrawal, over or under-eating, sleeping all the time or other changes in behaviour, he or she could be depressed. Your GP can refer your child to a paediatrician or child psychologist.

Be honest If your child's depression has been sparked off by a family trauma such as a divorce, be honest and keep him or her in touch with what is happening.

Provide the words Young children may not have the vocabulary to express feelings such as sadness, anger or confusion. Help your child to find the words he or she needs.

Provide a shoulder to cry on Let your child know that you are there to talk to. If your child does not want to talk to you, another parent, teacher or family friend may be willing to listen.

WHICH IMMUNIZATIONS AND WHEN

Here's a checklist of the immunizations that are routinely offered to all children in the UK, and the age at which they should ideally be given.

2 months
Diphtheria, tetanus, pertussis (whooping cough), polio and Haemophilus influenzae Type b (Hib – a bacterial infection that can cause severe pneumonia or meningitis in children) given as a 5-in-1 single jab known as DTaP/IPV/Hib (first dose)
Pneumococcal infection (first dose)

3 months
DTaP/IPV/Hib (second dose)
Meningitis C (first dose)

4 months
DTaP/IPV/Hib (third dose)
Pneumococcal infection (second dose)
Meningitis C (second dose)

Around 12 months
Meningitis C (third dose)*
Hib (fourth dose)*
*often given as a single jab

Around 13 months
Measles, mumps and rubella, given as a single jab known as MMR (first dose)
Pneumococcal infection (third dose)

3 years and 4 months, or soon after
MMR (second dose)
Diphtheria, tetanus, pertussis and polio (DtaP/IPV) (pre-school booster)

12–13 years
HPV (Human papilloma virus vaccine), which protects against cervical cancer (girls only) (three doses given within a six month period)

13–18 years
Diphtheria, tetanus and polio, given as a single booster jab, known as Td/IPV

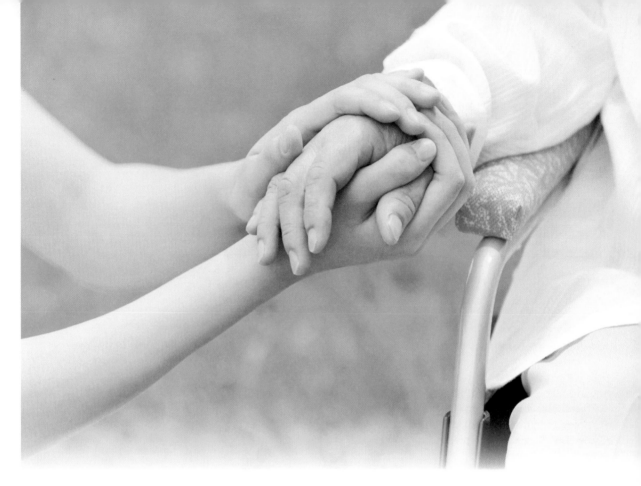

CARING FOR **OTHERS**

At some point in life most people have to look after someone else – whether it's a period of intensive short-term care as a friend or relative recovers from an accident or illness, or a much longer-term or even full-time commitment. Knowing that your efforts can help someone you love to recover can be its own reward. But effective caring can be demanding. It often requires patience and optimism, as well as nursing know-how.

● **Involve your GP** Your doctor can help you to get access to social, mental health or other services, and may be able to offer home visits if the person you are caring for does not find it easy to get to the doctor's surgery.

● **Think about your employment** If someone close to you is in need of long-term personal care, talk to your employer about reducing your working hours or organizing more flexible hours for the duration of the person's recovery.

● **Get a care assessment** Social services in England and Wales, social work departments in Scotland, and health and social services trusts in Northern Ireland can assess your needs and help you to obtain respite care, aids and adaptations for your home, financial assistance and emergency help.

● **Join a support group** For a long-term care commitment, becoming part of a support group can enable you to meet people in a similar situation. You can find information about local groups from Carers UK (www.carersuk.org).

● **Consider how you can maintain and demonstrate respect** It will help, for example, if you treat the person you are looking after as a partner in the care process, encouraging him or her to be as independent as possible and to play role in any decision-making.

● **Be alert for appetite and weight changes** They can be early signs of physical or mental health problems. If the person you care for has unexplained weight loss, arrange for a vistit to the GP.

● **Plan how best to handle bad news** It can be difficult to be the bearer of bad tidings – a poor medical prognosis or the need to consider residential care, for example. Your GP, community matron or nurse, counsellor or a carers' organization may be able to provide assistance.

● **Don't underestimate what it means to be a carer** Whether you feel that caring for someone is a duty or a privilege, it's vital to acknowledge that it's not necessarily easy. Enlist the help of friends and family and seek advice and additional support, if necessary, from your GP and local social services.

THE MAIN INGREDIENTS OF **GOOD NUTRITION**

If you're caring for someone who's ill, offering small, nutritious, home-cooked meals presented attractively can help to whet a feeble appetite and improve health. The following foods and nutrients are especially important.

• **Starchy foods and fibre** Bread, rice, pasta, cereals, pulses and potatoes provide vital energy, protein, vitamins, minerals and fibre to help prevent constipation and enhance digestive health. Avoid insoluble fibre in the form of bran, which can hinder the absorption of calcium and iron.

• **Iron** Red meat, offal, pulses, oily fish, eggs, bread, green vegetables and fortified breakfast cereals are foods that can help prevent iron-deficiency. Vitamin C aids iron absorption, so offer a glass of fruit juice with meals. Avoid serving tea with iron-rich meals, as it can block absorption of iron.

• **Vitamin C** This is a key nutrient for promoting resistance to infections and wound-healing. Encourage the person you care for to eat citrus fruits, green leafy vegetables, peppers, tomatoes, potatoes, fruit juices and fruit drinks with added vitamin C. Smoothies can provide additional vitamin C for someone who does not feel like eating solid food.

• **Calcium** Dairy products such as milk, cheese and yoghurt, canned fish with bones, such as sardines, green leafy vegetables (such as broccoli and cabbage, but not spinach), soyabeans and tofu are all good sources of this vital mineral, which can help strengthen bones.

• **Vitamin D** People whose poor health or poor mobility may limit their opportunities to go outside, can be short of vitamin D, which is made in the skin from sunlight and is also found in oily fish and dairy products. Try to encourage the person you are caring for to eat these foods, or ask the doctor or a dietitian about the advisability of supplements.

• **Water** A good intake of fluids is essential to hydrate the cells, maintain the tone and elasticity of tissues and ensure nutrients are absorbed. Experts advise consuming at least 1.2 litres of fluids every day (this includes any liquid in food). Fluid requirements may be higher if there is a fever, diarrhoea or vomiting. If the person you are caring for doesn't like plain water, offer tea, squash, milk, juice, smoothies and soups instead.

TAKE RESPONSIBILITY FOR MEDICINES

When you look after someone who is bed-bound, you'll probably have to take responsibility for administering medicines – especially if the person is drowsy or confused. In this situation you'll need to find out as much as possible about them.

- Check the leaflet in the medicine packet. It often has useful guidance on storage and what to do if a dose is missed or too many are taken.
- Don't guess or estimate doses for liquid medicines. Pharmacists can provide syringes, pots or spoons for precise measurement.
- All types of medicine have the best effect when taken at regular intervals. If the medicine is to be taken once a day, try to administer it at roughly the same time each day. For more frequent doses, ask the doctor if you should wake the person in the night to take medication or space the doses through the waking hours.
- If the information for a tablet says 'to be swallowed whole', it is important not to crush these tablets since stomach acid could make them less effective. People who have difficulty swallowing may need special help to take medication safely as choking or a fatal chest infection could result if a tablet becomes lodged in the windpipe.
- The best way to take medicines is standing or sitting up, with a small amount of cool or tepid (not hot) liquid from a cup or glass. If the person cannot take a medicine for any reason, consult the doctor.
- If the person for whom you are caring needs to go to hospital, be sure to take a copy of the most recent prescription or the medicines themselves if the prescription cannot be found so that the hospital staff are aware of what he or she is taking.

● **Encourage the recovering person to maintain a healthy weight** In some cases, someone recovering from a long-term illness may need to put on weight, but may not feel hungry. When preparing food, try to make sure that every mouthful contains plenty of calories and protein. Fortify food with melted butter, grated cheese or cream. You might also add some finely ground nuts or seeds to fortify smoothies and soups, or sprinkle over vegetables.

Offering six small meals a day instead of three large ones may achieve more successful results. You can also add full-fat milk and sugar to tea and coffee to provide extra calories, and choose high-fat options such as pastry and full-fat milk. If weight loss continues, ask the doctor whether supplement drinks might be advisable.

● **Create a healthy environment** Someone recovering from an illness may need to spend hours, or perhaps all day, in the same room. Thoughtful adaptations to create a healing environment can make a huge difference to a patient's state of mind and speed of recovery.
Lighten up Draw back curtains whenever possible. Mirrors can also increase the sense of light and space, but may not be suitable for rooms used by patients with dementia or mental-health problems, who can find them distressing.
Bring the outside in Adorn the room with plants or fresh cut flowers.
Be a colour therapist Colour affects mood. Pale shades are calming. Keep brighter colours for cushions and ornaments.

The best way to take medicines is standing or sitting up, with a small amount of cool or tepid liquid from a cup

Keep it dust-free and sparkling Vacuum carpets at least once a week and wipe over hard surfaces, sinks and taps daily. Having sparklingly clean windows can do wonders for the spirits.

Declutter Keep the room free of unnecessary objects. This is not only important for fall prevention; a clutter-free environment is a soothing place in which to spend time.

Make space for favourite things A bedside table for books, a portable TV, a radio or a laptop computer.

● **Follow good food hygiene** Wash your hands and clean work surfaces, utensils and chopping boards before and after use. Check use-by dates and adhere to them strictly. Heat chilled and frozen food until it's steaming hot throughout.

● **Avoid food poisoning** Bacteria such as salmonella and listeria are a risk for anyone with reduced immunity, especially people over the age of 60. Avoid raw or lightly cooked eggs (or products that contain them), raw or undercooked meat, soft cheeses such as Camembert and Brie, soft blue cheeses and pâtés, including vegetarian options.

● **Help the person to keep clean** Being clean and fresh is vital to wellbeing and self-esteem, but, for short periods, no damage is done if the ill person misses a daily bath or shower. Providing soap and a damp washcloth so that the person can wash their face, hands, armpits and genital area (in that order) is adequate for a couple of days.If the person is confined to bed for any longer, you may have to give a bed bath. If he or she is sufficiently mobile and the doctor agrees, you may be able to help him or her to wash. This may require safety equipment such as non-slip mats and grab rails.

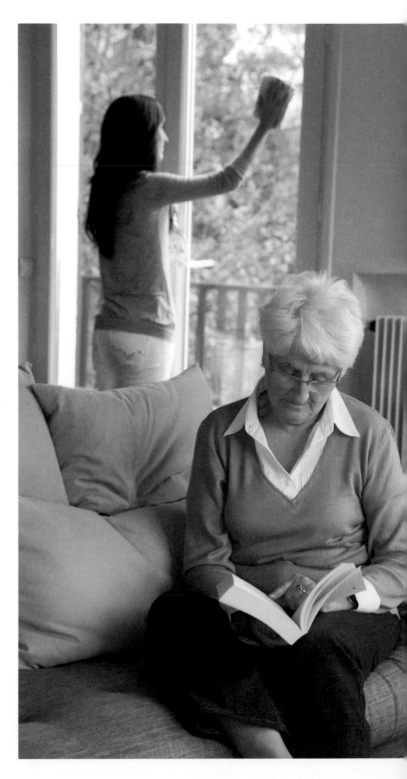

Knowing that your efforts can help someone you love to recover can be its own reward. But effective caring can be demanding. It often requires patience and optimism, as well as nursing know-how

● **Encourage activity** As a first step, discuss with your doctor whether any medicines may be affecting the person's ability to stand or walk – for example, by causing side effects such as fatigue, muscle weakness or dizziness – and if so whether a change of medication could help. Also check how any medical conditions are likely to affect mobility at a later date.

● **Consider walking aids** If you think walking aids may provide the reassurance your loved one needs to feel confident about regaining mobility, ask your doctor or physiotherapist whether a stick or walking frame might help. These are often available through local council social services departments.

● **Try 'chairobics'** As soon as the person you are caring for is able to sit in a chair, it's worth suggesting some gentle exercises using light weights to help build strength. Cans or small bottles of water can make ideal improvised weights.

Choose a chair that allows the person to keep their knees at 90 degrees when seated. During the exercise, it is important for the patient to sit tall and hold in the stomach muscles to maintain good posture. Each exercise should be repeated ten times.

Lateral raise With a weight in each hand, raise the arms up to the side to shoulder height and, slowly and with control, take them back down.

Biceps curls With a weight in each hand, elbows at the sides, palms facing upwards, curl the arms towards the shoulders, then slowly bring the hands back down to their original position.

● **Explore exercise options** Once the person has regained confidence and reasonable mobility, doing a course of tai chi, gentle yoga or Pilates can improve core strength and balance. Check at the local library for classes for people with restricted mobility. Age UK offers exercise DVDs and videos for older people. Its 'Be Strong, Be Steady' programme has chair-based and standing exercises that strengthen the muscles, increase flexibility and improve balance.

● **Treat toileting with tact** Toileting is a highly sensitive aspect of personal care that should be handled with tact and respect. A basically healthy person confined to bed with a short-term illness can usually get up to use the lavatory, as long as it is accessible. In such cases it may still be wise to stay close by in case of falls. If it's not possible for the person to walk more than a few steps, you may need to get a commode. Ask your GP, occupational therapist or social services department how to acquire one. For a person confined to bed, a bedpan may be the best option. You'll need advice from your medical team and training for helping the person on and off the pan.

9 most effective ways to survive as a carer

Being a carer can reinforce the love you feel for the person you are looking after and provide a satisfying sense of achievement, but it can also be physically exhausting and mentally draining. It's crucial that you care for yourself too, especially if your commitment is a long-term one.

1 CONSIDER YOUR OWN PEACE OF MIND

Take some time out every day for a little self-indulgence. For example, you could read a book or a newspaper, watch television, listen to your favourite music or simply relax.

2 DEAL WITH STRESS – HEALTHILY

A massage, a dance or yoga class, a walk in the country, a park or by the sea, or a visit to a spa if you can afford it, are all excellent ways to combat stress.

3 FIND EMOTIONAL SUPPORT

Your friends and relatives have different things to offer. Some who are no good at practical tasks may be able to offer a sympathetic ear. Try to find a confidant with an open mind who's a good listener. If you're religious, you may find help within your faith community.

4 MIND YOUR BACK

Caring for someone who is bed-bound can involve lifting. Ask your doctor for advice about acquiring special equipment.

5 KEEP YOURSELF WELL

Keep an eye on your own health. Eat sensibly and make time for exercise.

6 SEEK RESPITE

If you are caring for someone with a long-term condition, consider respite care. Residential care homes and nursing homes may offer short-term options. Organizations such as Macmillan Cancer Support and the Alzheimer's Society can also provide advice.

7 SLEEP TIGHT

Have a bedtime routine to help you wind down and pamper yourself at the end of the day.

8 A HEALTHY DIET

It's tempting to eat junk food or simply to snack and carry on, but try to make time to enjoy healthy food and relaxed mealtimes.

9 DON'T TRY TO DO IT ALL

You aren't superhuman. Ask for the help you need. Friends, family or neighbours often want to help and it's up to you to tell them how. This might include housework, gardening, shopping or sitting with your loved one.

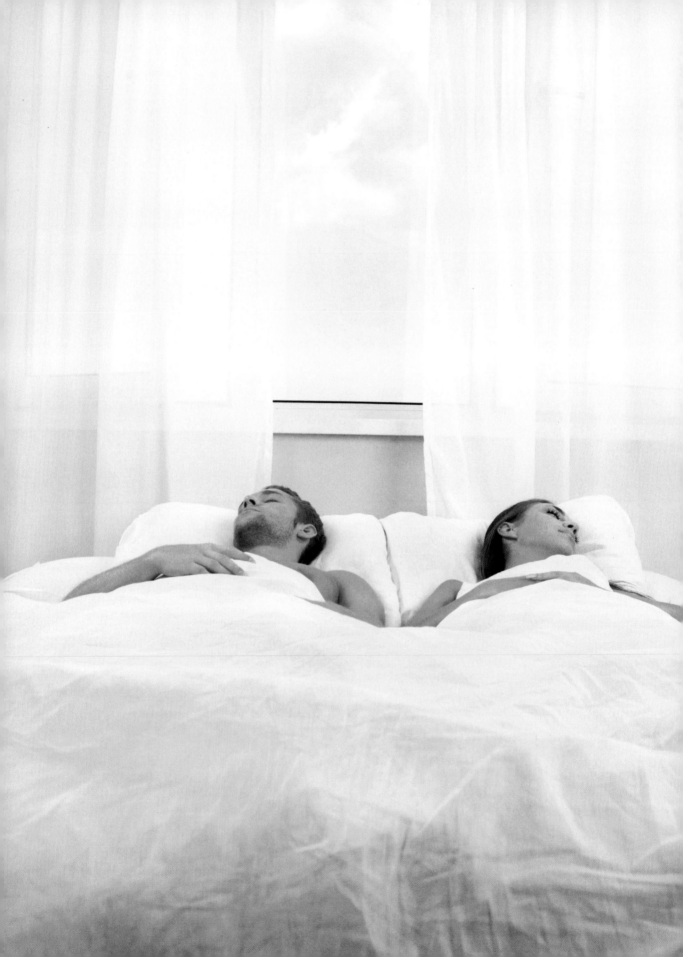

SLEEP
soundly

When you sleep well, you wake feeling bright and alert. When you don't, you're tired, your memory suffers and you can't concentrate. Whatever prompts it, lack of sleep is a common cause of stress. As stress also leads to sleeplessness, you can soon be caught in a vicious cycle of sleepless nights and anxious days that is damaging to health.

It doesn't have to be that way. This section's imaginative strategies can help you and family members to break a sleepless pattern and banish bad dreams. A good night's sleep has just become a much more achievable goal.

TOP TIPS FOR
GOOD SLEEP

One of the most beneficial things you can do for your health is to get a good night's sleep. Conversely, sleep deprivation can disrupt your levels of thyroid and stress hormones, potentially affecting everything from your memory to your immune system. The following steps will help to ensure that you fall asleep easily and stay asleep as long as possible.

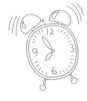

● **Monitor your sleepiness** There are three good ways to tell if you're getting enough sleep. First, do you need an alarm clock to wake up most mornings? Second, do you become drowsy in the afternoon to the point that it affects what you're doing? Third, do you doze off shortly after eating dinner? If the answer to any of these is yes, you need more sleep. And if you're getting enough sleep (about 8 hours) and still have these troubles, talk to your doctor about your low energy.

● **Establish a nightly routine** This should be something you do every night before going to bed. It could be as simple as turning out the lights, turning down the heating, washing your face and brushing your teeth. Or perhaps a series of yoga or meditation exercises. As you begin to perform your familiar activities, your brain will signal to the rest of your body that you are preparing for sleep.

● **Listen to a book on tape while you fall asleep** Just as a bedtime story soothes and relaxes children, a calming book on tape (try poetry or a biography, but stay away from horror novels) can have the same effect with us grown-ups.

● **Close the door on snoring pets** A 2002 research study found that one in five pet owners slept with their pets – and that dogs and cats created one of the biggest obstacles to a good night's sleep since the discovery of caffeine. One reason? The study found that 21 per cent of the dogs and 7 per cent of the cats snored.

● **Take a hot bath** Do this 1½ to 2 hours before bedtime. A study published in the journal *Sleep* found that women with insomnia who took a hot bath at this point – with the water temperature at about 40°C (104°F) – slept much better that night. The bath increased their core body temperature, which abruptly dropped once they got out of the bath, preparing them for sleep.

● **Keep your toes warm** Tuck a hot-water bottle between your feet or wear a pair of ski socks to bed in winter. Warm feet help your body's internal temperature to reach the optimal level for sleep. Essentially, you sleep best when your core temperature drops. By warming your feet, you make sure blood flows well through your legs, allowing your trunk to cool.

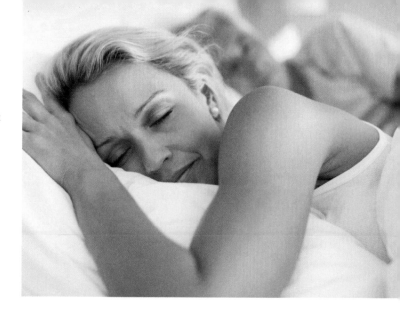

● **Get in tune with your rhythms** Do you ever find that you get really sleepy at 10pm, that the sleepiness passes, and that by midnight you're wide awake again? Some experts believe sleepiness comes in cycles. If you soldier on through a period of tiredness, you probably won't be able to fall asleep easily for a while. If you've noticed these kinds of rhythms in your own body clock, use them to your advantage. When sleepiness comes, go to bed. Otherwise, it might be a long time until you're ready for sleep again.

● **Exercise at the right time** Even mild exercise, such as 30 minutes of walking, can lead to sounder sleep. But when you take your exercise is also important. It's not something you should do just before getting into bed. Instead, plan to do some in the early evening – a few hours before bedtime as it can take this time for your body's metabolism and temperature to return to normal after exercising.

● **Give yourself a massage** Slowly move the tips of your fingers around your eyes in a slow, circular motion. After a minute, move down to your mouth, then to your neck and the back of your head. Continue down your body until you're ready to drop off to sleep.

Another option is to ask your partner to give you a massage – and suggest that the two of you could massage each other on alternate nights.

● **Wear pyjamas or a nightdress** Warm skin helps to slow down your blood's circulation, cooling your internal temperature and generally contributing to a deeper sleep. Just don't overdo it. Your body goes through a few cool–warm cycles as the night passes, so you want pyjamas, sheets and covers that keep you comfortable through these changes.

● **Sleep alone** One of the greatest disruptors of sleep is your loved one dreaming away next to you. He might snore, she might kick or cry out.

In fact, one study found that 86 per cent of women surveyed said their husbands snored, and half had their sleep interrupted by it. Men have it a bit easier: 57 per cent said their wives snored, while just 15 per cent found their sleep bothered by it.

did you know?

How to nap Naps can revive you when you blood-sugar levels are low, but keep them short. Studies show that even 'shut-eye' without sleep can be helpful. Here are three simple rules to ensure that your naps don't interfere with your night-time sleep.
• Get the timing right: a mid-afternoon siesta is ideal because our natural 12-hour sleep cycle means we're extra-sleepy at this time.
• Nap length should be 20–30 minutes, plus the time it takes to fall asleep (allow 10 minutes). A short nap such as this will stop you feeling groggy when you wake up.
• Allow 20–30 minutes after a nap before doing anything that requires attention, as your mental performance will be poor for a while (a condition called 'sleep inertia').

WINDING **DOWN**

Your meal is finished, the washing-up is done and you're looking forward a couple of hours before your body begins sending go-to-sleep signals. You could sit down passively in front of the television or your computer screen – or you could think of a fulfilling activity that will put you in a mood more conducive to sound sleep.

● **Go for an after-dinner walk** What better time for a hand-in-hand stroll through your neighbourhood? To make it more interesting, play a game of observing two new things about your neighbours on each walk.

● **Play a game with your partner or children** Try a board game, work on a puzzle or opt for a rousing game of cards. It will make those brain cells work hard. And the social bonding with your loved ones will contribute to your family's emotional and physical health.

● **Get in the mood for sex** Put your arms round your partner's waist and begin kissing him or her on the back of the neck. Hopefully, this will lead to something more. As well as the obvious benefits of sex, you'll also be raising your heart rate, sending immune-boosting endorphins to your brain – and extending your life. One study found that sexually active men lived longer than those who made love less often – a finding that's likely to apply to women too.

● **Change into nightclothes and slippers early in the evening** It will help separate the 'daytime you' from the 'evening you', and be a constant reminder throughout the evening to relax.

● **Lose yourself in a book** Rekindle your love of reading. It's so much more rewarding than watching television. And it's much healthier, because it keeps your brain active and engaged.

● **Savour a piece of dark chocolate** Gram for gram, chocolate contains more healthy antioxidants, which repair damage to cells and prevent cholesterol from oxidizing (making it stickier), than any of the other antioxidant champions, including tea, blueberries and grape juice. Plus it's well known for its ability to soothe a troubled mind.

Keep the chocolate dark – it has the most antioxidants – and plain. You don't need the extra sugar and calories from caramel and other sweets.

● **Give yourself a pedicure** Fill a basin with warm water and a few drops of peppermint oil. Soak your feet in it until the water cools, then pumice away the rough skin on your soles. Massage a perfumed lotion all over your feet, inhaling the lovely scent and feeling your skin soften with every stroke. Trim your toenails, push back your cuticles and, if you desire, polish your toenails in a colour you'd never dare wear on your fingernails. If you can, persuade your partner to give you a foot massage.

● **Ask your partner or a friend to wash your hair** Having your hair washed and your scalp massaged is an unexpected luxury that will help wash away the stress of the day.

● **Clean out one cupboard in your home** This chore takes no more than 30 minutes, and leaves you with a sense of accomplishment, yet without any added stress because the task is simple and unchallenging, yet satisfying.

● **Make a yoghurt smoothie** Put a banana, a pot of low-fat natural yoghurt, a handful of blueberries and a teaspoon of honey into the blender along with some crushed ice. Blend the mixture until it is thick and smooth. The combination of the antioxidants in the blueberries, the potassium in the banana and the live bacteria in the yoghurt will give you a health boost that no vitamin can match.

● **Write your diary for 10 minutes** Not sure what to write? Just try listing what you did that day. Write down five things that made you smile. Note five things that made you angry – and why. Numerous studies attest to the stress-busting power of regular diary writing. Plus, it's fun to leaf back through your diary and see what you were doing a year earlier.

● **Write a to-do list for the next day** It takes 5 minutes, yet the peace of mind it brings is priceless. Instead of running a to-do list over and over in your mind – transforming your responsibilities into daunting challenges – you can enjoy the rest of your evening and have a better shot at sleeping.

● **Play with your dog or cat for 15 minutes** Studies show significant stress-reduction benefits from pets, particularly those that, like dogs and cats, can interact with you.

● **Prepare for the next day** Make your (or your children's) packed lunch, lay out your clothes, check your briefcase and make sure the children's school stuff is by the front door. This will avoid the surge in stress hormones the following morning that comes from rushing around frenetically while screaming at the children, ripping your tights and spilling juice on your silk shirt.

● **Put on a CD and dance for 20 minutes** If you do it energetically, you'll burn as many calories as if you were jogging. Dancing improves coordination and can give you the benefit of some good stretches. Plus, it's a great way for younger parents to engage their children in physical activity.

Dancing helps you let go and gives you the benefit of some good stretches

CONQUERING FATIGUE

Feeling tired all the time is frustrating and dispiriting. You want to race like a thoroughbred, but you feel stuck in the mud. Changes in the way you eat, drink and exercise may be needed – or there may be a serious underlying health problem. Uncertainty still surrounds two related conditions – myalgic encephalopathy (ME) and chronic fatigue syndrome.

● **Boost bloodflow to the brain** Lie on your back and use pillows to prop your feet at a level higher than your head or, better still, lie on an adjustable exercise bench or other surface that slants. In India, yogis fight fatigue through such practices by encouraging bloodflow to the brain, which is thought to boost alertness.

● **Give yourself a pick-me-up** For a quick fix, put 2 drops of peppermint oil on a tissue or handkerchief, hold it to your nose and breathe deeply. If you have more time, try adding 2 drops of the oil to bathwater along with 4 drops of rosemary oil for an invigorating soak.

● **Eat several small meals a day** Try to limit the size of each meal to 300kcal. This will keep your blood-sugar levels steady and help to prevent your energy levels plunging.

● **Go easy on simple carbohydrates** Foods high in simple carbohydrates make your blood sugar rise rapidly, then crash just as quickly. If you indulge in too much French bread, spaghetti and cake, you'll end up feeling weak and tired.

● **Eat more high-fibre foods** These are rich in complex carbohydrates and help to stabilize blood sugar. They include whole-grain cereals and wholemeal bread.

● **Cut down on fatty foods** To boost the function of your adrenal glands, which affect the way you metabolize nutrients, ensure that saturated fats make up no more than 10 per cent of your diet.

● **Sip water all day long** Drink at least eight glasses. Don't wait until you're thirsty, because your 'thirst alarm' isn't always accurate. Even a little dehydration can make you feel tired.

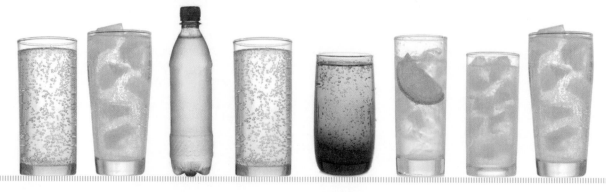

● **Get your engine moving** Try to do at least 30 minutes of aerobic exercise most days of the week. Not only does exercise help you to shed weight, it also gives you an energy boost. People who exercise regularly find that they also tend to sleep better.

Consider taking up yoga or tai chi. These ancient forms of exercise give you opportunities for physical activity and include relaxation components that can be reinvigorating.

● **Combat sluggishness** Try to do 10 minutes of low-level exercise whenever you feel sluggish. Usually people with fatigue have a decreased supply of adenosine diphosphate (ADP), an intracellular 'messenger' involved in energy metabolism. Translated, it means there's not enough 'spark' in the engine. Almost any kind of activity – singing, walking, stretching – will help.

● **Supplement your energy stores** Take a multivitamin and multimineral supplement daily to ensure that your body is getting the minimum amount of nutrients that it requires.
Ginseng Ginseng extract is an ancient cure for that rundown feeling. Take 100–250mg Panax ginseng or 300–400mg Siberian ginseng once or twice a day. It will stimulate your nervous system and help to protect your body from the consequences of stress.
Magnesium Take 150mg of magnesium (preferably as magnesium citrate) twice a day. This mineral is involved in hundreds of chemical reactions in the body. It plays a role in changing protein, fat and carbohydrates into energy sources.
Ginkgo Ginkgo improves bloodflow to the brain, which can make you feel more alert and less fatigued. Take 15 drops of ginkgo tincture in the mornings.

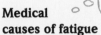

Medical causes of fatigue
Although poor sleep can lead to fatigue, there may be an underlying medical cause. If you haven't been able to resolve your sleep problems, visit your GP, who may suggest diagnostic tests. The most common causes of fatigue, apart from poor sleep, are:
• Lack of minerals such as iron.
• Hormonal disturbances. These may be related to the thyroid or adrenal glands or to diabetes.
• Recurring infections or lowered immunity.
• Gluten intolerance and coeliac disease.
• Heart, lung and neurological disorders.

● **Keep caffeinated drinks to a minimum** The caffeine in coffee and some colas can give you a short-term burst of energy, but following that rush, there's usually a 'crash'.

● **Limit alcohol consumption** Alcohol depresses your central nervous system. It also reduces your blood sugar level.

● **Always get up at the same time** Do this even at weekends. Your body will benefit from a regular sleep routine.

● **Clock off early** Go to bed earlier than normal if you need extra sleep. As long as you're getting up at the same time every morning, it's fine to have a flexible going-to-bed schedule.

Improving bloodflow to the brain can reduce feelings of fatigue

OVERCOMING INSOMNIA

Insomnia can become a real nightmare as the clock ticks on into the night and you're awake to notice. But you're not alone. At any one time, the problem affects around 15 per cent of the UK population. So what's the remedy? Have a go at counting sheep – it really can work. Even better, try some of the ideas suggested on these pages.

● **Go bananas** Have a slice of chicken or a banana before going to bed. These foods contain tryptophan, an amino acid that the body uses to make serotonin. And serotonin is a brain chemical that helps you to sleep.

● **Add carbohydrates** Carbohydrates help trytophan to enter the brain. Try a glass of warm milk (milk contains tryptophan) and a biscuit, or warm milk with a teaspoonful of honey. A sprinkling of cinnamon won't hurt and might add mild sedative properties of its own.

try it... **Hide your clock** Put it under the bed or on the bottom shelf of your bedside cabinet, where its glow won't disturb you. That way, if you do wake up in the middle of the night or have problems sleeping, you won't fret over how late it is and how much sleep you're missing.

● **Wake up at the same time each day** Aim to wake up at a set time in the morning regardless of how little sleep you had the night before. At weekends, don't have a lie-in. Follow the same routine so your body adheres to the same pattern all week. You'll fall asleep faster.

● **Every morning, go for a walk** Your walk doesn't have to be long but it should be outdoors. The presence of natural light tells your sleepy body it's time to wake up for the day. With your body clock set to natural daylight, you'll sleep better at night.

● **Avoid late meals and spicy or sugary food** You need 3 to 4 hours to digest a big meal, so if you eat a lot within 3 hours of your bedtime, don't be surprised if intestinal grumblings keep you awake. Spices can irritate your stomach and, when it tosses and turns, so will you. Having a lot of sugary food – especially chocolate, which contains caffeine – can make you feel jumpy.

● **Try not to snooze during the day** People who don't have insomnia often benefit from a short afternoon nap. However, if you nap during the day only to turn into a wide-eyed zombie at night, there's a good chance that the afternoon snooze is disrupting your body clock. If you must have a nap, limit it to no more than half-an-hour.

● **Let yourself go** Once you get into bed, imagine your feet becoming heavy and numb. Feel them sinking into the mattress. Then do the same with your calves and slowly work your way up your body, letting it all grow heavy and relaxed. The object of the exercise is to let yourself go, in gradual phases, all the way from head to toe.

● **Don't lie in bed worrying** If you simply can't sleep, don't lie in bed worrying about it. That will only make getting to sleep harder. Get up, leave the bedroom and grab a book, some knitting, a jigsaw puzzle or watch television. Don't read or watch anything too exciting, though, or you'll become engrossed and your mind will be even more wakeful.

● **Consult your doctor** If you've tried self-help strategies and still can't get a good night's sleep, talk to your doctor. This is especially important if sleep deprivation is harming your relationships, your work performance or endangering your life – as in causing you to fall asleep at the wheel. You may need to be evaluated overnight at a sleep clinic.

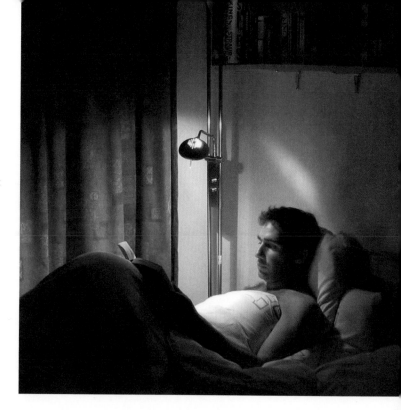

Don't read or watch anything too exciting – or you'll become engrossed and find it even harder to sink into a restful sleep

● **Avoid caffeine, alcohol and tobacco in the evenings** Caffeine's effects vary from person to person, but the stimulating effects can be long-lasting. And, while a tot of whisky might help you to fall asleep, the effects soon wear off and you're much more likely to wake up in the night.

If you smoke within 4 hours of going to bed, look no further for the cause of your insomnia. Nicotine stimulates the central nervous system, interfering with your ability to fall asleep and stay asleep.

● **Avoid exercising within 4 hours of bedtime** It's too stimulating. Instead, exercise in the morning or after work. An exception is yoga. A number of yoga postures are designed to calm your body and prepare you for sleep.

● **Brew up some lettuce** Simmer three or four large lettuce leaves in about 200ml water for 15 minutes. Remove from the heat, add two sprigs of mint, leave for a few minutes, then strain off the liquid.

Sip the brew just before getting into bed. Lettuce contains a substance called lectucarium, which acts on the brain in a similar way to opium.

● **Check the label** Be cautious about taking any over-the-counter painkillers before going to bed. Some of them, such as Anadin Extra, contain caffeine – a stimulant. In addition to caffeine, cold remedies like Sudafed may contain ingredients, such as pseudoephedrine, that rev up your nervous system and leave you unable to fall asleep. Look for a night-time formula.

WHAT **DRUGS AND SUPPLEMENTS** CAN DO

Sleeping pills and other sleep-inducing medications may help to promote sound slumber if you take them for short periods and in certain situations, but many such drugs have side effects such as a next-day feeling of grogginess and what's known as 'rebound insomnia' – and, if taken long term, they may lead to dependence.

● **Review your current medicines**
If you go to a doctor complaining of insomnia, he or she may not link your sleeplessness to one of your current medicines. Yet many drugs can interfere with sleep. These include beta blockers, thyroid medication, decongestants, some antidepressants, corticosteroids and medicines containing caffeine, such as many of the over-the-counter painkillers and cough and cold cures.

So, if you're consulting your doctor about insomnia, take along a list of everything you're using or have recently used and their dosages – including all over-the-counter medications and herbal and nutritional supplements.

● **Use antihistamines with caution**
Antihistamines, originally used to treat allergic reactions, are sometimes prescribed for insomnia.

Generally, the body breaks down antihistamines over several hours, so if you take them you may experience 'hangover' effects the morning after. It is not advisable to use them routinely.

● **Try a sedating antidepressant**
Antidepressants such as amitriptyline and dosulepin are often prescribed as aids to sleep. Hangover effects may occur, and some people may develop a dependence. Always follow your GP's instructions when taking these drugs.

● **Extend your dreams with 5-HTP**
5-HTP is derived from tryptophan, an amino acid responsible for the manufacture of the hormone serotonin. Used in supplement form to boost levels of serotonin in the brain, 5-HTP has been prescribed for decades for the treatment of depression and insomnia.

5-HTP has been shown in studies to promote sleep, and to improve the quality of sleep, by increasing the amount of time people spend in two key sleep stages: deep sleep and REM sleep (the dreaming stage). After dreaming for longer, those on 5-HTP wake up feeling more rested and refreshed.

Take a single 100mg dose half an hour before bedtime. Don't use for more than three months except on medical advice.

Tryptophan has been described as 'nature's tranquillizer'

● **Calm those restless legs** Do your legs throb or crawl with uncomfortable sensations just as you're drifting off to sleep at night, making you fully awake again? Does this phenomenon recur at intervals throughout the night? If so, you could have restless legs syndrome, and the answer to your poor sleep pattern could be as simple as a vitamin supplement.

In one study, researchers found that women who frequently experienced restless-legs syndrome, were often deficient in folic acid, a form of vitamin B_9 that is essential for proper brain and nerve function. Symptoms improved when these women were given a dose of folic acid. So try taking a supplement of between 400 to 800mcg folic acid a day, along with 50mg vitamin B-complex in order to avoid upsetting your body's vitamin B balance.

● **Beware of tolerance and addiction** Benzodiazepines, such as diazepam, and so-called 'Z drugs' (zopiclone, zolpidem, zaleplon) are sometimes prescribed for short periods to relieve sleeplessness. They work by affecting the way neurotransmitters send messages to brain cells. In effect, they decrease the excitability of many brain cells, which has a calming effect on various functions of the brain. These drugs often work well in the short term, but they should not be taken for more than 2–4 weeks. Otherwise, the medicine may lose its effect (you may become tolerant to it) and you may also become addicted to it. Each 'Z drug' has its pros and cons, so your GP will advise what's best for you.

● **Get enough of 'nature's tranquillizer'** The amino acid tryptophan, which is present in most protein-based foods, has been described as 'nature's tranquillizer' because it is responsible for the manufacture in our bodies of the hormone serotonin. Serotonin is a neurotransmitter – a chemical substance that transmits nerve impulses across the space between nerve cells – which plays a crucial role in the regulation of learning, mood and sleep.

High levels of tryptophan are found in cheese, meat, soya beans, sesame seeds, chocolate, oats, bananas, dried dates, milk and salmon. A diet low in tryptophan can lead to low levels of serotonin, which in turn can result in depression, poor sleep and poor concentration.

● **Ask your doctor about melatonin** Melatonin is a hormone produced by the pineal gland, a pea-sized structure in the brain. It is secreted only during the night and even this release can be blocked if light is present. Melatonin has an effect on our biological clock and in some cases it is sleep-inducing. Taken as a supplement, it is useful for controlling jet lag.

Melatonin and melatonin-like drugs may be prescribed by GPs in the UK only under special circumstances, though they are more freely available in the USA. Since melatonin is processed rapidly by the body, a hangover effect is rare.

High levels of tryptophan are found in salmon

9 most satisfying ways to drift off with herbs

Many people find herbal and other dietary supplements effective in the treatment of sleep disorders. If you have been prescribed any medications, consult your doctor before taking herbal preparations because they can interact with prescription drugs.

1 BANISH ANXIETY WITH VALERIAN

Valerian can help you to fall asleep faster without groggy after-effects. It calms the brain and body so that sleep can occur naturally. The herb itself stinks, so don't try to make it into a tea. Instead, take 250–500mg of the powdered extract in capsule or tablet form or 1 teaspoon of valerian tincture an hour before going to bed.

2 FALL ASLEEP NATURALLY WITH CAMOMILE

Camomile has a mildly sedative effect, but more importantly it also calms the body, making it easier for the person taking it to fall asleep naturally. Pour a cup of very hot (not boiling) water over 2 teaspoons of dried camomile flowers. Steep for 5 minutes and strain. Drink up to three cups a day or a cup at bedtime. Alternatively, try sprinkling some dried or fresh flowerheads or a few drops of the essential oil under your pillow, or add some to your bathwater.

3 SCENT YOUR SPACE WITH LAVENDER

Lavender is a mild tranquillizer. Dilute lavender oil in a carrier oil (5 drops per 10ml) and dab a little on to your temples and forehead before you go to bed. The aroma should help to send you off to sleep. You can also add lavender oil to a diffuser or vaporizer to scent your bedroom or place a lavender sachet near your pillow. Try a soothing aromatic bath before bedtime: add 5 drops of lavender oil and 3 drops of ylang-ylang oil to warm bathwater and enjoy a glorious soak.

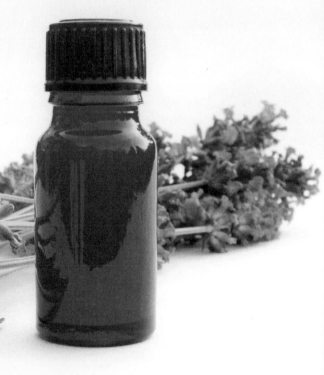

4 TRY JASMINE ESSENTIAL OIL

Put a drop of jasmine essential oil on each wrist just before you go to bed. One American study discovered that people who spent the night in jasmine-scented rooms slept more peacefully than people who stayed in unscented – or even in lavender-scented – rooms.

5 EASE CONGESTION WITH PEPPERMINT

There is evidence that peppermint reduces sleeplessness, particularly for those suffering from common colds, because of its decongestant properties. You can make a tea by steeping 1 or 2 teaspoons of dried peppermint leaves in 250ml of very hot water for between 5 and 10 minutes. Be sure to cover the cup to prevent the volatile oil from escaping. Drink up to four cups of peppermint tea a day.

6 EMBRACE PASSIONFLOWER

Passionflower is widely used as a mild herbal sedative. It can also be taken as a supplement in combination with valerian or chamomile, for example.

7 BANISH TENSION IN THE BATH

Add 3 drops of ylang-ylang oil, 5 drops of lavender oil, 2 drops of bergamot oil and a handful of Epsom salts to warm bathwater for an anxiety-soothing soak.

Alternatively, you can use dried herbs such as lavender and chamomile. For maximum benefit, tie a bunch of herbs in a piece of muslin or cheesecloth and hold this under the running tap while you fill the bath.

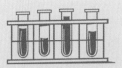

The power of aromatherapy

Many people swear by aromatherapy as an aid to sleep. This faith is reinforced by studies indicating that certain essential oils can help to relieve anxiety and depression, tame our reactions to stress and enhance energy. The scents of plants such as lavender, bergamot, geranium, marjoram and sandalwood have been shown to alter brain waves, inducing relaxation and sleep.

The benefits of essential oils can be enjoyed by inhaling the fragrance, soaking in water than contains an oil or massaging it into your skin, but an oil used for bathing or massage must always be diluted in a 'carrier' such as almond, grapeseed or sunflower oil. Essential oils can also be used to promote sleep associations.

Sleep associations work by fooling your brain into connecting certain sensations or routines with your body's need for sleep. For example, if you have trouble sleeping when you are away from home, try sprinkling geranium oil on your pillow at home for a week before the trip. Take the oil with you and sprinkle it on the pillow in the unfamiliar bedroom. Sleep should come easier because your brain associates the smell of the geranium with sleeping.

8 SEW A HOP PILLOW AND TAKE IT TO BED WITH YOU

Hops – flowers of a plant used in beer-making – release a mild sedative into the air, and for some people they induce sleep more rapidly than valerian, but avoid hops if you have depression as they many accentuate symptoms.

To make your own hop pillow, sew two 30cm (1ft) squares of fabric together along three sides to form a pocket. Stuff it full of dried hops and sew the fourth side shut. Put the pillow near your head so you can smell it at night.

9 MAKE A HERBAL INFUSION AND DRINK IT BEFORE BEDTIME

Other plants that are commonly used to promote sound sleep include California poppy, lemon balm, lime flowers, vervain and wild lettuce.

Add 200ml (⅓ pint) of boiling water to about 10g of your chosen dried herb or mixture of herbs, infuse for 10 minutes and strain. Drink before going to bed.

SLEEPING POSITIONS AND YOUR BEDROOM

If you're waking up sore and aching each morning, you need to re-evaluate the positions in which you're sleeping and the quality of your mattress and pillows. There may be other features of your bedroom that could be improved to enhance comfort and relaxation.

● **Try not to lie flat on your back** Lying in this position forces your spine into an unnatural position, which can strain your muscles, joints and nerves. Your spine isn't meant to be straight – it has three natural curves: one in your lower back, one in the middle of your back and one near your neck.

● **Adopt the foetal position** Lie on your side in the foetal position with your knees bent and a pillow tucked between your legs. This will take the most stress off your back and is particularly suitable for people with back pain.

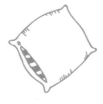

● **Put a pillow under your knees** If you must sleep on your back, prop a big, fluffy pillow under your knees to reduce the pressure on the sciatic nerve in your lower back.

● **Keep wrinkles at bay** One exception to the advice not to sleep on your back concerns wrinkle prevention. When you sleep on your side or on your front, you bury your face in the pillow, 'ironing in' wrinkles and crevices.

● **Think about neck support** If you find yourself tossing and turning as you try to get comfortable, consider buying a special neck-supporting pillow. They are specially designed for people who have neck pain or tension that prevents sleep.

One Swedish study found that neck pillows can enhance the quality of your sleep as well as reduce neck pain. The ideal neck pillow should be soft and not too high, provide neck support and be allergy-tested and washable. Alternatively, use an ordinary small pillow or a rolled-up towel under your neck as long as it doesn't push your chin too far forward.

● **Don't sleep on your front** Sleeping face down can exaggerate the arch at the base of your spine and cause strain. Try sewing or taping a tennis ball to the front of your nightdress or pyjama top. It will put an end to your stomach-sleeping days – unless you have sciatica, in which case lying on your front is the recommended position.

● **Ease heartburn** You can counteract the discomfort of indigestion, by raising the head of your bed 10–15cm with wooden blocks or old phone books. When you sleep tilted at an angle, gravity helps to keep acid in the stomach.

● **Cool your bedroom** Turn the central heating off (or at least right down) before going to bed. Most people sleep better when the air around them is cool and their bedding is snug.

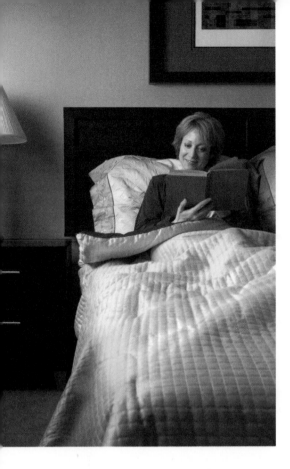

● **Buy a bigger bed** If you share a bed, consider buying a queen or king-size bed so that you and your partner don't keep each other awake. Some mattresses are designed so that when your partner moves you feel nothing. Or consider sleeping in separate beds.

● **Move your bed away from an outside wall** This will help to cut down on noise, which, according to a Spanish study, could be a significant factor in causing insomnia. If you are still bothered by noise even after moving your bed, try a white-noise machine or turn on a fan.

Remove the clutter from your bedroom – distractions stand in the way of a good night's sleep.

● **Paint your bedroom a soothing colour** First, remove the clutter from your bedroom – it provides a distraction and stands in the way of a good night's sleep. A soothing colour such as sage green provides a visual reminder of sleep, relaxing you as you lie in bed reading or preparing for sleep.

● **Switch to heavier curtains** Cover the windows if you find it hard to drop off. Even the light from street lamps, a full moon or your neighbour's house can interfere with the circadian rhythm changes that prompt you to fall asleep.

● **Change your pillow** If you're constantly pounding it, turning it over and upside down, your poor pillow deserves a break. Find a fresh new pillow from the linen cupboard, put a sweet-smelling pillowcase on it and try again.

● **Invest in a good mattress** If your mattress is ten or more years old, you need a new one. If your mattress is lumpy, ditch it. Another sign that your mattress needs replacing is waking up feeling sore or stiff, even if you haven't been physically active the day before. Although no single style of mattress works best for everybody, there are some guidelines to follow:
Size Make sure you buy one that's larger than you think you will need, especially if you sleep with someone else.
Firmness This is strictly an individual decision. But make sure you try out any mattress in the shop. Lie on it. Roll over. Get into your typical sleeping position.
Good-quality frame Make sure you get a sturdy, good-quality frame, one with at least ten slats.
Maintenance Turn your mattress over and upside down every three months.

BEST WAYS TO DEAL WITH **SNORING**

If you're the snorer in your household, you're probably getting a great deal more sleep than anyone lying next to you. Changing your sleeping position may be all it takes to resolve the problem, and preserve a harmonious relationship, but for many people a bigger project – namely, losing weight – is often the real key to tranquil nights.

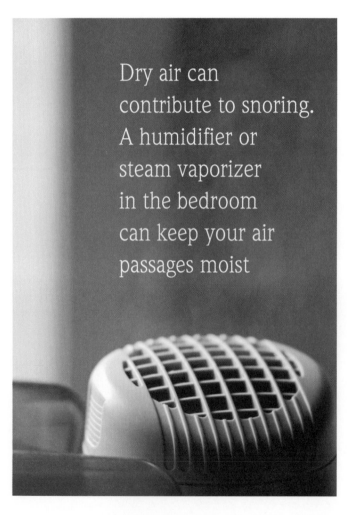

Dry air can contribute to snoring. A humidifier or steam vaporizer in the bedroom can keep your air passages moist

● **Don't eat or drink before bedtime** Avoid eating a heavy meal or drinking alcoholic beverages within 3 hours of going to bed. Either can cause your throat muscles to relax more than normal.

● **Give up smoking** Tobacco smoke irritates mucous membranes, so your throat swells, narrowing the airway. Smokers also have more problems with nasal congestion.

● **Review your medication** If you regularly take any kind of medication, talk to your doctor about alternatives. Some drugs can make snoring worse, including sleeping pills and sedatives.

● **Humidify the air** Dry air can contribute to snoring. A humidifier or steam vaporizer in the bedroom can keep your air passages moist; be sure to clean it regularly, following the manufacturer's instructions. Another tactic is to inhale steam. Just before bedtime, fill a bowl with hot water, drape a towel over your head, bend over the bowl so your nose is roughly 30cm (12in) from the water and breathe deeply through your nose for a few minutes.

● **Prop yourself up** Buy yourself a few extra pillows and prop yourself up in bed, rather than lying flat on your back. You'll prevent the tissues in your throat from falling into your air passages.

● **Shed a few pounds** Losing weight can reduce your snoring by easing constriction of the upper airway.

● **Raise the head of your bed** Place several flat boards under the legs at the top end of the bed. Alternatively, a couple of old telephone books under each leg should also raise the bed high enough.

● **Sleep on your side** Of course, there's no guarantee you'll stay lying on your side, but at least start that way, with your arms wrapped around a pillow. There's a good reason you don't want to sleep on your back: in that position, your tongue and soft palate rest against the back of your throat, blocking the airway.

● **Unblock your nose** If nasal congestion is causing your snoring, try taking a decongestant or antihistamine before you go to bed. But use these only as a temporary measure if you suspect that a cold or allergy is to blame. Prolonged use of either can be harmful.

● **Tape your nose open** You can do this with nasal strips, available at most pharmacies. Following the directions on the package, tape one of the strips to the outside of your nose when you go to bed. They work by lifting and opening your nostrils to increase airflow.

● **Get rid of allergens** To relieve nasal stuffiness, banish bedroom allergens (dust, pet dander, mould) by vacuuming floors and curtains. Change sheets and pillowcases often.

● **Gargle with a peppermint mouthwash** The effect is to shrink the lining of your nose and throat. This works particularly well if your snoring is a temporary condition caused by a head cold or an allergy. To make the herbal gargle, add 1 drop of peppermint oil to a glass of cold water.

● **Keep your chin up** It might sound extreme, but some snorers have used a neck brace – the kind people with whiplash injuries wear – to stop their snoring. It works by keeping your chin extended so that your throat doesn't kink and your airway stays open.

● **Drink nettle tea** If your snoring is a seasonal problem – and you know you're allergic to pollen – try drinking nettle tea. Herbalists recommend it for soothing inflammation caused by pollen allergies. To make the tea, pour a cup of boiling water over 1 tablespoon of the dried leaf. Cover the tea and let it steep for 5 minutes. Strain and drink. Drink up to three cups a day, one just before bedtime.

did you know?

Are you suffering from sleep apnoea? Loud, excessive snoring can signal sleep apnoea, a potentially dangerous condition that requires treatment. Contact your doctor if you're a loud snorer who stops breathing for short periods when you're asleep. You should also notify the doctor if you sometimes wake up gasping for breath, if you wake up with headaches, or if you're sleepy during the day. Sleep apnoea can reduce levels of oxygen in the blood, eventually leading to elevated blood pressure and an enlarged heart.

In addition to lifestyle modifications (losing weight or changing your sleeping position), some doctors recommend a continuous positive airway pressure (CPAP) device to use at night. Surgery is also possible.

CHILDREN AND SLEEP

Having a young baby in the house is bound to disrupt your sleep, and irregular sleeping habits in older infants can cause problems for children and parents alike. Establishing a simple and soothing bedtime routine is the first step in avoiding or resolving sleep problems.

● **Let your baby doze off** To encourage healthy sleeping habits, it's wise to put babies in their cots when they are tired but before they are fully asleep. Don't rock them to sleep all the time. They have to learn to doze off unaided.

● **Lie babies on their back** The relatively recent move towards doing this rather than placing babies on their front to go to sleep has markedly reduced the incidence of cot death.

● **Don't worry about noise** Babies don't need complete quiet. It's good for them to learn to sleep anywhere. But avoid sudden loud noises.

● **Establish a pattern** Help your baby to wind down every evening with a regular and enjoyable routine – a bath followed by a feed, for example. Then put your baby to bed and say goodnight.

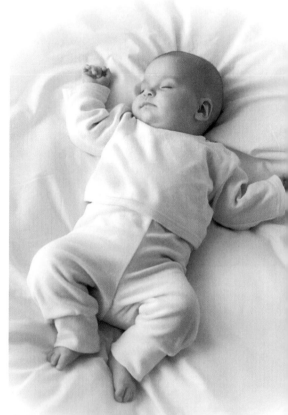

● **Don't be reluctant to seek help** Living with a baby who never seems to stop crying can test your patience to the limit, especially if nights of broken sleep have left you exhausted.

If you feel that you can't take any more, it's vital to seek help. Ask your health visitor or doctor about local support for parents of crying babies or call a telephone helpline.

● **Take it in turns** As far as possible, share the night-time burden of attending to a young baby with your partner, and use the times when your are not 'on duty' to catch up with your sleep.

A breastfeeding mother will inevitably do the lion's share of caring during the early weeks and months of a baby's life, but even she can have some respite by arranging for her partner to bottle-feed the baby with expressed breast milk.

● **Sleep when your baby sleeps**
When your baby is asleep during the day, seize the opportunity to have a nap yourself. Don't worry about housework or chores.

● **Keep it low-key** If your baby needs attention at night, make sure you keep the interaction low-key. Your baby needs to learn that night-time is not for having fun. It's for sleep.

● **Be firm about habitual crying**
If your older infant habitually cries after you have left the room or wakes up repeatedly during the night, there are several things you can do.

Wait a couple of minutes before going back into the bedroom. Say goodnight again and reassure your child, but make it clear that the child is expected to stay in bed. If your child is standing, tuck him or her in again, but keep any conversation to a minimum. Be firm and do not pick the child up.

Repeat the process for however long it takes, leaving longer intervals before your return each time.

● **Deal with nightmares and night terrors** Children who have nightmares need plenty of comfort and reassurance. Nightmares are not usually an indication of emotional disturbance, but if they occur often it may be a sign that your child is anxious or upset about something.

Children who experience night terrors may give out piercing screams or cries of fear. You will probably find the child sitting up in bed and staring in terror, but still asleep, and not aware of your presence. The best thing to do is not to wake the child, but to stay until he or she falls back into a calm sleep again. By the morning the dream will have been forgotten.

try it... **Reaching crisis point** If your baby is crying and you feel that you can no longer cope, hand him or her to someone else to hold. If you are alone, put your baby down in a pram or cot straight away. Make sure he or she is safe and close the door. Go into another room and calm yourself down before going back. Leaving your baby to cry for a short time will not do any harm.

● **Devise a bedtime routine**
Creating a bedtime routine for your child, and sticking to it, is a good recipe for household harmony, and should help all the family to sleep soundly.
• Decide what time you wish your child to go to bed – and give a warning when that time is approaching.
• Give your child a bath around the same time each night. Allow a little play but no stimulation such as television or noisy games before bedtime.
• Offer a milky drink or snack. If your child asks for food or drink once in bed, give the drink or snack in the bedroom.
• Brush your child's teeth – or make sure that he or she brushes them.
• Spend some quiet time with your child. Chat about the day's events, give cuddles, then put the child to bed before he or she falls asleep.
• Read a bedtime story.
• Tuck up your child and kiss goodnight.
• Leave the bedroom before the child falls asleep.
• Leave a night light on or leave the door open if your child is afraid of the dark.

● **Don't get angry** If your child repeatedly gets out of bed and comes downstairs or into your room, try not to get angry or give in. Say firmly that the child has to go to bed and take him or her back. Ignore any crying. Repeat this process until your child gets the message that you mean what you say.

Try to share with your partner the burden of getting up at night to care for your baby

10 steps to finding true calm

If you have tried numerous strategies and tactics for getting a better night's sleep but haven't seen much improvement, it may be that you are suffering from stress. The best way to deal with this – and to find true calm – is to reassert control over your life.

1 DEFINE YOUR ROLE IN LIFE

Be sure you understand your own role and responsibilities, at home and at work. Delegate tasks if you can, both at home and at work.

2 WRITE IT DOWN

When bad things happen, sit down and write out what you might have done differently. If you get a bad evaluation at work, say, don't blame the boss. Instead, be honest with yourself about what you could have done differently – getting into work on time, meeting all your deadlines, etc. – to get a better result. Understanding your role in the situation will help you to realize that the world is more controllable that you might think.

3 BUILD IN CONTINGENCIES

Imagine, for example, that you have an outdoor party planned for 20 people but it rains on the day. You can't control the weather, but you can control where you hold it (move it inside), when you hold it (postpone it) and how it's held (if you were planning a barbecue, prepare a couple of large dishes of lasagne instead).

4 TAKE UP A NEW HOBBY

Mastering a new skill, whether it's paddling a kayak or learning to knit, will return a sense of control to your life.

5 CREATE A PERCEPTION THAT YOU'RE IN CHARGE

Research shows that the perception of being in control is more important to an individual than the actual fact of being in control. For instance, people are able to tolerate a hot room if they know they have the option of turning down the heat. So, if you can identify in your mind some small changes that you could confidently make, it will make your apparently chaotic situation seem more manageable.

6 TAKE TIME TO DE-STRESS

Put your feet up, do some relaxation breathing, have a cup of tea. Calming yourself down is something you can do for yourself to help you to feel in control.

7 DISTINGUISH WHAT YOU CAN'T CONTROL FROM WHAT YOU CAN

You'd be amazed at how many people still think they can control the traffic, the weather, their boss's mood or the stock market. Make a list of all the things in your life that you can't control, no matter how hard you try, and stick it on your fridge and your computer. Then accept it. Of course you can care about these things and try to influence their outcome. But it's essential that you untie your emotional wellbeing from those things that you cannot alter.

8 PRACTISE POSITIVE SELF-TALK

It would be great if someone else did this for you, but often you have to do it for yourself. Self-talk means saying things like, 'I'm going to be OK', 'I'll get through this' or 'Right now, I have to give myself a few minutes, then I can begin coming up with a plan to handle this.'

9 DO ONE THING

When life feels chaotic, choose one thing to work on where you can make a difference. For example, start an exercise programme, write in your diary one day a week, balance your bank account or make sure you take your car in for a scheduled service.

10 MAKE A LIST

Nothing puts more control back into your hands than taking hold of all the 'to-dos' swirling through your head and writing them down. Now plan how you will accomplish each one. If one of the things on your list is Christmas shopping, say, set yourself a date, a time and a time limit to do it. If another item on your list is to clean the whole house, break it down into smaller, more manageable parts. So on Monday you clean the kitchen, on Tuesday the bathroom and so on.

Is stress causing your **sleep problems?**

Tick any of the following that apply to you and check the results at the end.

- Are you putting on weight around your 'middle' – that is, in your abdominal region?
- Do you find that you have a 'short fuse', are more sensitive, irritable or easily frustrated than you used to be?
- Do you have a general feeling of being overwhelmed by everything you're dealing with right now?
- Do you find yourself always feeling overtired or exhausted?
- Have you experienced notable weight gain or weight loss recently?
- Do you feel muscle tension, especially in neck, back and jaw?
- Do you find that you are ill more often than usual?
- Do you find it more difficult to make decisions and concentrate, and do you forget things more often?
- Do you often feel anxious about things you can't control?
- Has your libido decreased or are you often just too tired for sex?
- Do you experience tension headaches?
- Do you find yourself eating to copy with annoyances, or craving sweet or salty food more often than usual?
- Do you find yourself drinking more alcohol to relax, smoking to deal with stress, or becoming dependent on illegal drugs or prescribed medication?

If you have ticked more than three questions, stress may be affecting your sleep – in which case, the next section, on relaxation, will be of particular relevance to you.

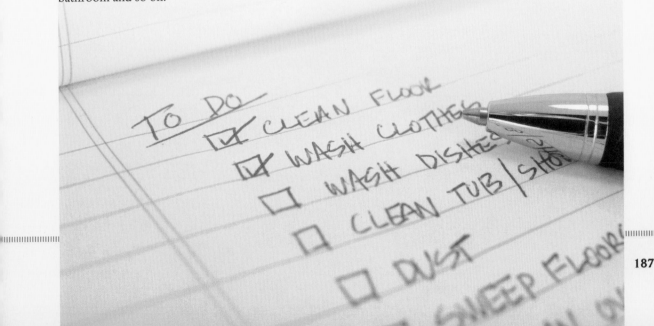

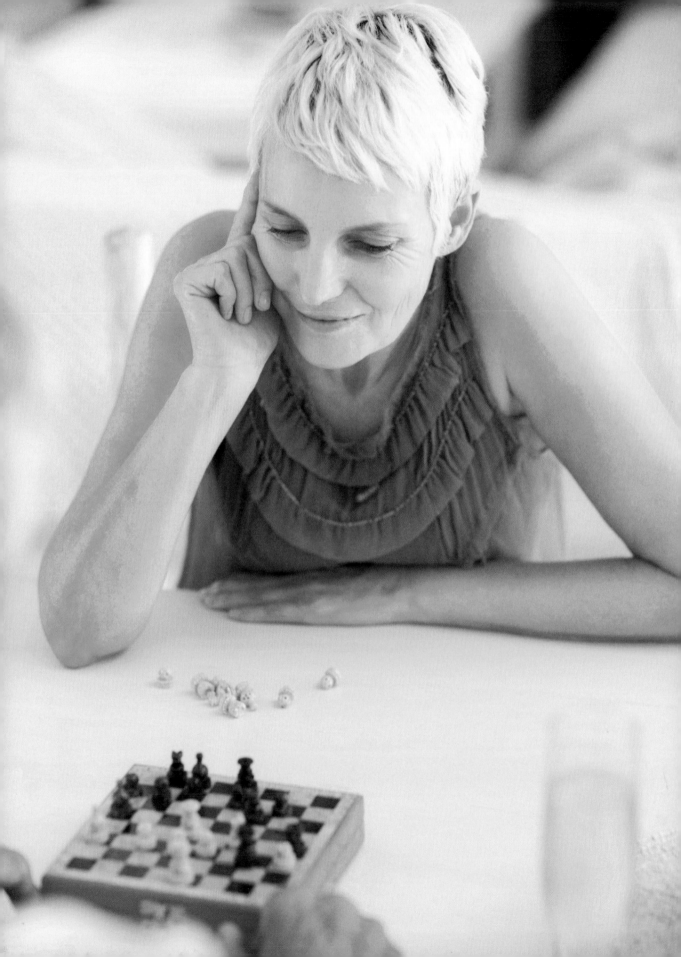

RELAX
and banish stress

Nothing has a greater impact on your wellbeing than the way you treat yourself. Thinking and acting positively is one of the best ways to maintain both physical and mental health. Calm resistance to the adverse influences of stress, hostility and hopelessness can work wonders in the fight against heart attacks and strokes.

As you'll discover from the advice in this section, friendship, laughter and an outgoing, optimistic attitude are also golden tickets to a longer life. Learning to relax is key and the single skill that will help you to banish stress, take control of your life and enjoy it to the full.

LEARN HOW TO
REDUCE STRESS

Stress can be a stimulus to act which some people take in their stride, but others become tense, angry or tearful, lose concentration or reach for 'comfort foods', alcohol or cigarettes. None of these is beneficial to health. Indeed, undue stress is one of the key indirect causes of illness.

● **Take care of yourself** Make sure you get plenty of sleep, eat a healthy diet, stop smoking and don't drink too much. Not only can stress interfere with your sleep, but also not getting enough sleep can add to your stress levels. (See pages 166–87 for advice on sleeping well.) A healthy diet helps to keep your immune system and metabolism functioning well and protects you from the effects of stress.

● **Talk about it** Cultivate a support network. You might find it hard, but start sharing your feelings on a regular basis with at least one family member or trusted friend. And then listen to your confidant's problems.

● **Let it out** If stress accumulates to such a degree that you feel like crying, take heart. Emotional tears are quite different from the sort you produce when you're in pain or peeling an onion. Scientists think that a good cry actually clears out stress-related chemicals produced when we're under pressure. Some doctors speculate that this is why men, who cry less often, are more at risk of stress-related diseases than women.

● **Take charge of your destiny** Recognize that in most situations you do have a choice, if only about how to react, and it is your own choices that largely determine what happens to you. So, at times of uncertainty, repeat to yourself: 'I have a choice.' People with what psychologists call a high 'locus of control'– who feel themselves in charge of their own destiny – have a 25 per cent lower risk of heart attack than those who feel buffeted by random forces beyond their control. They are generally happier and less likely to become depressed.

● **Be more decisive** Work at becoming more decisive and developing problem-solving abilities. People who adapt well to stress are 25 per cent less likely to suffer a stroke than those who don't.

great idea!

Attend a 'laughter yoga' class For those who want to combine getting fit with having fun, there is an international laughter movement that runs 'laughter yoga' classes. This gives you a chance to get together with other people and simply laugh. It's an excellent aerobic workout, combining the physiological benefits of laughter with yogic breathing, which delivers more oxygen to the body and brain.

● **Try to enjoy your work** If you wake up each morning full of dread at the thought of having to go to work, seriously consider searching for an alternative source of income.

● **Laugh away your troubles** Laughter is a great way to relax and release tension, which would suggest that a lively sense of humour can boost your cardiovascular health. Research has shown that laughing out loud – whether it's helpless giggles or a full-blown guffaw – expands the inner walls of your blood vessels, boosting blood flow by 25 per cent. That's equivalent to the physiological impact of a stroll in the park or even being on a course of cholesterol-lowering drugs. It's so good for you that heart experts recommend you aim for 15 minutes of laughter every day.

Simply thinking about humour has been shown to benefit health. The anticipation of watching a favourite comedy show reduces levels of stress hormones such as cortisol and increases levels of stress-relieving endorphins, the 'feel-good' and pain-relieving hormones produced naturally by the body.

● **Know when to say 'no'** Living entirely for others is a major cause of chronic stress.

● **Set limits** Find a way to prevent other people's hurtful behaviour from upsetting your peace of mind.

● **Do aerobic exercise regularly** It's easiest to do if you find an exercise you thoroughly enjoy. Gentle exercise, such as yoga or Pilates, has been shown to reduce stress.

UNDERSTANDING **STRESS**

When we experience an event or situation as stressful, our body's defence mechanism against danger – the 'fight or flight' response – kicks in. This leads to an increased release of adrenaline and other stress hormones, causing the heart to beat stronger and faster, raising blood pressure and breathing rate, promoting sweating (in anticipation of intense activity, as sweat helps to regulate body temperature), and shutting down digestion and other non-essential functions. This response would have been helpful to ancient humans facing the threat of attack by a wild animal; it is much less so in the face of irritating, automated telephone-answering systems and traffic jams. Persistent stress can lead to high blood pressure and a raised clotting tendency – a risk factor for both heart attack and stroke. Stress also prompts the body to release a hormone called cortisol, long-term exposure to which has been linked with abdominal obesity, high blood pressure and Type 2 diabetes. A sudden rise in blood pressure, stimulated by acute stress, can also trigger haemorrhagic stroke (bleeding in the brain).

● **Run up and down stairs** Physical activity is one of the best stress-busters and one of the best exercise aids is easy to use and almost universally available – a staircase. When daily life starts getting on top of you, run up and down stairs a couple of times or, if you can spare 10 minutes, go for a brisk walk around the block in the fresh air.

● **Focus on deep breathing** Regular deep breathing is a simple but highly successful stress-buster. You can teach yourself or learn how to do this from a yoga teacher or in a special relaxation or meditation class.

Heart experts recommend 15 minutes of laughter each day

TAKE CONTROL
OF YOUR LIFE

As well as knowing how to deal with sudden stress, you can devise a longer-term plan for a calmer existence. Taking control will help you to feel more positive about yourself and to keep feelings of frustration and anger at bay. It will also make you feel happier and allow you to share that happiness with others. All of these things are good for your health.

● **Make a place for you** Try to designate one place in your home that's truly 'yours', where you can retreat when you need to get away from it all. Keep it free of clutter and make it as calming as possible – with, for example, a favourite chair and a few objects you find visually pleasing. We all need to be able, on occasion, to stare out of the window, read a book or enjoy a lazy, luxurious bath.

● **Learn to meditate** When scientists measured the amount of atherosclerosis in arteries of volunteers with high blood pressure, they found a significant reduction after nine months among those who'd learned to meditate. Choose from hundreds of guided meditations that can be downloaded from the internet. Thanks to the iPod or MP3 Player, you can lose yourself in centuries-old wisdom while travelling on a jam-packed train on the way home from work.

● **Stop anger in its tracks** Recognize the warning signs of anger – rising irritation, a faster pulse or breathing rate, for example – and react to them by taking a break while you get things in perspective. Take deep breaths and give

Optimists have a highly beneficial effect on their own health

try it...

Learn how to relax
Getting into the habit of progressive muscular relaxation can really help to alleviate the effects of stress on your body. It doesn't take long and it is really simple to do.

Lie down comfortably on your back on the floor with your legs straight. Close your eyes. Start by tensing the muscles in your feet, then relax. Then work your way up your body doing the same thing in sequence from your feet to your head. Sometimes it's only by experiencing muscle tension like this and letting it go that we become aware of just how much tension our bodies are retaining.

yourself a vital few seconds to release tension. Regular exercise and relaxation will make you less prone to angry outbursts and more able to brush aside the little things that used to bother you.

If you have a serious problem with anger, think about doing an anger-management course – it could improve your life as well as save it.

● **Be happy** Feelings of happiness counteract the effects of stress. When scientists tested men and women taking part in a major study of heart disease risk, levels of cortisol were almost a third lower among people reporting their happiest moments during the day. Regardless of age, you can start feeling happier straightaway by being more extrovert and energetic in your activities.

● **Share your pleasure** The effects of happiness are stronger between friends of the same sex and can be seen at three degrees of separation – your friend's friend's friend's happiness affects your own. In general, a key determinant of human happiness is the happiness of those around you. Similarly, students with a mildly depressed roommate are more likely to become depressed themselves. Statistics show that each happy person you know increases the likelihood of your own happiness by 9 per cent.

● **Think furry** Pet-owners have better than average survival rates after a heart attack, and a lower risk of succumbing to cardiovascular disease in the first place. And older people who own pets are generally healthier and happier than those who don't. According to a study at Queen's University, Belfast, having a dog does more for your heart than having a cat – dog-owners had lower than average blood-cholesterol and blood-pressure readings, possibly because of the extra exercise they get while walking their pets.

● **Be optimistic** If you are an optimistic person, you are lucky. Optimists have a highly beneficial effect upon their own health – and are much less likely than pessimists to die of cardiovascular disease, according to a study of older people in the Netherlands.

● **Take a view** Nature is a great stress-reliever. Studies have shown that patients experience less pain after surgery if they have a view of trees rather than a brick wall. And tests on students given a stressful task showed that their heart rates returned to normal faster when they gazed at a real fountain rather than at a digitally created image of the same thing.

● **Spread the warmth** If you want someone to warm to you, give him or her a hot drink, say scientists. In one study, volunteers rated characters in a story as 11 per cent 'warmer' (more generous and caring) after holding a cup of hot coffee than they did after holding a cup of iced coffee. Holding something warm also makes people feel warmer and more generous themselves since physical warmth promotes trust between people.

● **Never stop learning** You may be aware that by continuing to be mentally active you can help to stave off the decline in cognitive function that often accompanies the onset of late middle age and reduce your risk of dementia – in fact, mental exercise, just like physical exercise, seems to be protective. But did you know that exercising your mental muscle may also help to stave off cardiovascular disease?

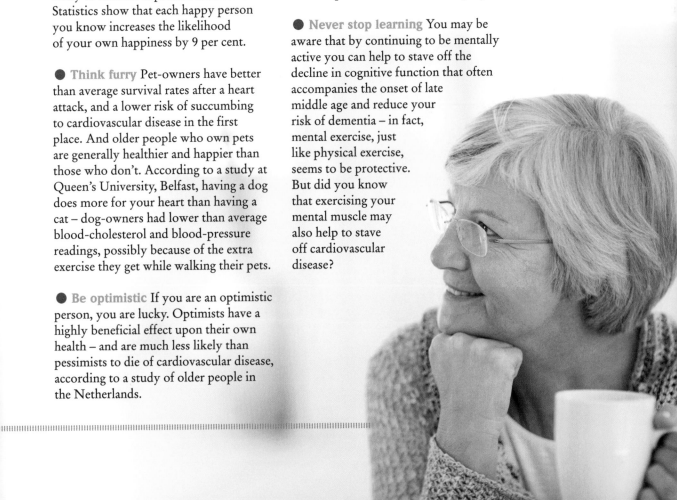

11 great ways to loosen up

Here are some simple loosening and unwinding movements that you can use daily, or whenever you feel the need, to restore a sense of calm. Do them while waiting for a kettle to boil, sitting at your desk, or travelling on a bus, train or plane – the leg and ankle exercises are especially useful during air travel. Don't strain or push your body any further than is comfortable.

1 ARM RELEASE

Stretch your arms out sideways, at right angles to your body, and then bend your wrists, pulling your hands backwards. This releases tension when you've had your arms and hands in fairly static positions for a long time, perhaps holding the telephone, using a keyboard, driving or gripping a pen for hours on end. This stretches out all the nerve fibres, as well as the muscles.

2 ARM ROTATION

Stretch your arms out to the sides and circle them backwards eight times, then forwards eight times. This vigorous movement helps you to breathe more deeply – as though your breath has been released from tight bands constricting your middle. It also releases the upper back muscles, and helps prevent curvature of the spine caused by poor posture.

3 ARM SWING

Swing your arms up to shoulder height in front of you and then let them drop – just let them go – registering the sensation of letting your arms drop down naturally. Keep swinging them for a few moments – up and drop, up and drop – and enjoy this carefree, rhythmical movement. This is very relaxing for the arms, where a great deal of tension accumulates during the day.

4 NECK STRETCH

Turn your head to the right, as if you're trying to see someone standing behind you. Hold for a count of six and feel the stretch on the opposite side. Now do the same to the left, looking over your left shoulder. Repeat about six times each side, always holding for a count of six. Keep your body facing forwards, and don't clench your teeth.

5 NECK TILT

Tip your head towards your left shoulder as if you were trying to touch your shoulder with your ear. Keep your head facing forwards and don't let your shoulders hunch up. Hold for a few seconds and feel the stretch in the opposite neck muscles. Now do the same to the right. Repeat six times or more.

6 SHOULDER DROP

Drop your shoulders and breathe out in a long sigh. Then pull your shoulders down a little further towards your hips, breathing deeply into your abdomen at the same time. Hold your shoulders down for a second or two, then just let them go and breathe out slowly. Your shoulders will bounce back into their natural relaxed position, and your breathing should be calmer. Keep breathing slowly into your abdomen.

7 SHOULDER ROTATION

Circle your shoulders regularly to keep them supple and relaxed. Circle backwards for six rotations, and then forwards for six. End with a few backwards circles to leave the shoulders in a good position.

8 LEG STRETCH

Push your heels away from you and feel the releasing stretch in your calf muscles. Then point your toes downwards and stretch the shin muscles (if you suffer from cramp, don't hold this movement for too long). Do this when you've been sitting still for long periods.

9 ANKLE ROTATION

Circle your ankles and rotate your feet, first in one direction for a count of ten, then in the other. This improves circulation in the legs when they have been still for some time. This exercise is crucial for older people, who can develop leg ulcers if circulation becomes too sluggish.

10 BODY SWING

Swing your shoulders round to the right and then the left several times, letting your arms flop and fold loosely around you as you swing. Don't use any effort to swing your arms – just let them go limp and loose, as if they were ribbons hanging from your shoulder joints. This childlike, carefree movement is excellent for releasing tension.

11 LEG SHAKE

Stand up if possible, and shake your legs one at a time – the way you see swimmers and athletes limbering up before a race. Shake your legs vigorously and feel the wobble going all the way up into your thigh muscles.

CREATING A PERSONAL SANCTUARY

Your surroundings can have a marked effect on your emotions, your moods and even the way you view the world. Most people need a personal sanctuary in their lives – a place of peace and calm where they can divest themselves of negative thoughts and relax and recharge at the end of the day or at weekends. Your home can be that sanctuary, but there are hurdles to be overcome and also key ingredients for success.

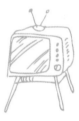

● **Clear out your clutter** One of the greatest obstacles to feeling relaxed and peaceful at home is clutter. Paperwork, books, newspapers, letters, bills, clothes and shoes scattered about, or randomly balanced in untidy piles, are not conducive to calm. Overcrowded surfaces and overflowing cupboards create a psychological burden that you'd be much better off without. Even if you have to do it gradually, sort through your clutter and get rid of what you don't want.

● **Keep up the good work** To maintain your calm and harmonious space once you've cleared the clutter, create some simple rules for yourself and other family members. For example, allocate 10 minutes at the end of each day for tidying and putting things back in their designated place. Or promise yourself that you'll tidy your main living area before you go to bed: straighten cushions, take any glasses, cups or plates into the kitchen, put books back onto the bookshelves, tidy magazines or papers, and move items of clothing, shoes or toys to their proper 'home'.

● **Negotiate the allergy minefield** If you suffer from allergies, you need to keep your home as fresh and dust-free as possible. The more dust, the more food there is for dust mites, which are a major source of allergies.

● **Open your windows** Opening windows and doors to ventilate your home – especially in winter – is one of the best things you can do to improve the air quality. This is particularly vital in modern, energy-efficient homes, which are designed to keep the heat in, often at the expense of fresh circulating air. Good ventilation is crucial to a healthy indoor environment. Even opening windows for as little as 10 minutes a day will help.

● **Bathe stress away** When you have time for a luxurious soak, make it extra special by using scented candles – bathing by candlelight is a lovely way to relax – or just dim the lights if you can, to create a soothing atmosphere. The bathroom is the place to indulge your senses; add scented oils to your bath, or warm aromatic essential oils in an oil burner.

Use colour to influence mood

Individual colours affect our physical, emotional and spiritual wellbeing in different ways, often at an unconscious level. In colour counselling, a popular therapy, practitioners work with people's instinctive response to colour to help them deal with crises. The colours you choose in your home can create a distinctive atmosphere, so it's worth getting to know their purported properties and powers.

Grow your own air filters

Cultivating plants that act as natural air filters, such as gerbera, ivy, lady palm, spider plant and peace lily, is an effective way to improve air quality. Research by NASA in the 1980s, investigating how to keep the air fresh inside space capsules, showed that these plants, among others, help to combat the damaging effects of the three most harmful household pollutants: benzene (found in polystyrene foam, and used in making an enormous range of products including computers, cooking utensils and household fabrics), formaldehyde (found in shampoos, bubble bath and household cleaners, for example) and trichloroethylene (sources include aerosol products, paints, varnishes and air fresheners).

Add texture

Textural elements such as rugs, upholstery, curtains or blinds, bed linen, cushions and throws all add to the ambience of a room. Interesting and creative accessories help to make a home your own, which is key to relaxation. Choose fabrics that are soothing to touch, such as velvet and suede, or add a little luxury with a few silk cushions that shimmer with reflected light. Wool or cashmere throws that you can snuggle under on cold winter evenings will make you feel extra cosy and comfortable.

AN OUTDOOR **HAVEN**

If you're lucky enough to have a garden, you can create a tranquil and beautiful outdoor haven in which to relax. Since it puts you in touch with the slower-moving natural world, gardening itself is a stress-reducing activity.

• Think about installing a water feature or a pond with a small fountain in the centre; moving water produces health-giving negative ions, as well as preventing the build-up of algae.

• Plant sweet-smelling, easy-care plants. Honeysuckle and jasmine both give off a heady scent, especially at night, and only need occasional pruning.

• A small statue, half hidden in a border, or proudly positioned on a plinth, can add an artistic element, and a well-placed mirror can give the illusion of a larger space.

• Try to grow some herbs, including parsley, mint, lemongrass, rosemary, basil, thyme or coriander, either in pots or alongside your flowers. As well as scenting your garden, they will enhance your culinary efforts.

• If your garden is large enough, create a restful, secluded area by screening it off with a trellis – you can use it to train a climbing rose to beautiful effect. Here you can place a wooden bench or arbour seat, creating a special place in which to enjoy tranquil moments.

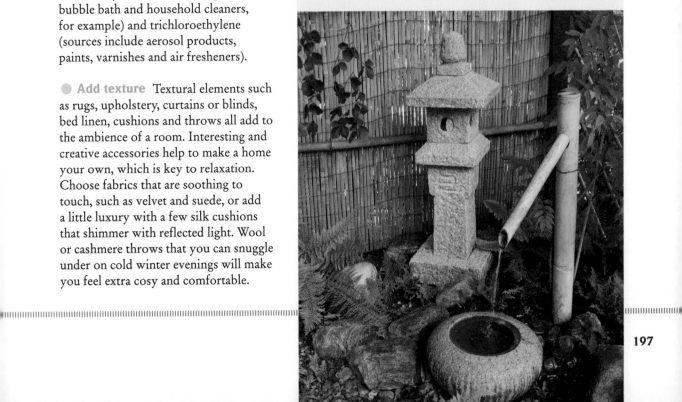

COPING WITH STRESS AT WORK

Problems at work are more strongly associated with health complaints than any other cause of stress. For example, among many similar research findings, a link has now been established between back pain and people who feel unfairly criticized in their jobs. Here is a wealth of health-boosting tips to help you to cope with stress at work.

● **Do one thing at a time** Multi-tasking can be exhausting, inefficient and highly stressful. So, instead of constantly checking emails, having two or three documents open on your screen, or returning emails as they come in, try to concentrate on one thing at a time.

● **Work in short bursts** It is hard to work intensively on one task for long stretches. Rather, our brains work in cycles of creativity, then take a rest. So, after an hour of focused work, get up for 5 minutes, walk around and do some stretches. Not only will this help the quality of your work, but also, by the end of the working day, you'll have done 30 minutes of stress-reducing exercise.

● **Say no to coffee** A study sponsored by the British Economic and Social Research Council found that when men drank coffee while working together in a group, it tended to make the group less effective. The study also found that just the perception that the drink contained caffeine – whether or not it actually did – also increased the men's feelings of stress and their heart rates.

● **Keep a holiday file on your desk** Fill it with brochures of places you'd like to visit. When you're feeling stressed, daydream your way through it. It will remind you of one reason you're working, and provide a brief virtual holiday.

● **Make a display** Include pictures of your spouse, children and/or pet, a photograph of yourself doing something fun, plus a memento that reminds you of a special occasion. When you feel yourself getting overwhelmed and stressed out, take 5 minutes and simply stare at the display. Recall the day each picture was taken. Hold the memento and return in your mind to the place where you got it. Now you're ready to return to work.

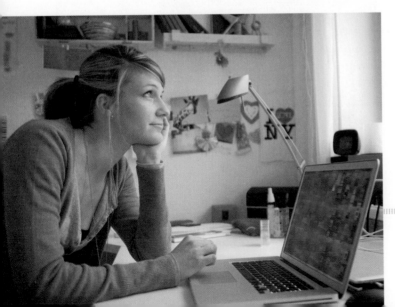

Manage your emails Read your emails once and answer them quickly. Then delete the messages, if possible, or move them to appropriate folders. Overflowing inboxes are depressing and take too long to read and sort. Don't waste time acknowledging receipt of email. Also, don't email and phone with the same message. Use the automatic signature function in your email so that people can phone you or send you information via snail mail. Use the 'rule of three': if you've gone back and forth three times on a topic and you're still confused, pick up the phone.

Never send an email if you're angry. You can write it (either as a draft, or preferably in your word-processing program) then save it and look over it when you feel calmer.

Listen to music A study by Sheffield University found that listening to music in an office environment put workers in a more positive mood, which they believe improved their overall work performance. It was important that the workers were able to choose the music themselves.

Talk to your best friend at work Studies find that social support at work is associated with lower blood pressure during the working day and smaller blood pressure surges even during work-related stressful moments.

Walk and talk more slowly This tricks your body into thinking that things are calmer than they actually are.

Munch on a handful of pumpkin seeds A useful source of iron and micronutrients, pumpkin seeds taste delicious and are a healthy way of providing a distraction from stressful moments in the working day.

great idea! **Keep a work diary** This is a diary you keep in your desk drawer (preferably locked). Write in it whenever you feel your temper rising or your despair increasing. You can write down all the things you'd like to say to the boss/client/colleague so you get your frustration out of your system without losing your job.

Rub a drop of lavender oil on your wrist The aroma of lavender is a known relaxant. Close your eyes, hold your wrist to your nose and sniff deeply, picturing as you do a field of lavender in Provence, the purple stalks waving in the breeze.

Eat peppermint chocolates Treat yourself to some peppermint chocolate – particularly if it's dark chocolate. The chocolate itself is stress relieving, the peppermint provides a burst of minty energy, and the tiny sugar rush might be just enough to get you over the hump.

Offer feedback As they say, it's better to give than to receive. Provide praise and recognition to others at work whenever it is appropriate. You will feel good by making others feel good, and the good feeling will tend to spread.

Get out more Suggest a once-a-week lunch gathering with colleagues where you can talk about a particular work issue. Use the collective brain to figure out how to do something better, improve your work facilities, perhaps, enhance productivity or improve relationships.

Structure your day Start your day by blocking out 2 hours for uninterrupted work. During this time, don't answer your phone or check emails. Then check messages and respond to all at once.

LESS STRESSFUL AIR TRAVEL

Modern air travel involves missed and cancelled flights, tightly packed cabins and long security procedures – any of which can send stress levels soaring. Add the physical tolls exacted by the dry cabin air and hours of sitting in a narrow seat, and you'll realize why caring for yourself before and during the flight is so crucial.

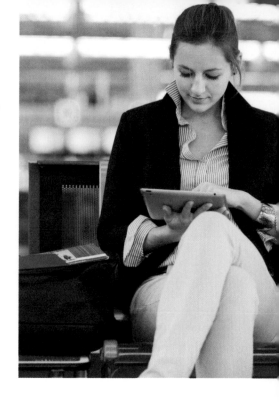

● **Bring healthy snacks** Even if you are taking what's expected to be a short flight, bring a bag of healthy snacks in your hand luggage, and buy a bottle of water once you're through security. Not only do fewer airlines serve complimentary food these days, but also unexpected delays (such as sitting on the tarmac for 90 minutes while the wings of the plane are de-iced) can send your blood sugar plummeting.

● **Keep your shoes on** Resist the temptation to remove your shoes during the flight. You'll end up with swollen feet due to the low air pressure in the cabin, and your shoes will be uncomfortable when you have to put them back on.

● **Dress in layers** Planes are often too hot or too cold. Stay in control of your own body temperature by wearing layers that you can put on or take off.

● **Keep your nasal passages and ears clear** Take a decongestant as directed for 24 hours before your flight. This will shrink the membranes in your sinuses and ears, reducing the painful pressured sensation flying can often produce.

● **Chew or swallow during takeoff and landing** Chew some gum, swallow vigorously or yawn widely when the plane is taking off or landing. This will equalize the pressure in your middle ear.

● **Drink herbal tea** Pack camomile tea bags in your hand luggage. During the flight, ask for a cup of hot water and dunk a tea bag in it. The tea will soothe any travel jitters and relax you enough to get some sleep on the plane.

● **Don't sit with your legs crossed** Instead, prop up your feet on a carry-on bag to make yourself more comfortable.

Herbal tea will soothe travel jitters and help you to sleep

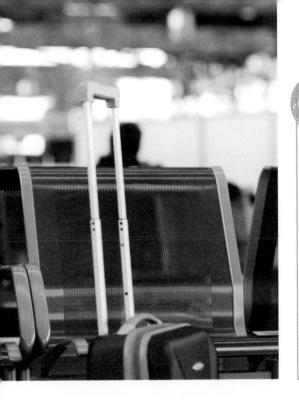

Reduce the effects of jet lag Nothing's worse than arriving at your holiday destination only to spend the first three days feeling like you've been hit by a truck as you try to recover from jet lag. There are several things you can do to make recovery easier.

For example, if you're flying east, book an early flight; if you're flying west, book a later flight. Begin preparing for time changes a few days before your departure by getting up an hour earlier or by going to bed later (depending on where you're going). When you get on the plane, adjust your watch to the time of your destination. If it's night-time, try to sleep.

When you reach your destination, use sunlight to reset your body clock. After flying west, spend a few hours outdoors in the afternoon; after flying east, take a half-hour walk outside in the morning.

● **Don't drink alcohol** The air in the plane is dry enough; drinking alcohol during the flight will simply dehydrate you even more. The same goes for caffeinated drinks. Water is the best drink to have on a plane.

● **Take a light backpack** This will allow you to use the stairs in the airport instead of the lift or escalator. You'll probably have the stairs all to yourself, and it's a wonderful way to stretch your legs and burn a few calories before you board the plane.

● **Buy a pair of flight socks** You can purchase special flight socks (also called compression stockings), which improve blood flow during the journey, helping to relieve aching legs and prevent deep vein thrombosis (DVT).

Make sure you choose the correct size, not just for your foot, but for your ankle and calf. The socks should not be too loose or restrictive or cause you any discomfort or pain.

● **Do exercises to guard against thrombosis and stiffness** Here are six exercises that you can perform every half-hour while sitting in your seat. They will keep your blood flowing during the flight and help to prevent stiffness.
• Raise your shoulders and rotate them front to back, then back to front.
• Drop your chin to your chest. Nod yes, then shake no, pointing your chin to one shoulder, then the other.
• Clasp your fingers together, palms facing each other, then stretch your arms out straight in front of you, palms facing out.
• With your heels on the floor, pull your toes up as far as possible. Hold for a few seconds, then release.
• Lift one foot slightly off the floor and make small circular motions in each direction with your foot. Repeat with the other foot.
• Lift one heel as high as possible while keeping your toes on the floor. Hold for a few seconds, then release. Repeat with the other foot.

ACHIEVING A BETTER
WORK–LIFE BALANCE

British people work some of the longest hours in Europe, and more than half of us admit that pressure of work disrupts our private lives, causing friction with our partners. Medical research links stress at work to an increased cardiovascular risk, so a better work–life balance will improve your health as well as your relationships.

● **Manage your time more effectively** If you are someone who neglects your own needs because you're always doing things for other people, you may need to educate those around you to give you some extra space. Accept offers of help from others and ask them to do tasks that are not strictly your responsibility. Don't try to cram too much into your schedule, and avoid taking on anything else until you've completed the task in hand. Say 'no' sometimes when asked to do extra work. Don't give reasons – just say that you're not able to do it.

● **Ask to work flexi-time** Flexible working arrangements should allow you to travel outside peak hours. As long as you get the work done, most employers are sympathetic.

> **try it...** **Monitor how you spend the day** Make a careful note of how long you spend doing tasks in the course of a day. Other members of your household may be surprised when you show them the results, and it may be the motivation you need to cut the time you spend doing chores.

● **Stop doing what doesn't need to be done** Don't let your conscientious instincts get the better of you. Not every item of laundry needs to be ironed, for example. Ask yourself if it's essential to wash the car as often as you do.

● **Set goals** Be clear about what you want to achieve. Having set yourself goals, take steps to make them happen. Do something each day towards reaching your bigger goals. If you feel stuck, break the goals down into small steps that are more manageable.

● **Make detailed plans** Plan what you will do during each day or week at home or at work. Accept that you can switch from one task to another as long as you undertake to spend a set amount of time on each during the day.

● **Look after yourself** Exercise each day, even if it's simply a matter of using the stairs rather than the lift. Eat more fruit and vegetables, and stop eating junk food. Take a healthy packed lunch or choose a healthy meal if you eat in your workplace canteen or restaurant.

● **Make a clear division** Aim to establish a clear division between your home life and your work life. Leave work on time. Don't take work home. And don't check your work email account out of hours or while you're on holiday.

● **Share out what needs to be done** Tell your family that the household routine needs to change so that some tasks are shared, and that they'll be involved in deciding who does what (they're more likely to do tasks if they choose them themselves).

● **Find a better way** If it's essential that you do certain tasks (for example, because you're the only driver in the family), find a more efficient way to do them. Could you share some with a friend, taking turns each week, for instance?

● **Make specific commitments** Find a way to do the things that you never usually have time to do. Be aware that it's better to do something for half an hour daily than to wait for that elusive 'free' day. Too often, the excuse for not doing something is, 'I'll do that when I have time.' The reality is that you'll never find the time unless you make specific commitments to do what you want to do.

● **Carve out a space for yourself** Discuss your need for personal space with family and friends and decide where it will be. It must be a place where you can shut the door and spend time undisturbed when you need to.

● **Exercise on your way to work** Cycle or walk part of the way to work, for example, or visit the local swimming baths or health centre once a week, early in the morning. You'll burn up stress hormones and get some exercise.

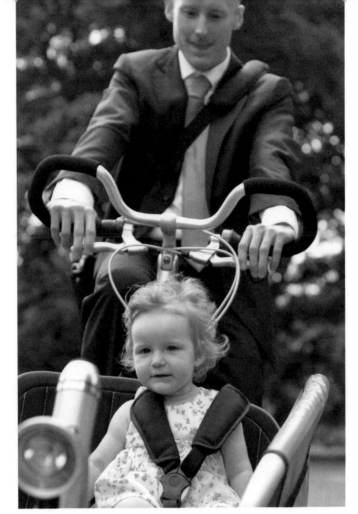

● **Settle for less than perfect** Work at 90 per cent of your capacity rather than 110 per cent – and delegate. If you tend to overload yourself at work, delegate some of your tasks to members of your team.

● **Exercise at your desk** If you spend most of your time at work sitting at a desk, do some exercises to ease the strain.

● **Have a proper lunch hour** Always stop work during your lunch hour and, preferably, have a change of scenery. Try not to discuss work during the break.

● **Learn how to prioritize** Make lists of the tasks that you need to perform and do the most important ones first.

9 effective ways to work with **a life coach**

If you'd like to have more control in your life but you're not getting far by yourself, a few sessions with a life coach may be useful. A life coach is similar to, but different from, a counsellor or therapist. Here are some ways in which a coach might help you to set and achieve your goals.

1 FIND A BETTER BALANCE

The aim is to help you to reduce the amount of time you spend working, if this is a cause of your stress, or to take time out for yourself from other stressful obligations such as childcare or looking after an ageing relative. You will be coached in learning to say 'no' when asked to do extra work, especially if it's outside your normal working hours, and on how to delegate responsibilities.

2 GET HELP IN A CRISIS

An important lesson in stress reduction is asking for help when you feel a crisis point looming, whether you approach a friend or family member or pay someone to help lighten your load.

3 LOOK AFTER YOUR BODY

Many life coaches will suggest that you think about how to improve your diet. You'll often feel much less stressed if you change your habits and start to eat fresh, healthy food without additives or sugar and keep to low-fat foods. Similarly, you will be urged to avoid smoking and consuming excess alcohol, and to keep your body flexible and de-stressed by taking regular exercise.

4 STOP DOING WHAT DOESN'T HAVE TO BE DONE

A life coach will help you to step back and examine why you're doing some of the things that you do. Maybe there is no longer any reason for performing certain tasks, but it's become a habit that needs to be stopped. You will also be encouraged to prioritize tasks and not to spend an excessive length of time on jobs that could be completed more quickly.

5 DELEGATE

Learning to delegate certain everyday tasks is crucial to psychological equilibrium. Perhaps a colleague could take on some work tasks, or family members be asked to help more with domestic chores. You may be able to share or swap some tasks with a friend – join forces to alternate doing the school run or supermarket shopping, for example. If you can afford it, sometimes it's worth paying someone to take on difficult or time-consuming tasks, such as decorating, cleaning or gardening, whether on a one-off or a regular basis. You will be coached in how to explain clearly what you want and how you want it done, and to leave the other person to get on with it while you go off and do something else.

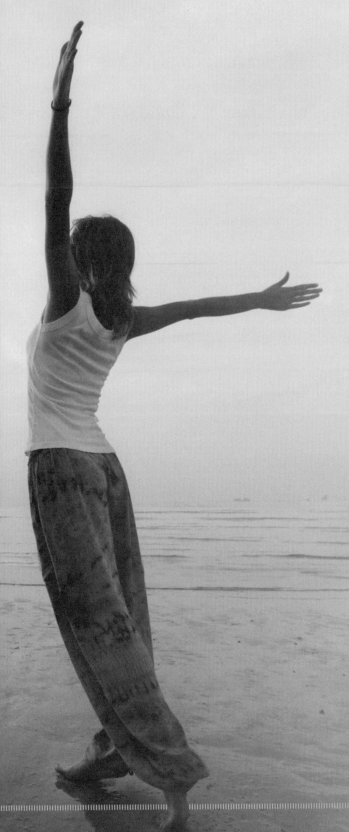

6 BE MORE ORGANIZED

A life coach will help you to appreciate how much less stressed you feel when you know where everything is. Tidying up your workspace, garage, wardrobe or kitchen is a good start. You will also learn that it's counter-productive to hoard stuff just in case you might need it some day. Throwing stuff away if you haven't needed it for several years or if it's broken or out of date is liberating.

7 NURTURE YOUR SPIRIT

This is crucial in becoming a well-rounded, balanced person, so you may be encouraged to connect with nature each day, to watch the sunrise or the stars, to make time for your spirituality, however you view it, through formal or informal religion or otherwise.

8 CARE FOR YOUR MIND

You'll often be urged to reinvigorate your mental faculties – by keeping up to date with current events, reading regularly, attending concerts or going to the theatre or cinema, and/ or by doing puzzles – both as a way to relax and to keep your brain active. Enjoyable mental stimulation can keepy our mind off other problems and reduce your stress levels at the same time.

9 KEEP IN TOUCH WITH SUPPORTIVE FRIENDS AND FAMILY

They say that blood is thicker than water. Love them or hate them, your family matters, and family members will often rally round to help in a crisis if you explain your problems, as will true friends. However, you may need to cut back on seeing anyone who makes excessive demands or saps your spirit. A life coach can help you to find out the level of contact with friends and family that works for you.

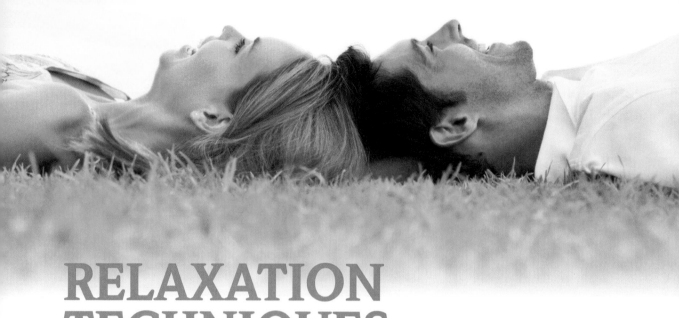

RELAXATION TECHNIQUES & STRATEGIES

You may be able to relieve feelings of stress, anger or unhappiness simply by letting off steam, but popular relaxation techniques such as meditation, visualization and massage are likely to offer more effective solutions. Any physical activity will reduce stress levels and improve your mood. Longer-term benefits may be gained from consulting an expert in hypnotherapy, acupuncture or cognitive behavioural therapy.

● **Let off steam** When events or people wind you up, or when you feel frustrated or tense, try one of the methods of release below (some of which are best done in private), or devise your own. Once you've let off steam, perform a relaxation technique or two, so that your body's functions can return to normal.

• Stamp your feet vigorously and loudly on the floor, in the manner of a toddler having a tantrum.

• Turn up the music on your radio and sing along loudly.

• Run up and down stairs a few times, or go for a brisk walk around the block.

• Write down exactly what is upsetting or stressing you. This can be a positive way of getting it all out of body and mind, enabling you to gain a little distance and look at the problem more objectively.

• Start a cleaning task that you've been avoiding for ages – and revel in being utterly miserable. You'll feel so much better once that chore is behind you.

• Punch a pillow or cushion to release pent-up tension, anger and frustration.

● **Escape in your mind** Visualization – which requires no more than imagination – can be highly beneficial for people who feel anxious, hostile or angry. You simply sit, close your eyes and conjure up a favourite scene – a beach perhaps, where you can feel the sun on your face, see the seagulls swooping, taste a salty tang. Just be there ... until you unwind.

● **Don't neglect your sex life** We are programmed to enjoy sex, but we often give it a low priority, so it simply doesn't happen. This is to ignore one of nature's great relaxants and a joyful de-stressing activity that burns calories, too.

Think about how to create a romantic ambience. Buy an oil burner, to produce a sensuous fragrance, and give your partner a relaxing massage in a candlelit room, using aromatic oils such as jasmine, rose or bergamot. Put on soothing music, and take time to slow down. Enjoy simply being with your partner.

Being touched reduces stress – as well as alleviating pain and helping to heal injuries. Taking time for those intimate moments also soothes us, uplifts us (due to the release of mood-enhancing endorphins), and gives a sense of belonging and security.

● **Try deep relaxation** Deep relaxation isn't just a pleasant sensation – it's also vital in assisting the body with all the renewal and repair processes necessary to maintain health. Many of us don't relax properly even when we're asleep, often grinding our teeth all night or simply not letting go of the tension in our muscles. As a result, we don't feel refreshed when we wake up.

Learning deep relaxation will help you to add a restorative period to your day, and allow you to sleep better as you become more practised at letting go.

● **Learn how to meditate** Meditation slows down the heart rate, lowers blood pressure, reduces anxiety and, as a result, relieves stress. Studies have found that athletes who meditate improve their performance. In one trial, participants on an 8 week stress-reduction programme based on mindfulness meditation experienced significant reductions in reported daily irritations (24 per cent), psychological distress (44 per cent) and medical symptoms (46 per cent), and the benefits were maintained at a follow-up session three months later.

You can practise meditation in a group or by yourself. Start by getting comfortable. Wear loose-fitting clothes and pick a quiet corner of your home where you can relax – in an easy chair, perhaps, but don't slump in it as a straight posture helps breathing and keeps you mentally alert. Look at your watch or a clock and decide to distract yourself for 10 or 15 minutes. Then choose a word or sound like 'om' on which you can focus while you meditate.

Focus on breathing. You can close your eyes or keep them open, whichever feels most comfortable and helps you to concentrate. Breathe deeply and repeat your chosen word or sound in your head every time you exhale, making sure you consciously direct your mind away from other thoughts and back to the sound.

Keep everything else outside this little bubble of peace that encloses you. Focus only on the sound and on your rhythmic breathing; this will boost the oxygen supply to your body and help you to relax. Your goal is to be awake and alert but not at all tense.

Deep relaxation is vital in helping the body to renew and repair itself

Simply going for a walk in the park has been found to boost both attention and memory, as well as improving sociability

● **Develop your spirituality** Both formal religious practice and other forms of spiritual comfort have been found to be beneficial for health and wellbeing. For instance, church attendance may increase life expectancy, according to a study published in the *International Journal for Psychiatry and Medicine*. It can help to counter stress and emotional problems and appears to protect against heart, respiratory and digestive diseases, possibly due to the support and moral guidance received from belonging to a like-minded community.

Similarly, creating green spaces around housing estates seems to reduce levels of aggression and violence. Simply going for a walk in the park has been found to boost both attention and memory, as well as improving sociability.

● **Tap into your subconscious through hypnosis** Hypnotherapists induce in their subjects a deep state of relaxation, during which they suggest beneficial behavioural changes.

Although you will remain aware of your surroundings while under hypnosis, you may not remember afterwards all that was said to you; your subconscious mind, however, will register what was said, so the hypnotherapist's suggestions will remain with you and help to make you feel more relaxed.

A group of students at Imperial College Medical School in London, who were taught self-hypnosis to cope with the stress of exams reported increased calmness and higher energy ratings, and were also found to have improved measures of immunity.

● **Indulge in a massage** It's very soothing to experience a massage, and may be even more relaxing if aromatherapy oils such as lavender or ylang-ylang are incorporated. In a small study of eight hospital patients in Sussex, England, six reported improvements in anxiety and depression scores following a weekly aromatherapy massage for six weeks. The best thing about massage is that if you and a friend or partner learn the basics, you can both give each other treatments for free. There are plenty of books and DVDs available, or you could attend a workshop or take a course.

● **Try acupuncture** This ancient Chinese procedure involves having very fine needles inserted just under the skin along so-called acupuncture points. According to Chinese medicine, these points are situated on meridians (channels) along which a life force called chi or qi flows, and are believed to connect your internal organs. It has been shown that acupuncture has beneficial effects on stress, causing the release of endorphins, among other things. In one study in Leicester, England, 94 per cent of volunteers reported reduced stress ratings after four brief acupuncture sessions, with an average 44 per cent fall in stress scores. Several treatments are usually recommended; your acupuncturist may then suggest continuing treatment to top up the effects of the initial sessions.

● **Discover biofeedback** Biofeedback derives from the principle that being aware of how your physiology changes when you are stressed – for example, your heart rate increases – will help you to control it. It is usually best to learn the techniques from an expert, but you can buy biofeedback equipment to use at home. This works non-invasively and displays your body's responses, to help you to monitor these changes and learn how to respond differently.

● **Explore cognitive behavioural therapy (CBT)** This therapy is based on the belief that you can alter the way you react to stressful situations by changing the way you think and behave. Courses are usually between 5 and 20 sessions; CBT can also be learned from a book or computer program. Practitioners ask their clients to talk about the goals they want to achieve, then help them to deal with undesirable situations in a calm and logical way. One study in Sweden showed that four months of CBT produced major improvements in self-rated stress, stress-related behaviour, anger, exhaustion and quality of life, accompanied by improved measurements of blood pressure, heart rate and stress hormones.

● **Consider other psychological therapies** Although the most widely used therapy is cognitive behavioural therapy (CBT), your doctor may advise you to try other psychological therapies, depending on your circumstances and the resources available in your area. These might include other forms of behaviour therapy, interpersonal therapy, problem-solving therapy and short-term psychodynamic psychotherapy.

If you have a problem keeping your anger under control, anger-management courses will help you learn how to deal with your own emotional outbursts and those of others.

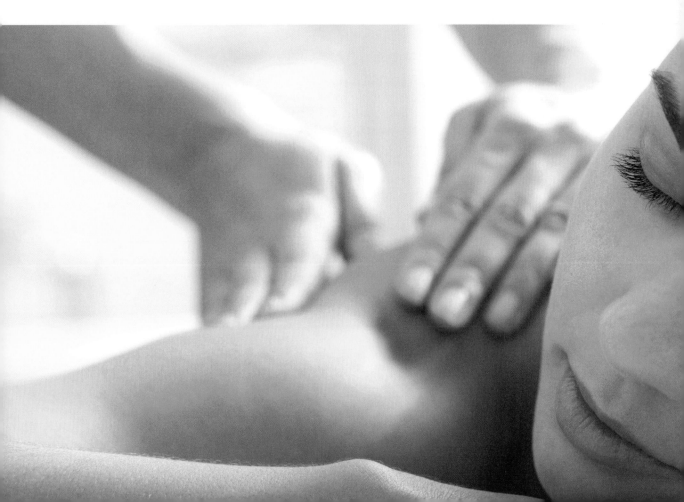

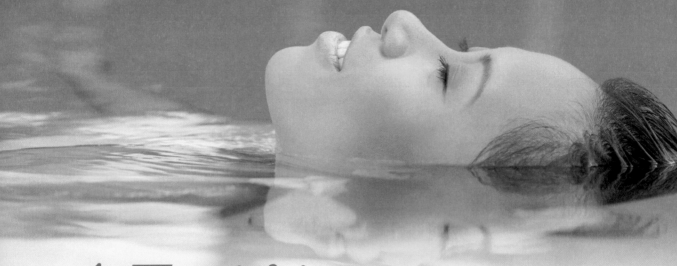

15 satisfying steps to total relaxation

Practise this routine three days a week for about half an hour and you'll soon become skilled at 'letting go'. Then use it whenever you're tense, when life feels overwhelming, when you can't sleep at night, or simply to restore energy levels. You could ask your partner or a friend to read out the steps as you work your way through them.

1 LIE DOWN ON A FIRM BED OR FLOOR MAT

Place a small cushion under your head and a large cushion or pillow under your thighs, to take the strain off your abdomen and ease the small of your back. Make sure that you are warm.

2 BECOME AWARE OF YOUR LEGS

Push your legs down into the support, hold them there for a few seconds, and then let go. Now let your legs fall apart a little more. Feel them sinking down more heavily into the support. Let go a little more and feel the relaxation flowing through all your leg muscles.

3 LET YOUR FEET FLOP OUT

Stretch your toes and hold for a moment, then let your feet flop out sideways. Feel your feet in contact with the support.

4 WORK YOUR SHOULDERS

Pull your shoulders towards your feet. Hold them there for a few seconds, then let go. Now feel as if your shoulders are tipping backwards towards the support you are lying on.

5 STRETCH YOUR FINGERS

With your hands supported, stretch out your fingers and thumbs. Hold for a few seconds.

6 BE AWARE OF YOUR ARMS

Move your arms away from your sides and bend the elbows outwards. Let your hands rest apart from each other on your lower abdomen or on either side of the body. Push your arms down into the support, hold for a moment, then stop pushing. Feel your arms sinking down heavily into the support. Tell yourself to let go through all the muscles in your arms.

7 RELAX YOUR ABDOMINAL MUSCLES

As you breathe out, let the muscles below the waist feel loose, limp and easy. Now feel your buttock muscles letting go. Feel the whole of your lower body being supported more fully and relaxing more completely.

8 BE AWARE OF YOUR DIAPHRAGM

Feel as if the part of your body just above the waist is expanding slightly. Let go all around your middle, and feel how you breathe naturally into your diaphragm area as you relax. Be aware of your middle expanding as you breathe in, and then feel yourself letting go even more as you breathe out. As you breathe out, say to yourself 'let go', and feel this letting-go all through your body.

9 FEEL YOUR BODY GETTING HEAVIER

Press your body down a little more heavily into the support, hold for a few seconds, then stop pushing and let go. Feel your whole body relaxing deeply.

10 BECOME AWARE OF YOUR EYES

Let your eyelids be lightly closed; let your eye muscles relax. Don't focus on anything. Simply let your eyes rest.

11 IMAGINE A SCALP MASSAGE

Imagine those gentle hands smoothing up over your head, gently massaging your scalp. Feel as if your head is expanding a little, as you let go of any tension in your scalp. Imagine the tension floating away.

12 THINK ABOUT YOUR FOREHEAD

Imagine that gentle fingers are smoothing it outwards from the centre to the temples. Feel as if it is widening out. Imagine all the worry lines being smoothed away. Now imagine it being gently smoothed upwards. Feel as if your forehead is becoming higher.

13 TURN ATTENTION TO YOUR MOUTH AND JAW

Make sure your top and bottom teeth are slightly apart, not clenched together. Let your tongue rest near the bottom of your mouth behind your lower teeth. Let your lips touch lightly.

14 IMAGINE THE START OF A SMILE

Starting from your mouth, let the smile spread slowly out into your cheeks. Feel as if your cheeks are widening a little, so that the whole of your lower face feels relaxed and calm.

15 ENJOY THE FEELING OF BEING DEEPLY RELAXED

Rest in the calm that comes with letting go completely. Stay in this relaxed state, and rest your mind by picturing a beautiful place that feels safe and calm. Rest here for a few minutes. This is your inner sanctuary, where you can return for rest whenever you choose. When you're in a state of deep relaxation, hold the awareness that all the repair mechanisms of the body are enhanced, and the immune system is boosted.

GIVE YOURSELF A
SOOTHING MASSAGE

A self-massage will help to reduce muscle tension in many ways, including increasing blood flow to your muscles. Some research shows that a regular massage may also boost your immunity by stimulating the production of white blood cells. A massage may also make you more productive at work by reducing stress.

● **Hammer out the kinks** Every morning and evening, hammer out the kinks. Using your fists, gently thump the outside of your body, starting with your legs and arms, working from top to bottom. Then move inwards to your torso and thump from bottom to top. Pummelling your muscles and bones will help to strengthen your body, stimulate blood circulation and relax nerve endings. Done in the morning, this self-massage technique will waken and prepare your body and mind for the day ahead. Done before bed, it calms down the mind and beats out the stress and tension of the day.

● **Rub your stomach after every meal** Most of us do this instinctively, especially after overeating. Place one or both palms on your abdomen and rub it in clockwise circles. This is the same direction that food naturally moves through your intestine, so your circular massage will help to stimulate digestion.

● **Give yourself a bear-hug** The aim here is to dissipate shoulder tension. Cross your arms over your chest and grab a shoulder with either hand. Squeeze each shoulder and release three times. Then move your hands down your arms, squeezing and releasing until you get to your wrists.

● **Rub yourself down before and after exercise** Massaging your body before cardiovascular or strength training increases blood flow to the muscles. Massaging your muscles after exercise may help to encourage waste removal and speed muscle recovery. Before exercise, use a pummelling motion with your fists to bring blood flow to your leg and arm muscles. After exercise, rub along your muscles with your palm or fist, moving in the direction of your heart.

 great idea!

Roll on a tennis ball If your foot feels tense, stand with one hand on a wall for support and place the arch of the foot on top of a tennis ball. Gradually add more body weight over the foot, allowing the ball to press into your arch. Begin to move your foot slowly, allowing the ball to massage your heel, forefoot and toes. If the tennis ball seems too big for your foot, try a golf ball instead. You can also lie on the ball to get at that hard-to-reach spot between the shoulder blades or to soothe tension in your lower back.

● **Massage your hands** Do this whenever you put on hand lotion. Start with the bottom of your palms by clasping your fingers and rubbing the heels of your palms together in a circular motion. Then, with your hands still clasped, take one thumb and massage the area just below your other thumb in circular motions, moving outwards to the centre of the palm. Repeat with the other hand. Then release your fingers and use your thumbs and index fingers to knead your palms, wrists and the webbing between your fingers. With one hand, gently pull each finger of the other hand. Finish by using your thumb and index finger to pinch the webbing between your other thumb and index finger.

● **Give your eyes some heat** When your eyes feel tired from staring at your computer screen all day long, give them some heat. Rub your hands together vigorously until you feel the skin on your palms begin to warm up. Then cup one hand over each eye, feeling the heat from your hands relax your eyes.

● **Give your feet a break** If your feet are sore after a long day of standing, take off your shoes and socks, wash your feet and give them a rub-down. Sitting on a comfortable couch or chair, thread the fingers of one hand through the toes of one foot, spreading out your toes and placing the palm of your hand against the bottom of your foot. Use your palm to rotate the joints of your forefoot forward and back gently for 1 minute. Then remove your fingers from your toes, hold your ankle with one hand, and gently rotate the entire foot with the other hand, starting with small circles and progressing to larger circles as your ankle warms up. Change directions, then repeat with the other foot.

● **Relieve a headache** When you have a headache, stand up, bend forward from the hips and place your forehead on a padded chair. The chair will put gentle pressure on your head as you relax in the bend. Hold for 30 seconds. When you rise, sit down and spread your fingers through your hair, making a fist. Gently pull the hair away from your head. Hold for 2 or 3 seconds, then release. This stretches the fascia, the fibrous tissue, along your scalp, releasing tension. Continue to grab different clumps of hair all over your head, working from the top front of your head, progressing to the sides, and then to the back.

● **Give your arms a pinch** After tennis, cycling, rock climbing and other arm-tiring sports, give your arms a pinch. Place your right arm across your chest with your elbow bent. Reach across your chest with your left arm and pinch your right arm's triceps, near the shoulder, with the thumb and index finger of your left hand. Hold for a few seconds, release, then pinch again an inch lower on the arm. Continue pinching and releasing until you've made your way to your elbow. Then pinch your right arm's biceps near your armpit and work your way in the same way down to the elbow. Change arms. This will release tension in your muscles and help to improve blood flow.

Massage your muscles before and after exercise

THE BENEFITS OF YOGA

As well as improving muscle tone and physique, regular yoga practice enhances happiness and tranquillity, among other psychological benefits. It can also relieve symptoms of chronic illnesses such as cancer, arthritis and heart disease. You may wish to join a yoga class, but here are a few simple poses to get you going.

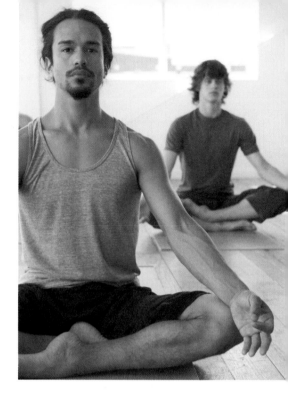

● **Be well grounded: Mountain Pose** Stand straight with your feet hip-width apart and your hands either at your sides or in prayer position in front of your chest. Raise your toes and spread them wide, then place them back on the floor. Your weight should be distributed evenly across the bottom of each foot so that you feel grounded, and you are not leaning forwards or back. Exhale.

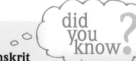

Yoga means 'union' in Sanskrit
Traditional Eastern medicine uses holistic systems such as yoga to treat your mind and body as one. Even the term 'yoga' is a Sanskrit word for 'union', implying the experience of oneness with your inner being. There are several types of yoga, with the most common type practised in the West being hatha yoga. This combines physical exercises and postures, breathing techniques and meditation. Its goal is to achieve perfect physical and mental health, happiness and tranquillity.

● **Expand your chest: Overhead Reach** Starting in mountain pose, inhale as you sweep your arms out to the sides and high overhead until your palms are together. Stretch up, allowing your chest to expand fully, then arch backwards and look up at your hands. Stay in the pose for a few seconds, holding your breath and keeping your eyes focused and your mind silent. Exhale gently.

● **Bend from the hips: Forward Fold** Exhale as you gently bend forwards from the hips, keeping your palms together, tucking in your head and keeping your back straight and long.

When you have bent as far forward as comfortably possible, grasp the backs of your legs (anywhere from the ankles to the thighs), bend your elbows and very gently tuck your chin to your chest and move your upper body towards your legs. Hold for a few breaths. Release and slowly swing up to standing position. Rest and repeat.

● **Stretch calves, hamstrings, chest and spine: Downward-dog Pose** Kneel with your palms on the floor under your shoulders and knees under your hips. Spread your fingers as wide as you can, with the middle fingers pointing forward.

With feet hip width apart, tuck your toes under, coming onto the balls of your feet. Roll your shoulder blades away from each other, bringing the creases of your elbows towards each other.

Lift your tail bone. Then exhale as you extend your legs and lift your hips towards the ceiling, forming an upside-down V shape with your body. Relax your head between your arms. Press into your palms to bring more body weight back into your legs. Continue to roll your shoulder blades away from each other and the inner creases of your elbows towards each other. Hold for five to ten breaths. Rest and repeat.

● **Play dead – and come back to life: Corpse Pose** Lie on your back with your arms at your sides and palms facing up. Place your heels slightly apart and allow your feet to fall naturally to the sides. Starting with your feet, progressively contract (or flex) and then relax all of your muscles – in other words your toes, then your ankles, calves, knees, thighs and so on to the top of your head. When you've finished, relax and breathe deeply.

● **Try the snake: Cobra Pose** Lie face down with your feet together, your toes pointed behind you and your hands, palms down, just in front of your shoulders. Lift your chin and gently raise your head and chest so that your torso is supported on your forearms. Keep your shoulders back and down. Hold for 30 seconds and rest. Repeat several times. Remember to breathe deeply throughout.

The purpose of yoga practice is to achieve perfect physical and mental health, happiness and tranquillity

● **Boost circulation around your heart: Spinal Twist** Lie on your back with your knees bent, your feet flat and your arms at your sides.

Slowly lower your knees to the left while simultaneously extending your arms to the right as far as comfortably possible. Keep your shoulders in contact with the floor or bed. Repeat on the other side, holding each position for 15 seconds.

● **Strengthen your lower back muscles and tone your abdominals: Locust Pose** Lie on your front on the floor, an exercise mat or your bed, with a small cushion or folded towel under your head and your arms by your sides.

As you inhale, slowly lift up one leg as far as is comfortable, keeping the leg straight. Hold for a moment, then exhale as you bring your leg back down, and repeat with the other leg. Alternate, raising each leg about four times. Then, if you are able, lift both legs together four or six times.

If you feel strong enough, try lifting your upper body at the same time as both legs and hold for a count of six. This will help to tone slack abdominal muscles.

● **Lengthen and stretch: Prayer Pose** Kneel with the tops of your feet on the floor or bed and your toes pointed behind you. Sit back onto your heels, then lower your chest to your thighs. Extend your arms and rest your palms and forehead on the floor or on a soft support. Hold for at least 30 seconds. Rest and repeat.

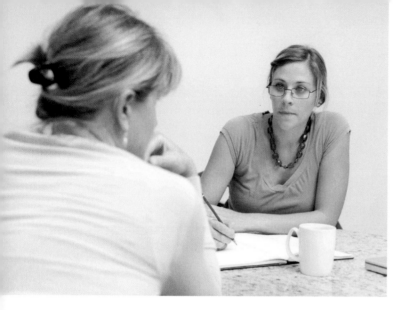

DEPRESSION
AND ANXIETY

Depression manifests itself in many ways, from temporary unhappiness to serious mental illness. Anxiety likewise ranges over a wide spectrum, from a feeling of general unease to terrifying phobias. There are often self-help measures you can take to alleviate the symptoms.

● **Be aware of your thoughts** Stand back and try to observe what's going through your head. This will allow you to spot unhelpful patterns of thinking that may be causing you to feel depressed.

● **Stay in touch** Don't let worries isolate you from loved ones or enjoyable activities. Social interaction and caring relationships can help to keep your worries in the background rather than letting them dominate your thoughts.

● **Get help** Whatever the severity of your depression, don't suffer in silence. Share your feelings with family, friends or a health-care professional. The right support and treatment can help to stop depression taking over your life.

● **Join a group** People who are experiencing similar problems can offer great support. Your GP should have a list of what is available in your area.

● **Look after yourself** Pay attention to simple physical needs such as eating, sleeping and exercise, which can all help to alleviate mild to moderate depression.

● **Do what you enjoy** Make a big effort to do what you like doing. Buy yourself something new, listen to music, watch a film, have a massage.

● **Try something new** A new hobby or activity or an evening class will get you out of the house. How about joining a book club, a knitting circle or having a go at the local pub quiz? Social activities such as these can help to break the vicious circle of loneliness.

● **Take a multivitamin every day** A daily multivitamin will ensure you consume the recommended amount (200mcg) of folate, an important B vitamin that may help to lift depression.

Folate and other B vitamins help to maintain nerve and blood cells, used in brain reactions and essential for the production and function of a number of mood-boosting brain chemicals. In a Finnish study, participants with the lowest folate consumption were found to be at the highest risk of depression. Another study found that this vitamin helps to enhance the effectiveness of antidepressant medication.

● **Cultivate close friendships** Spend at least 1 hour each week with a close friend. In a British study, when 86 depressed women were paired with a volunteer friend, 65 per cent of the women felt better. In fact, regular social contact worked as effectively as antidepressant medication and psychotherapy. Regular contact with a close friend may boost self-confidence and encourage you to make other positive changes that will help to lift depression, such as starting an exercise programme.

● **Put it on paper** Writing down your thoughts and feelings can help prevent half-formed but emotionally powerful thoughts from getting out of proportion in your mind. The physical process of writing may help to distance you from your thoughts so you can examine them in a more detached way.

● **Play with a dog** When non-pet-owners played with a dog for just a few minutes a day as part of a US study, blood levels of the brain chemicals serotonin and oxytocin – both mood-elevators – rose. You don't need to own a dog to experience these feel-good effects (although dogs are great antidotes to the kind of chronic stress that can result in depression). Pet your neighbour's dog, offer to take it for walks, or volunteer at an animal shelter for some furry one-on-one therapy.

● **Endure an all-nighter** Staying up all night for one night – and therefore depriving yourself of sleep – has been shown to lift depression for as long as a month. Although researchers aren't sure why it works, they speculate that one night of sleep deprivation may reset the sleep clock, enabling people who are depressed to sleep better.

BOOST MOOD WITH FOOD

A healthy balanced diet is the best way to ensure that you get all the nutrients you need for good mental health.

Eat more whole grains Foods such as brown rice, whole-grain couscous, whole-grain pasta, buckwheat, oats and other complex carbohydrates give your brain a steady supply of glucose – the brain's main fuel. Whole grains also contain B vitamins, which are linked with better mood.

Stimulate the release of tryptophan High-carbohydrate foods encourage the amino acid tryptophan to flood your brain, boosting levels of serotonin, a mood-enhancing neurotransmitter, or chemical messenger.

Always eat breakfast Ensure that your brain has nutrients and glucose to see you through the morning. Try eggs with whole-grain toast and some fruit, or a bowl of whole-grain breakfast cereal, such as muesli with fruit.

Eat protein at every meal Protein, for example from meat, fish, lentils, beans or tofu, supplies the building blocks for endorphins and other neurotransmitters.

Eat more oily fish Omega-3 essential fatty acids found in oily fish, such as salmon, mackerel and sardines appear to be especially important for a healthy brain.

Avoid processed foods Trans fats (also known as hydrogenated or partially hydrogenated fats) found in some biscuits, pastries and ready meals, can interfere with the brain's uptake of healthier fats. Processed foods are also high in sugar, which can cause fluctuations in blood glucose, triggering a mood roller-coaster.

● **Have a good drum** People at a retirement home who took a drumming class felt less depressed six weeks after the class than before they started it. Researchers think that drumming helps to relax your body. Beating out a rhythm on your desk may help, but joining or starting a weekly drumming circle may be even more effective because it offers the opportunity for social interaction, which also helps with depression.

● **Make yourself smile** Look in the mirror and force your lips into a smile. Research shows that the physiology of smiling actually makes you feel happy. If you need a little extra help in the smile department, watch a funny film, read a comic or a humorous book, or ask a friend to tell you a joke every day.

● **Sleep in a different bedroom** Many people with depression also have insomnia. Changing your sleep location can help. You can also reduce insomnia by getting up at the same time every day, never napping for more than 20 minutes, avoiding caffeine after 3pm and relaxing for an hour before bed.

● **Walk frequently in winter** Aim to take a 30-minute walk three times a day in winter. Many people feel depressed during the winter months, when they travel to and from work in darkness and don't get enough natural sunlight. But physical exercise encourages the release of hormones and neurochemicals that boost mood. Walking outside during the day will give you a few short doses of sunlight, which has also been shown to improve mood.

great idea!

Name your fears If you are anxious about your son/daughter/partner getting hurt or killed in a car crash, for example, discuss it – at least with yourself. Look up the statistics on driving and injury to ease your mind. Do the same for whatever else worries you, whether it's terrorism, cancer or a type of phobia. Once you name your fears and learn more about them, you can take steps to minimize your risk. You'll also find that the fears you name and tame are far less menacing than the fears left to lurk in the shadows of your imagination.

● **Drink one or two cups of coffee or tea each morning** Regular, modest caffeine intake cuts the risk of depression by more than 50 per cent, but don't overdo it: too much caffeine consumption increases agitation and anxiety.

● **Break out of your routine** If you are stuck in a rut, change your daily routine. Book a day off from work to explore a nearby town. If you usually eat in, go out to a restaurant for dinner. Choose a different route to work, wear something that's totally 'not you', or take your camera and go on a photography ramble.

● **Don't be too hard on yourself** When something goes wrong, resist the urge to beat yourself up mentally. When you catch yourself berating yourself for some supposed failing, replace your negative thoughts with the phrase, 'I am doing the best I know how to do. When I know a better way and can do it, I will.'

● **Read about it** Some people find that reading about depression or anxiety helps them to deal with their problems. Much has been written, for example, about the effectiveness of various therapies.

● **Share anxieties with a confidant** It's a good idea to find someone who can help you to understand why you worry too much. If appropriate, try to play the same role for that person. We are usually better at putting someone else's worries in perspective than we are our own.

● **Stay positive** Try to replace 'negative self-talk' with 'coping self-talk'. When you catch yourself thinking something negative such as, 'I can't do this, it's just too hard,' try changing it to a more positive thought, such as, 'This is hard, but I can get through it.'

● **Lift your spirits with lemon balm**
Lemon balm – taken as a tea, a tincture, or rubbed on the skin in the form of an essential oil – can significantly improve calmness and increase memory and brain function. Research shows that it can help people suffering from depression and anxiety, and can even improve the emotional and mental state of those with dementia. Unsurprisingly, it has been known for centuries as the 'calming herb'.

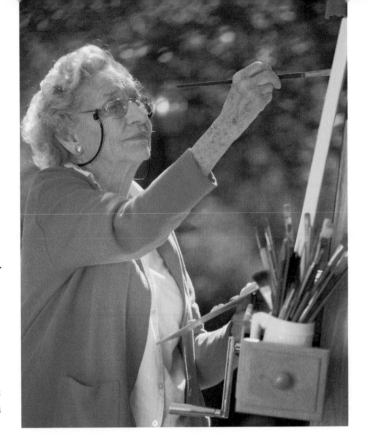

● **Refocus your attention** Distracting yourself by paying attention to what is going on around you can be an effective strategy for coping with anxieties. For example, if walking down a crowded street or sitting in a packed train makes you anxious, try looking for certain items in shop windows or identifying objects in the landscape you are passing through.

● **Expose yourself to it** It may seem like the last thing you want to do, but there is evidence to show that, if you expose yourself to the situation or thing you fear in small doses, your fear will gradually recede. Exposure therapy sessions are available for many of the more common phobias, such as fear of flying or of certain animals.

● **Record it** Keep an anxiety diary. Rank your anxiety on a 1–10 scale. Note the event during which you felt anxious. Jot down any feelings or thoughts you had just before you got anxious. Keep track of things that make you more or less anxious.

● **Talk to yourself** Remind yourself about how you handled similar situations in the past, your strengths and how long you will need to get through it. Convince yourself that this anxiety is manageable as well as time-limited.

● **Entertain yourself** Take up oil painting (or some other hobby), visit a museum or see a film. People who are bored tend to score higher on tests designed to measure levels of anxiety.

● **Watch a funny DVD** Let yourself laugh out loud. The act of laughter stimulates endorphins that help to blow stress hormones (which contribute to that feeling of anxiety) out of your system in the same way that a good thunderstorm can blow away hot, humid weather.

● **Concentrate on relaxation** Avoid conversations likely to increase your anxiety when you're tired, overwhelmed or stressed. For instance, tell your children you're not available for problem solving after 8pm. Try to maintain a 'trouble-free' time, especially before bed, when you don't address difficulties but focus on pure relaxation.

BETTER BREATHING

Most of us breathe too shallowly and too fast. Our lungs and hearts would prefer longer, slower, deeper breaths. This is true for your general health, and it is also true for managing stress. Deep breathing sends a signal to your brain to slow down, which results in hormonal and physiological changes that slow down your heart rate and lower your blood pressure.

● **Time your inhalations** In general, inhale slowly and deeply through your nose. A healthy inhalation should take about 5 seconds.

● **Empty your lungs** In general, exhale slowly through your mouth. Empty your lungs completely. Good breathers focus more on thorough exhalation than on inhalation.

● **Use your diaphragm** For good deep breathing, engage your diaphragm – the sheet of muscle along the top of your abdomen that pulls your lungs down to draw in air, then pushes your lungs up to expel carbon dioxide. With a good inhalation, your lungs inflate as your diaphragm contracts and flattens. As you exhale, your diaphragm relaxes and rises. You may not feel the muscle moving but you can tell if you're using it as your abdomen will swell a little as you inhale.

● **Breathe deeply** In a stressful situation, stop what you are doing and take four or five deep breaths, inhaling so that your abdomen rises. A team from Birmingham University, England, has shown that deep breathing counteracts the physical effects of stress. When volunteers had to perform a mental maths test, blood pressure increased and heart rate variability (HRV) decreased. (HRV is an important indicator of heart health; reduced HRV is associated with an increased risk of heart attack.) When the volunteers engaged in a paced breathing exercise, blood pressure decreased and HRV increased. It is almost impossible not to calm down when you breathe slowly and deeply.

● **Make fewer inhalations** Work towards taking just six or eight deep breaths a minute. Most of us breathe more than 20 times a minute.

● **Breathe away anxiety** Proper breathing is particularly important during moments of great anxiety. At times like these, many people resort to the type of big, desperate inhalations and exhalations that make you rapidly puff up and deflate your chest. To re-establish healthy breathing during periods of anxiety, lie on the floor and place your hand on your chest. Using your hand as a gauge, try to reduce the amount of chest movement, while continuing to breathe normally. You don't want your chest to move; you want the other parts of your body to take over the breathing – using your diaphragm instead of the big chest inhales and exhales. Do this for 5 minutes.

● **Keep breathing while you exercise**
Many people unintentionally hold their breath when they exercise, then suddenly feel breathless and tired. Oxygen is invigorating, and muscles need it to create energy. So, as you inhale, bring the air to the deepest part of your lungs by expanding your ribs outwards and your abdomen forwards and inhale for a count of three. Then exhale fully through your mouth, also to a count of three.

Our lungs and hearts would prefer longer, slower, deeper breaths. Oxygen is invigorating, and muscles need it to create energy

HOW TO BREATHE
DURING A PANIC ATTACK

Extreme emotion alters our natural breathing pattern, making us breathe shallowly, in the upper part of the chest. The following technique helps to return breathing to normal, and restores a sense of calm and ease. Use it if you suffer from panic attacks or whenever you become stressed in any way.

• **Breathe out** Let your breath out in a slow sigh. Now breathe in slowly, feeling your diaphragm (just above your waist) expand outwards. Now breathe out again slowly, saying to yourself, 'Let go.'

• **Breathe in again** As you do so, feel your ribcage on either side of your body expand sideways. Now slowly exhale, making your out-breath a little longer and a little slower than your in-breath.

• **Repeat by inhaling slowly** Think to yourself 'low and slow', and direct your breath low down into your diaphragm. Feel the middle of your body expanding and your ribs spreading sideways, as your lungs fill up with oxygen. Never hold your breath once you have inhaled – just let your breath out again in a slow sigh.

• **Pause for a second** Then breathe in again, feeling the expansion in the middle of your body. Now breathe out again slowly.

• **Persevere** Even if your breathing still feels too high in your chest, maintain this pattern. Your breathing will soon drop down to your diaphragm as you relax.

• **Continue this rhythm for a few minutes** Concentrate on breathing 'low and slow', and always let your out-breath be a little longer and slower than your in-breath. This is our natural breathing rhythm. Remember: it's the exhalation, or out-breath, that relaxes you.

NURTURING LOVE AND FRIENDSHIP

Love and friendship are crucial ingredients of psychological wellbeing. While most couples come together expecting their relationship to remain as warm and intimate as it was at the start, this won't happen by chance. Successful relationships depend on mutual respect, trust, loyalty and appreciation. Friendships, likewise, need careful nurturing to survive.

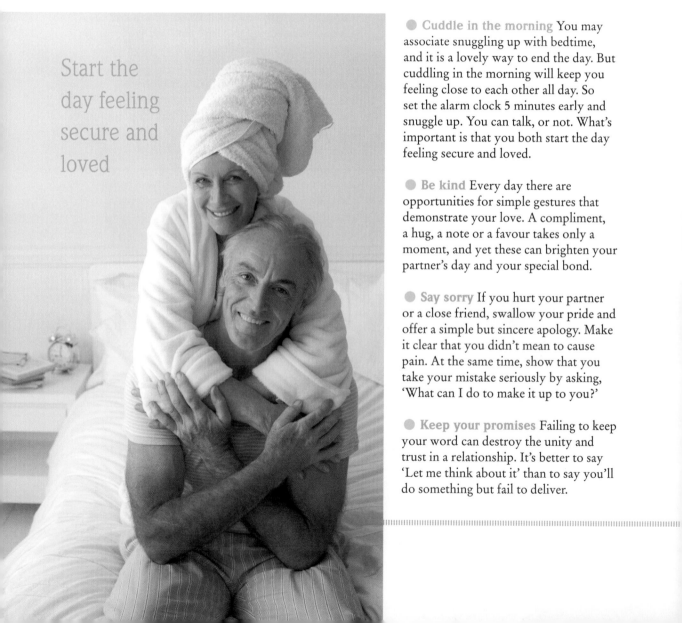

Start the day feeling secure and loved

● **Cuddle in the morning** You may associate snuggling up with bedtime, and it is a lovely way to end the day. But cuddling in the morning will keep you feeling close to each other all day. So set the alarm clock 5 minutes early and snuggle up. You can talk, or not. What's important is that you both start the day feeling secure and loved.

● **Be kind** Every day there are opportunities for simple gestures that demonstrate your love. A compliment, a hug, a note or a favour takes only a moment, and yet these can brighten your partner's day and your special bond.

● **Say sorry** If you hurt your partner or a close friend, swallow your pride and offer a simple but sincere apology. Make it clear that you didn't mean to cause pain. At the same time, show that you take your mistake seriously by asking, 'What can I do to make it up to you?'

● **Keep your promises** Failing to keep your word can destroy the unity and trust in a relationship. It's better to say 'Let me think about it' than to say you'll do something but fail to deliver.

● **Give a full pardon** When your partner has hurt you, being forgiving frees you from the bitterness that can eat away at your relationship. But don't think you have to forgive him or her instantly. Forgiveness is a process, rather than an event, so be as kind as you can be to your partner while you heal.

● **Play the newlywed game** Do something for your partner that you did when you were newlyweds or first got together. Make a special meal. Send some flowers after a night of lovemaking. Tuck notes in unexpected places or leave sexy messages on your partner's mobile phone.

● **Treat your partner well in public** Whether you're at a party, a business meeting or just strolling down the street, treat your partner with respect and admiration. And never, ever, make fun of your partner in public.

● **Share your passions** Take turns in choosing an arts or cultural event to attend together each month. The point is to show your partner what you love, so that he or she can experience it as you do. To make this work, both of you have to be flexible: you may have to attend a football match, and your partner may have to go to the theatre with you.

● **Get active together** Are you both a few pounds heavier than when you first met? Engaging in a physical activity that you both enjoy can be as good for your relationship as it is for your body, and can reinforce the fact that you're a team of two. You needn't run a marathon together (although training for one could provide a lot of couple time). How about tennis? Golf? Swimming? Even gardening can be a good workout, if you're landscaping the garden or tending a large vegetable plot.

> **try it…**
>
> **Be a better listener** It can be the hardest thing in the world simply to listen as your partner or friend pours out their troubles or seeks your opinion, but it's worth the effort.
>
> • Keep eye contact. Offer nods and murmurs to show that you understand the other person's point of view.
> • Don't finish the other person's sentences. If you catch yourself planning your response while your partner or friend is still talking, gently remind yourself to focus.
> • Minimize distractions – don't write or read emails, open the post or watch television while you're on the phone to your partner or friend. He or she will hear the lack of interest in your responses.
> • Be careful with advice. Allow the person to let off steam rather than offering him or her a plan of action.

● **Schedule time for lovemaking** Yes, you're both busy. But don't let it stand in the way of an activity that's so crucial to a loving relationship. It may not be as spontaneous as you'd like, but there's something nice about looking forward to a night (or morning, or afternoon) of sex.

● **Make time for friendships** Nothing makes closeness fade away more than never talking to or seeing each other. While some bonds of friendship may be strong enough to span long silences, most aren't. If you cherish a person's friendship, make time for him or her, whether it's just the occasional phone call, email or a weekly get-together.

● **Be constant** A true friend doesn't flee when changes occur. Nothing is sadder for new parents than to find that their single friends have abandoned them because of the baby. A good friend is one who stays true through it all – marriage, children, new job, new home, any losses. Just because a situation's changed, it doesn't mean the person has.

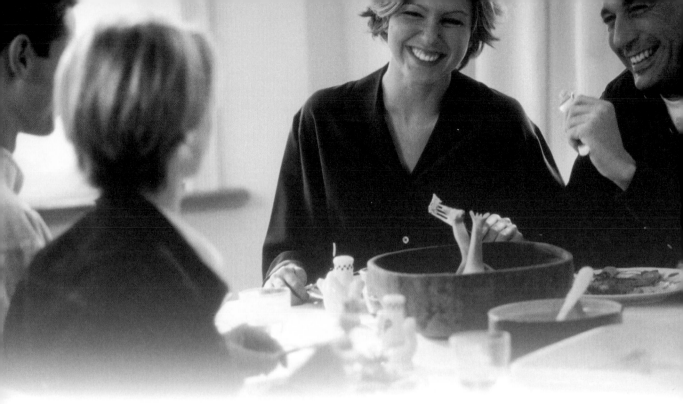

FORGING A
LASTING BOND

As your children grow and develop, so must your relationship with them. You need to be supportive but not intrusive; offer emotional back-up without interfering in their lives; and hope they make wise choices, while understanding that those choices are theirs to make. A difficult relationship with your children can put serious strains on your psychological health, so do what you can to forge lasting bonds.

● **Have dinner together** There is something enormously comforting about a family gathered round the dinner table, perhaps because the tradition of eating together is disappearing. Yet the evening meal is often the one time of day when the family can assemble in one place. So always strive to make dinner a family affair, even if you're just having a takeaway. Use the time to share news of your day, make weekend plans and enjoy one another's company. Research shows that adolescents who dine with their family several times a week are less likely to smoke and use drugs, and they tend to get better exam results.

● **Back off, but stay close** It's usual for adolescents to want to spend more time with friends than parents. But this doesn't mean your job as a parent is diminished. Find ways to stay involved in your child's life. For example, while tea parties may be a thing of the past, you can still get to know your children's friends by making them welcome after school. Staying involved may be more challenging, but it's an important way of enhancing your relationship with your child.

● **Share your own feelings with your teenager** Of course, spare the intimate details of very personal subjects, but confiding that you, too, occasionally feel angry, insecure or awkward shows your teenager that you're not just a parent – you're human. Not only will your child feel closer to you, but he or she may feel safe enough to disclose uncomfortable issues or feelings when they arise.

● **Seek your children's opinions** Young adults have opinions about everything, and they aren't shy about sharing them. So allow them to make some independent decisions. For instance, let them decide when and where to study, what to wear, what after-school activity to pursue. But keep in mind that some rules are non-negotiable. Parents need to set limits that protect their child's health, safety and wellbeing – at every age. These might include curfews, decisions about drinking and sexual activity, issues around study and university.

● **Trust your children to make wise choices** Of course, they'll make the wrong ones occasionally. But, especially if they're over 18, give them the chance to work out solutions to problems on their own. Didn't you want the same from your parents at that age?

● **Phone before you drop in** If you have an adult child, always call before you go to his or her home, unless it's absolutely necessary. If you're the parent of a teenager, knock before you enter his or her room.

● **Accept their holiday absences with grace** Yes, you may be disappointed that your children – and their children – spend Christmas without you. But don't nag or complain about it. You may win a battle over which in-law's house they visit for Christmas, but end up losing your child's respect – and an enduring relationship.

● **State your views, then invite reaction** 'Does that seem fair to you?'; 'Can you think of a better way to deal with this?'; 'What would you do in my position?' You're more likely to find a middle ground that you can both accept.

● **Respect your child's privacy** Don't read your child's diary, eavesdrop on phone conversations or badger him or her with questions. If any behaviour is troubling you, address it directly, using five little words: 'Can we talk about it?' Here's an example: 'You seem very quiet lately, and I'm worried about you. Can we talk about it?'

● **Be honest** Many parents offer praise when they shouldn't, as well as when they should. That simply undermines trust. If both your praise and criticism are heartfelt and valid, your children will learn to trust you.

● **Cultivate love, but demand respect** Don't try so hard to be your children's friend that you fail to set limits and earn their respect. You can be friends long after your children are grown up as long as you are the parent first.

ENJOYING A MATURING RELATIONSHIP

If your parents still treat you like a child even when you are a parent yourself, it can be irritating. Don't forget that, as we age, we all face new challenges – retirement or career changes, health issues, worries about the future. Part of that evolution means adjusting to a new relationship, between mature adults rather than between 'parent' and 'child'.

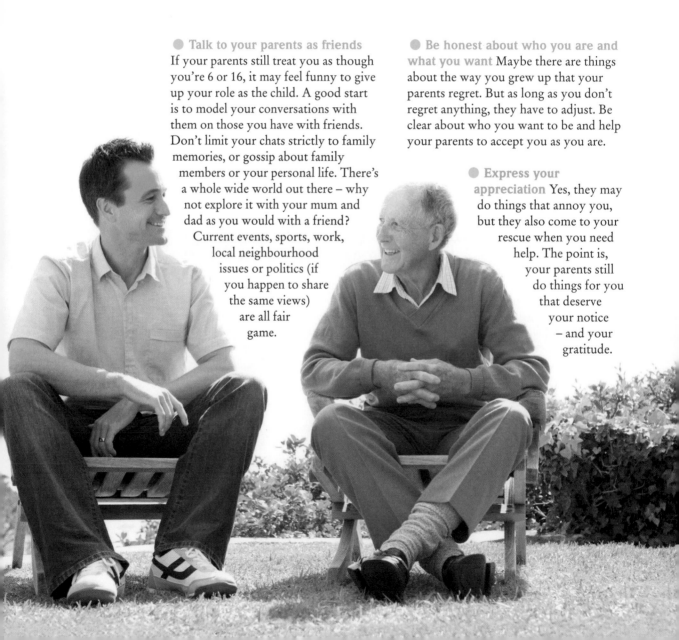

● **Talk to your parents as friends** If your parents still treat you as though you're 6 or 16, it may feel funny to give up your role as the child. A good start is to model your conversations with them on those you have with friends. Don't limit your chats strictly to family memories, or gossip about family members or your personal life. There's a whole wide world out there – why not explore it with your mum and dad as you would with a friend? Current events, sports, work, local neighbourhood issues or politics (if you happen to share the same views) are all fair game.

● **Be honest about who you are and what you want** Maybe there are things about the way you grew up that your parents regret. But as long as you don't regret anything, they have to adjust. Be clear about who you want to be and help your parents to accept you as you are.

● **Express your appreciation** Yes, they may do things that annoy you, but they also come to your rescue when you need help. The point is, your parents still do things for you that deserve your notice – and your gratitude.

● **Keep your sense of humour**
When you're dealing with your parents, laughter can be a lifesaver – both to help you to handle the stress of dealing with sometimes crotchety individuals and to help you to bond together. Tell a few jokes you know they'll enjoy, share some cartoons from the paper, watch a comedy programme together. If you can laugh together, you're doing OK.

● **Don't ask your parents' advice or opinion** Sometimes, asking for a parent's advice is really a way of asking for approval. If so, remember that you're an adult now, perfectly capable of choosing a living room carpet or a car on your own. If your parents are bent on offering you advice whether asked for or not, smile, nod and take it in. Then, make your own choice – without guilt.

● **Tell your parents what bothers you**
If you love your parents but they drive you mad, your resentment can eat away at your relationship. Don't seethe silently. Communicate, with gentleness and respect. So if your mother keeps ringing you at work, tell her that your boss is starting to notice and, while you love talking to her during the day, it's affecting how well you do your job. Arrange a call at a mutually convenient time.

● **Grant them their independence too** Sometimes it's the grown-up child who doesn't want to cut off the nurturing relationship. If you are older than 25 and still find it necessary to talk to your mother every night, or immediately turn to your father for a house repair rather than your partner, or automatically assume your parents will look after the children whenever you need to go out, then you may be the problem, not your parents. They deserve freedom too.

● **Don't ask your parents to bale you out of a financial crisis** While you may depend on their emotional support, relying too much upon their resources, rather than your own, can lead to mutual resentment. So get used to solving your problems on your own. You'll be amazed how good doing it all by yourself can make you – and them – feel.

● **Create opportunities for reliving old times** If your parents are older, look through their photo albums with them, asking them for stories about the people in the photos. You can help your parents to discover the meaning in their lives by encouraging them to talk about their accomplishments, the high points, and their joys and sorrows.

● **Rediscover and share mutual interests** When you were a child, did you and your dad share a passion for a particular football team? Did you and your mum spend time each summer making jam? Make these happy memories the foundation for new, shared activities.

try it... **New beginnings** Think of imaginative ways to get closer to your parents.
• Teach older parents to use email or surf the internet.
• Introduce your parents to your friends, and include them in social gatherings when appropriate.
• Eat out together. Explore a cuisine that you've never tried before.
• Join a book club together. Read the same books and talk about them in your own book club.
• Start a new family ritual involving the grandchildren, such as once-a-month picnics.
• Challenge your parents to a round of golf or a hand of bridge or gin rummy.
• Go bike riding or walking together.

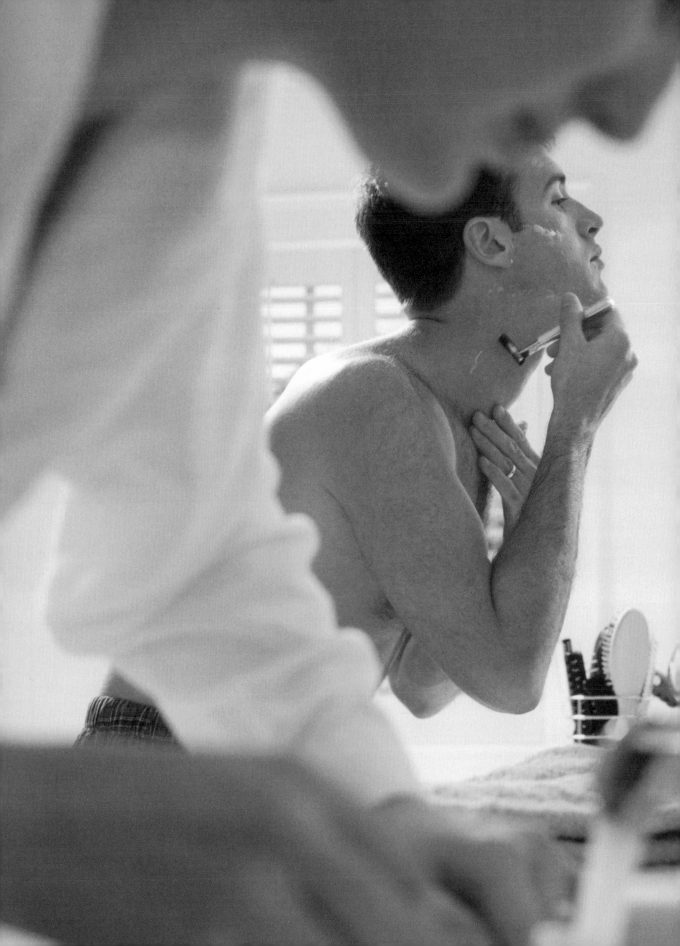

SHINE:
look and feel your best

The face we show to the world really does count. Healthy skin and shining, well-groomed hair announce clearly that we value and care about ourselves. Even more importantly, appearance is an excellent barometer of health, revealing both our physical and mental state.

So here are some simple hints and tips that are easy to work into everyday life. These strategies and routines will help you to protect your hands, nails, hair and complexion, and also combat any problems that arise. A little personal attention repays the effort; looking good makes you feel great.

BEST WAYS TO LOOK AFTER **YOUR SKIN**

Ageing causes the skin to become thinner and drier. While you can't control your age, you can control other factors affecting your skin, such as a poor diet and cigarette smoking. The skin is the first layer of your immune system, serving as a shield against a legion of germs, but it is vulnerable to environmental factors such as sunlight.

● **Make your showers short and cool** Skip long, steamy showers and opt for shorter, cooler sprays. Long, hot showers strip skin of its moisture and wash away the protective oils. So limit your showers to 10 minutes and keep the water cool.

● **Treat your neck and chest like an extension of your face** Your neck and upper chest area is covered by very sensitive skin, making it a prime spot for telltale signs of ageing such as dryness. To keep this area youthful, use facial cleansing creams that hydrate and cleanse gently rather than deodorant soaps, which can be drying.

● **Avoid skin destroyers** Shun smoking, tanning salons and sunbathing. All three will age your skin prematurely.

● **Apply olive oil** Smooth a couple of drops of olive oil over your face, elbows, knees and the backs of your arms every evening. The oil contains monounsaturated fat, which refreshes and hydrates the skin without leaving a greasy residue.

● **Hang room-darkening blinds in your bedroom** They will help you to avoid sleep disturbances or insomnia caused by ambient light. Sleep is critical to your skin's health because most cell repair and regeneration occurs while you are asleep.

● **Moisturize at night** For soft, young-looking hands and feet, put on plenty of moisturizing cream before you go to bed, then slip on thin fabric socks and gloves while you sleep.

● **Build collagen** Start the day with a glass of orange juice to help to build collagen, which keeps the skin smooth and youthful. Orange juice is rich in vitamin C, essential for the manufacture of collagen. Other foods with an abundance of vitamin C include guava, kiwi fruit and red peppers.

great idea!

Place rough, dry elbows on grapefruit halves First exfoliate your elbows in the bath or shower, then cut a grapefruit in half and rest one elbow on one half and one on the other, letting them soak for 15 minutes. The acid in the grapefruit provides extra smoothing power.

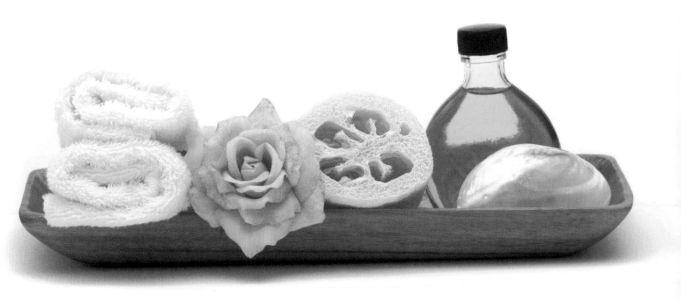

● **Use a loofah every day** This will keep ingrown hairs and scaly skin under control. While you're in the shower, gently scrub bumpy or scaly skin with a circular motion to remove dead cells.

● **Take a multivitamin every day** Many nutrients are vital to healthy skin, including vitamins C, A and B. The most reliable way to get them all is to eat healthily, as well as taking a daily supplement, if needed.

● **Apply vitamin C cream** For double protection, apply a cream containing vitamin C to your face over your sunblock. The cream helps to prevent facial skin damage, dehydration and wrinkles. Also try creams containing vitamin E or beta carotene.

● **Use unscented baby powder** Baby powder is very effective at keeping areas where skin meets skin – such as the inner thighs, the area under the arms and the area under the breasts – clean and dry. This helps to prevent intertrigo, an irritating skin condition that occurs when such areas remain moist, allowing bacteria or fungi to grow.

● **Cook with garlic every day** A 1996 Danish study found that skin cells grown in a culture dish and treated with garlic had seven times the lifespan of cells grown in a standard culture. They also tended to look healthier and more youthful than untreated cells. Plus, garlic extract dramatically inhibited the growth of cancerous skin cells.

● **Eliminate toxins through sweat** Go for a run, ride your bike or work in the garden on a hot day – anything to get you sweating. Sweating is nature's way of eliminating toxic chemicals that can build up under the skin. Plus, regular exercise maintains healthy circulation and blood flow throughout your body, including your skin. If you're exercising outdoors, remember to wear a sunscreen on your face that protects against ultraviolent A and B (UVA and UVB) rays, or a moisturizer with sunscreen protection.

● **Drink iced tea** Brew a pot of tea, chill it, then store it in the fridge and drink it throughout the day. Tea is a great source of antioxidants, molecules that fight the free-radical damage caused by sun exposure and cigarette smoking.

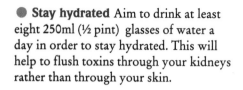

● **Stay hydrated** Aim to drink at least eight 250ml (½ pint) glasses of water a day in order to stay hydrated. This will help to flush toxins through your kidneys rather than through your skin.

● **Never rub your eyes** Apply compresses instead. The skin on your face is extremely delicate, especially under your eyes. So use a very light touch on your face at all times. If your eyes itch, apply a cold compress or cloth to the area, or try a cotton-wool pad moistened with toner or witch hazel.

Cut the end off of an aloe vera leaf, split it open and spread the gel on the dry area

● **Smooth aloe vera gel over extra-dry skin** The acids in aloe vera eat away at dead skin cells and speed up the healing process. Buy a pre-prepared product or cut the base off of an aloe vera leaf, split it open and spread the transparent gel contained in the leaf on the dry area.

● **Get rid of pollutants** Clean your face and neck with a natural cold cream and follow with a rose water and glycerine rinse twice a day to remove skin-damaging pollutants.

● **Keep your hands away from your face** Since your hands touch so many surfaces, they are a repository for dirt and germs. If you rub your eyes, stroke your chin or cup your cheek, you will transfer everything that is on your hands on to your face.

● **Use only one brand of skincare products** If you buy and use lots of different skincare products, some will probably contain the same ingredients, thus making them redundant. And some brands aren't compatible with others, though you have no way of knowing that until you've already paid for and opened them. You'll get better results if you use products that are formulated to work together.

● **Protect your skin from the sun all year round** Use a sunblock that has an SPF of 30 or greater. Just because there's snow on the ground doesn't mean your skin can't be damaged by the sun. Time outdoors is time well spent, but be sure to keep your skin either well covered or well protected with sunblock. In particular, the sun is at its most damaging between 11am and 3pm.

● **Banish bruises with an onion**
You've just tripped over and an unsightly bruise is taking shape on your knee. Take a slice of onion and hold it against the bruise for 15 minutes. The substance in onions that makes your eyes water – allicin – will help to flush away the excess blood in the damaged tissues that leads to bruising. But this 'cure' only works if the onion is applied just after an injury.

If you're too late to try it or it just isn't working for you, dab on some witch hazel. Then hold an ice pack, or some ice wrapped in a clean cloth, over the bruise for 5 minutes. This will constrict the blood vessels, reducing bleeding into the tissues and speeding up healing.

● **Beat athlete's foot with bicarb**
Dry your feet thoroughly after a bath, then sprinkle some bicarbonate of soda on your feet and between your toes. The bicarb absorbs moisture, so it helps to combat the fungus that can develop into itchy, unsightly athlete's foot if the skin is wet or sweaty. It will also help to freshen up and deodorize your feet.

If athlete's foot has already taken hold, try using garlic, which contains ajoene, a powerful antifungal agent. Stir 6 crushed cloves into 2 tablespoons of olive oil, then cover and leave for a few days. Strain the oil and apply it to the infected area once a day.

● **Repel insects with vitamin B** A mosquito bite can be more than an itchy nuisance; in tropical and subtropical countries it could also involve the transmission of a deadly disease such as malaria or Dengue fever. When visiting such places, always consult a doctor first; the usual precautions are a prescribed course of anti-malaria pills. To avoid getting bitten in the first place, pack the insect repellent and don't forget to use it.

● **Dab yoghurt on cold sores** Most cold sores are caused by the common herpes virus. This will live quietly in your body until you experience something stressful, which activates it and triggers a cold sore. Get rid of the sore by smearing a teaspoon of cultured yoghurt over it, two or three times a day. The active micro-organisms in the yoghurt will attack the virus, reducing the itching and helping the cold sore to heal faster.

● **Soothe jellyfish stings** Jellyfish stings are strongly alkaline, which explains why washing with an acidic solution is the best approach. Pour an acid liquid such as vinegar or lemon juice into the area to reduce pain. If these are not available, urine may also be effective. Remove any tentacles by rinsing or peeling off with a gloved hand and seek medical advice promptly.

● **Glue that splinter** Your child has been running around barefoot and picked up a large splinter. A quick and pain-free way to solve the problem is to put a large blob of PVA glue over the splinter site. Let it dry, then quickly peel it off – the splinter should come away too.

● **Neutralize bee and wasp stings**
Dab vinegar or lemon juice (acid) on the skin to counteract wasp stings, which are alkaline. Apply bicarbonate of soda (alkali) mixed with a little water to bee stings, which are acidic. If the sting remains in the skin, remove it as soon as possible. Scrape it out with a clean fingernail or a flat, smooth edge, such as a credit card – don't try to pull it out with tweezers as this is likely to squeeze more poison into the skin.

Skin acts as a shield against germs

10 great ideas for creating beauty treats

Whether your skin is oily, dry or somewhere in between, here are some simple but highly effective ideas for making your own cleansers, moisturizers and exfoliaters for softer, healthier skin.

1 GIVE YOUR SKIN A MILK BATH

The lactic acid in milk exfoliates dead skin cells and may also increase the skin's ability to hold in moisture. Soak a flannel in cold milk. Lay the flannel on any area of skin that is particularly dry or irritated. Leave it there for 5 minutes, then rinse off the milk gently, so that some of the lactic acid stays on your skin.

2 HOLD ON TO THAT YOUTHFUL LOOK

Mix together 60ml (2fl oz) of whipping cream, ½ teaspoon of olive oil, 2 tablespoons of ripe, mashed avocado and 1 teaspoon of calendula petals. Leave on for 5 minutes, then rinse. Avocado oil significantly increases the collagen content in skin, maintaining its youthful look. Not only does the oil in avocado act as an emollient, but the fruit also contains moisturizing vitamin E.

3 MAKE A CLEANSING, MOISTURIZING FACE MASK

Mix 1 tablespoon of plain yoghurt with a few dashes of sesame oil. Apply the mask to your face, avoiding the eye area. Leave on for 15 minutes before rinsing off.

4 MOISTURIZE DRY SKIN

Mash a banana well and mix with a little honey. Apply the mask to your face, avoiding the eye area. Leave on for 15 minutes, then rinse.

5 MAKE A TONER FOR OILY SKIN

Add 1 tablespoon of peppermint, yarrow, sage or hyssop leaves to 1 cup of boiling water. Steep for 30 minutes, strain and cool before dabbing it on.

6 REJUVENATE SKIN CELLS

Add a teaspoon of grapeseed oil to your toner. The oil acts as an anti-ageing serum by helping your skin cells to repair and rejuvenate themselves.

Fabulous **bath soaks**

To treat dry, rough, itchy skin, try adding these various combinations of ingredients to your bath and luxuriate in the warm water for 5 to 10 minutes.

- 225g (8oz) of sea salt and 450g (1lb) of sodium bicarbonate. Bathe until the water is cool to detoxify your skin and soothe the itch.
- 250g (9oz) of Epsom salts. In addition to soaking in it, while your skin is still wet, rub handfuls of Epsom salts on rough areas to exfoliate the skin.
- A few bags of your favourite tea. The tea provides antioxidants as well as a delicious scent.
- 100g (3 ½ oz) of uncooked oatmeal tied into an old stocking or muslin bag. Oats give your skin a healthy glow, leaving a thin film on the surface that seals in water.
- 115g (4oz) of powdered milk mixed with 1 tablespoon of grapeseed oil. The lactic acid in the milk will exfoliate your skin, and the grapeseed oil will provide a powerful dose of antioxidants.

7 CLEANSE AND TIGHTEN YOUR PORES

Mash peeled mango flesh until it turns soft and pulpy. Then massage it into the skin and leave on for a few minutes before rinsing.

8 PREPARE A HOMEMADE OAT SCRUB

Oats moisturize and exfoliate your skin at the same time. Grind 40g (1½oz) of rolled oats in a food processor or coffee grinder. Mix with 45g (1¾oz) of ground sunflower seeds, ½ teaspoon of peppermint leaves and 4 tablespoons of ground almonds. Mix 2 teaspoons with a little double cream. Scrub your face and neck with the mixture, then rinse well with cool water.

9 TONE WITH PEPPERMINT SAGE AND WITCH HAZEL

Sage helps to control oil, peppermint creates a cool tingle, and witch hazel helps to restore the skin's protective layer. Witch hazel contains tannins, which have an astringent effect, making the pores tighten up as they dry.

Combine 100g (3½ oz) of witch hazel with a teaspoon each of sage and peppermint leaves and steep for one to three days before application.

10 MAKE A HERBAL SPRAY

Use a spray of rose, sandalwood or bergamot essential oil mixed with water. All these oils are great for hydrating the skin. To create a herbal spray, mix a few drops of essential oil with water in a small spray bottle and spritz on your face whenever your skin needs a little boost.

Your skin is more pliable when it's hydrated, so a spray helps to stave off frown lines and general movement wrinkles. The hydrator also acts as a protection against pollutants and retains your skin's natural lubricants. As an added bonus, if you apply make-up after a herbal spray, it will stay on for longer and look more natural.

KEEP SMILING

Your teeth not only help you to talk and chew; they can also make or break your appearance. Although aesthetics are important, of even more concern is the health of your teeth and gums. In the past few years, researchers have found a connection between periodontal (gum) infection and an increased risk of heart disease.

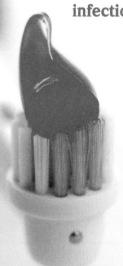

Grip the toothbrush like a pencil so that you won't scrub too hard

● **Grip your toothbrush like a pencil** Does your toothbrush look as if it's been used to clean the car? If so, you're probably brushing too hard. Contrary to what some scrub-happy people think, brushing with force is not the best way to remove plaque. The best way is to place your toothbrush at a 45-degree angle against your gums and gently move it in a circular motion, rather than a back-and-forth motion. Grip the toothbrush like a pencil so you won't scrub too hard.

● **Replace your toothbrush often** Throw away your toothbrush or change the head of your electric toothbrush at least every two to three months. Otherwise, you're just transferring bacteria to your mouth every time you brush.

● **Follow the rules** Brush your teeth twice a day, floss at least once a day, and see your dentist for a thorough professional clean every six months.

● **Hum while you brush** To get rid of all the bacteria-packed plaque in your mouth, you need to brush your teeth for at least 2 minutes. Use your watch or keep a timer in the bathroom and set it for 2 minutes. Or find a tune that lasts about 2 minutes and hum it to the end.

● **Use alcohol-free mouthwash to rinse away bacteria** Most over-the-counter mouthwashes have too much alcohol, which can dry out the tissues in your mouth, making them more susceptible to bacteria. Some studies even suggest a link between mouthwashes containing alcohol and an increased risk of oral cancer. To be safe, be a teetotaller when it comes to choosing a mouthwash.

● **Drink a cup of tea every day**
Flavonoids and other ingredients in
tea seem to prevent harmful bacteria
from sticking to teeth, and also block
production of a type of sugar that
contributes to cavities. Tea also contains a
lot of fluoride.

● **Clean your tongue with a tongue
scraper** Do this every morning to
remove tongue plaque and freshen your
breath. A major cause of bad breath is
the build-up of bacteria on the tongue,
which a daily tongue scraping will help to
banish.

● **Use a flattering lipstick** Choose a
medium-coral or light-red lipstick. These
colours make your teeth look whiter,
whereas lighter-coloured lipsticks tend to
bring out the yellow in your teeth.

● **Even if you're an adult, avoid
sugary foods** Sugar plus bacteria equals
oral plaque. Plaque then leads to bleeding
gums, tooth decay and cavities. Plus, the
acid in refined sugars and carbonated
beverages dissolves tooth enamel.

● **Brush with sodium bicarbonate
once a week** This will remove stains and
whiten your teeth. Use it as you would
toothpaste. Or use salt as an alternative
toothpaste. Also, if your gums start to
feel raw, brush with salt every other day.

● **Eat a pot of fat-free yoghurt every
day** Think of your teeth as external
bones; just like your bones, they need
adequate calcium to remain strong.

● **Numb those gums** To soothe gum
pain and reduce swelling, rinse your
mouth for 30 seconds with salt water
(1 teaspoon salt dissolved in a glass of
warm water).

**What you
eat shows up on
your teeth** If you're drinking a lot
of red wine and black tea, or smoking
cigarettes, expect the results to show
up as not-so-pearly whites. Other
culprits include colas, gravies and dark
juices. The plain fact is that, if it's dark
before you put it in your mouth, it
will probably stain your teeth, so take
action to counteract this.
• Brush your teeth immediately after
consuming foods that stain.
• Regularly use a good bleaching
agent, either from the chemist or your
dentist.
• Be conscious of tooth-staining foods
and drinks, and have them only when
you have a toothbrush to hand –
otherwise, have an apple for dessert.

● **Don't use your teeth as tools**
Keep a bottle opener and a small pair of
scissors in your bag or desk drawer. If
you have the right gadgets to hand, you
won't be tempted to use your teeth as
tools, which can damage them. In fact,
you should never use your teeth as tools
for anything except eating.

● **Don't chew hard foods** Suck – don't
chew – very hard foodstuffs such as hard
sweets or ice. Chewing hard foods creates
tiny fractures in the enamel of your teeth
that, over the years, combine to result in
major cracks.

● **Eat 'detergent' foods** These are firm
or crisp foods that help to clean the teeth
as they're eaten. They include apples,
raw carrots, celery and (unsweetened)
popcorn. For best results, make
'detergent' foods the final food you eat in
your meal if you know you can't brush
your teeth straight after eating.

HEALTHIER, MORE BEAUTIFUL HAIR

Considering it's technically dead tissue, we spend a great deal of time, money and energy on our hair. In addition to being fun to style and colour, hair serves a valuable purpose, keeping heads warm and helping to regulate body temperature. The typical hair cell stays with us for three to five years until it falls or grows out.

● **Smell extra-sweet** Mix a few drops of your favourite fragrance into your hair gel before applying. You'll end up with hair that not only looks good but smells great too. Another aromatic option is to transform ordinary shampoo into a herbal experience by adding a few drops of an essential oil. Dilute a 250ml (9fl oz) bottle of shampoo by half with water and add 20 drops of essential oil of lavender.

great idea!

Fight dandruff with Listerine
That antiseptic mouthwash in your bathroom cabinet has a secondary use that you may not be aware of: it is a wonderful cure for dandruff. Combine one part mouthwash with nine parts water and apply the mixture to your scalp after shampooing. Leave it on for 5 to 10 minutes, then rinse thoroughly.

If you dislike the antiseptic smell of Listerine, follow each treatment with a mint rinse – which needs to be prepared in advance. Crush a handful of fresh or dried leaves in a bowl, then pour over enough vodka to cover them. Leave for a day, then strain. Add about ½ teaspoon of water at a time to the mixture until it becomes cloudy. Apply to the scalp after shampooing and leave on for at least 5 minutes before rinsing thoroughly.

● **Encourage natural highlights** For soft, natural highlights, squeeze some lemon juice on your hair before going out into the sun. Or use shampoos and styling products that contain citrus fruits.

● **Prevent split ends** After washing your hair, and while it is still wet, wrap it gently in a towel and let the cotton absorb the moisture for a few minutes instead of rubbing. If you are prone to split ends, get your hair trimmed at least every six weeks, which will help to eliminate them.

● **If you're going bald, go short** One of the worst mistakes balding men make is the comb-over. A sexier, more modern style is to keep it closely trimmed. As a bonus, your hair will be easy to maintain.

● **Wash your hair in botanical oils** Available at health-food shops, olive, jojoba and sweet almond oils are all great hair elixirs. If your hair is thick and heavy, coconut oil works wonders. Dampen your hair and apply small amounts of the botanical oil until your hair is thoroughly covered. Cover with a shower cap and warm towel for half an hour, then rinse and shampoo as usual.

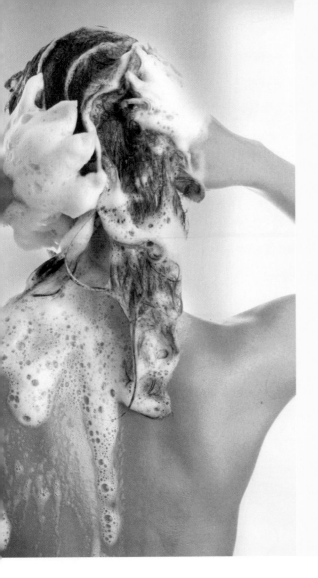

TOP TIPS FOR PERFECT
SHAMPOOING

Few people realize that there's a correct way to shampoo. Yet proper shampooing not only improves the look of your hair but also helps to slow down hair loss and promote healthier hair growth.

• Before you step into the shower, brush your hair from front to back with a stiff boar-bristle brush. This will stimulate the circulation and prevent the build-up of styling products.

• Wet the hair with warm water. (Hot water can strip your hair of protective oils.)

• Apply shampoo at the nape of the neck and shampoo the hairline first, then do the top of your head.

• Massage your entire scalp at least three times to push nutrients into the hair bulb and free your hair follicles of clogging deposits.

• After rinsing your hair thoroughly, apply conditioner. If you're doing all this outside the shower, wrap a 'steam towel' (a wet towel that's been microwaved for 2 minutes) round your head and leave it on for 30 to 60 seconds. The steam allows the conditioner to be absorbed more evenly.

• Finish with a cool-water rinse, which helps to tighten scalp pores, firm hair fibres, reduce limpness and increase sheen.

● **Brush up on brushing** Use a brush with natural bristles rather than synthetic ones. Synthetic materials generate static electricity, which will make your hair more brittle. First brush the ends to remove tangles. That way, you won't pull and break your hair when you take full strokes with the brush. After you've brushed the ends, make long, full strokes all the way from the roots of your hair to the ends to spread the hair's natural oils.

● **Strengthen your strands with supplements** B vitamins can make your hair stronger. Take a 50mg B-complex

supplement twice a day with food. The mineral selenium is also helpful for maintaining healthy hair. To add lustre to your hair, try taking 1000mg of evening primrose three times a day with meals.

● **Check the plughole** The typical person loses between 50 and 200 hairs a day. So it's normal to have a small clump of hair left in the plughole after washing. But, if that amount starts to increase, see your doctor about it. It could mean that you have a scalp infection, that baldness is starting to set in or, more rarely, that you have a nutritional deficiency.

Make your own conditioner Mix 200ml (7fl oz) olive oil and 200ml aloe vera gel with 6 drops each of rosemary and sandalwood essential oils. Olive oil is a natural emollient, aloe vera hydrates, while rosemary adds body and softness to hair. (The sandalwood, which is optional, adds fragrance.) Leave the mixture on for an hour or two before rinsing it out.

● **Shampoo grey hair with a blue-coloured shampoo** Do this every day. By the very nature of its light colour, grey hair gets duller, dirtier and drier than darker shades, which is why it's so important to shampoo and condition it daily. The bluish shampoo helps to hide any yellowish tinge, which can be ageing.

● **Use moisturizing conditioner** Condition your hair two to three times a week. This is especially important if you have fine, thin hair. Many people think conditioners will flatten thin hair, but, actually, using a moisturizing conditioner a few times a week will help your hair to block out humidity, which itself can make the hair flat.

When you use a conditioner, first apply it liberally to the ends, where hair is the driest. Then work your way towards your scalp.

● **For dry hair, try an avocado solution** Avocado moisturizes hair shafts and loads them with protein, making them stronger.

Thoroughly mix together a ripe, peeled avocado with a teaspoon of wheatgerm oil and a teaspoon of jojoba oil. Apply the avocado moisturizer to freshly washed hair and work it all the way to the ends. Cover your scalp with a shower cap or a plastic bag, wait 15 to 30 minutes, then rinse thoroughly.

● **Change the rinse cycle** If you have oily hair, rinsing your hair with water is fine, but you'll get even better results if you use a strong rosemary tea. Wonderfully aromatic, this herb contains essential oils that help control overproduction of oil on the scalp.

To make the rinse, pour a cup of boiling water over 2 tablespoons of dried rosemary. Steep for 20 minutes, strain, cool and pour into an empty plastic bottle. Keep this in the bathroom and splash your hair with the tea after the final clean water rinse. There's no need to rinse off the tea afterwards, as long as you like the fragrance.

● **Add interest with eye shadow** Create effective, instant highlights by applying champagne or gold-hued eyeshadow to your hair using an ordinary make-up sponge.

● **Zigzag your parting** If you have dyed hair and you want to hide your growing roots while trying a new hairdo at the same time, zigzag your parting.

● **Space out your colour treatments** Allow at least four weeks between single-process colour treatments and at least eight weeks between highlight or lowlight treatments.

● **Humidify your night air** Use a humidifier at night in your bedroom, especially in cold weather. Your central heating probably keeps the air very dry, which can dry out your hair.

● **Stay in condition** If you use a shop-bought conditioner, pick one with a 'thermal protector' ingredient such as dimethicone or phenyl trimethicone. These protect your hair from heat, which is especially important if you blow-dry.

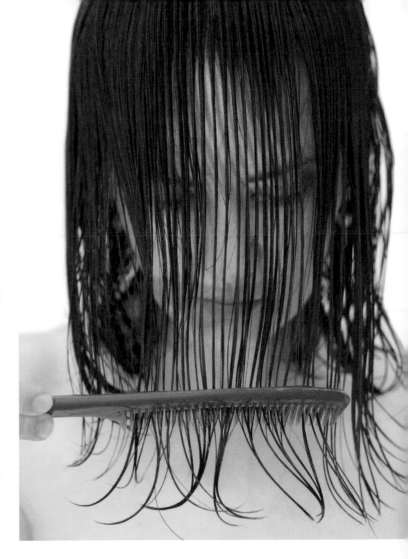

● **Do the natural thing** Let your hair dry naturally in the air whenever possible. If you must use a hair dryer, use it sparingly. The same goes for curling tongs, straighteners or hot rollers. When you apply heat, it's like drying out a leaf in sunlight – you're inviting brittleness.

● **Go acidic** Another way to reduce oiliness in your hair is to apply lemon juice. Blend juice from 2 lemons into 2 cups of distilled water and pour into an empty shampoo bottle. After washing and rinsing your hair, blot it dry and apply the mixture to your scalp. Leave it on for 5 minutes, allowing the acidic lemon juice to work on the oil. Then rinse with cool water. Vinegar, which is also acidic, is an alternative to lemon juice. Mix a cup of vinegar with a cup of water, then pour it over your hair as a final rinse.

● **Go for a light colour** Pick a hair colour that's just a few shades lighter than your complexion, which tends to lighten as you age. Highlight or bleach grey hair to give your hair a more uniform look and make your skin appear brighter.

● **Give your hair a rest** If you wear your hair in a ponytail, take it out for a few hours a day to give your hair a break. Also, try not to pull hair back too tightly. Never sleep with accessories in your hair.

● **Use conditioner before swimming** Comb conditioner through your hair before going swimming to protect it from the harsh chemicals. Do the same before going to the beach.

● **Revive your hairstyle** Flip your head over, spray the underneath layers of your hair with hairspray, and shake it out to style your hair instantly without having to re-wash and blow-dry.

Let your hair dry naturally in the air whenever possible. If you must use a hair dryer, use it sparingly

● **Banish frizz** In a frizz emergency, use a little bit of hand lotion and diffuse it smoothly and evenly through dry hair.

● **For oily hair, use a gentle shampoo** Ironically, harsh shampoos can actually lead to more oil because your scalp tries to compensate. Use a shampoo that's gentle enough for everyday use.

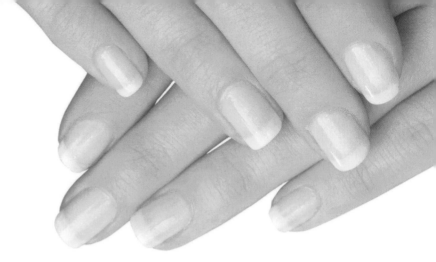

TIP-TOP **NAIL CARE**

No one knows why we have nails on our hands and toes but, whatever the reason, they make it easier to do many things, such as pick up small items. They also provide an external sign of health: weak, brittle nails often signal a nutritional deficiency. Ignore them and you could end up with painful ingrowing nails or a fungal infection.

● **Rub in petroleum jelly** To keep your nails hydrated, rub a small amount of petroleum jelly into your cuticle and the skin surrounding your nails every evening before you go to bed or whenever your nails feel dry. Not a fan of petroleum jelly? Substitute castor oil. It's thick and contains vitamin E, which is great for your cuticles. Or use olive oil – it also works to moisturize your nails.

● **Wear rubber gloves** Wear rubber gloves whenever you do housework or the washing up. Most household chores, from scrubbing the bathroom to washing the dishes, as well as gardening, are tough on your nails. To protect your fingers from dirt and harsh cleaners, cover them with rubber gloves at chore time. For extra hand softness, apply hand cream before you put on the gloves.

● **Trim your toenails straight across** The purpose of this is to avoid ingrowing toenails – particularly important if you have diabetes.

● **Don't clip your cuticles** When you do this, you remove your nail's protective barrier. Fungi and bacteria find it easier to get a grip around the base of the nail after the cuticle has been removed.

● **Combat nail fungus** Tea tree oil, a powerful antiseptic, can help to make nail fungus disappear. In one study it proved to be as effective as a prescription anti-fungal medicine. Once or twice a day, apply a drop or two to the discoloured nail. A good time to do it is after a bath or a shower, when your skin is softest. Alternatively, use an antifungal powder that absorbs moisture, preventing fungus.

● **Dry hands and toes thoroughly** After doing the washing up, dry your hands for at least 2 minutes. And dry your toes thoroughly after swimming or showering – leaving them damp increases the risk of fungal infection.

● **Air your work boots and athletic shoes after use** Better still, keep two pairs of each and alternate between them so you're never putting your feet into damp, sweaty shoes, which may lead to fungal infections. If your feet are sweaty when you get home, change into a fresh pair of socks straight away.

● **Wear 100 per cent cotton socks** Cotton socks are the most efficient option for absorbing dampness, thereby preventing fungal infections.

● **Take biotin for strong nails** The secret that vets have long kept under wraps is that biotin (also known as vitamin B_7) helps to strengthen horses' hooves, which are made from the same substance as human fingernails – keratin. A team of Swiss researchers confirmed this by giving a daily biotin supplement to a group of people with brittle nails. After six months their nails were on average 25 per cent stronger and thicker.

Biotin should not be taken in very large doses. About 250mcg three times a day should be enough to markedly improve the condition of your nails.

● **Try evening primrose oil** If your nails are brittle or flaking, try getting more omega-3 essential fatty acids. Evening primrose oil is a good source of omega-3s. Take 1000mg three times a day with meals.

● **Look out for a zinc deficiency** If your nails have white spots, you may be deficient in zinc. Increase your intake of zinc by eating beef, liver, poultry, eggs and seafood. It is also found in cheese, beans, nuts and wheatgerm.

● **File your nails correctly** To keep your nails strong, avoid filing in a back-and-forth motion – go in one direction only. Never file just after a shower or bath – wet nails break more easily.

● **Massage your nails** This will keep them extra-strong and shiny. Nail buffing increases blood supply to the nail, which stimulates the matrix of the nail to grow.

● **Polish your nails** Even a clear varnish will protect your nails. If you prefer colour, use a base coat, two thin coats of colour and a top coat. The colour should last at least seven days but should be removed after ten days.

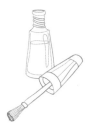

● **Use acetate-based polish removers** Avoid polish removers containing acetone or formaldehyde, which are drying to the nails. Use acetate-based removers instead.

great idea!

Freeze-dry your nails Using a quick-drying nail polish may seem like a good idea, but such products often contain large amounts of alcohol and formaldehyde, which can cause your nails to dry up and split. So stick with 'slow' varieties and try this fast-dry solution. Empty a tray of ice cubes into a bowl, add enough cold water to cover, then dip your freshly painted nails in for 1 to 2 minutes after applying each coat.

If your nails have white spots, you may be deficient in zinc

BETTER GROOMING

Few of us want to spend hours in front of the mirror primping or spend hundreds of pounds at a salon. So here are some easy grooming tips that will help you to look polished, refined and youthful – without investing a lot of money or time. Some are for both women and men, some for women only, and some for men only.

● **Limit your grooming time** Keep track of the amount of time you spend 'grooming', and stop at 45 minutes. That's the most it should ever take to shower, take care of your skin, apply make-up and style your hair. Any longer, and you need to get an easier haircut, use less make-up and cut down to one skincare product.

● **Have regular manicures and pedicures** Schedule a weekly manicure and a monthly pedicure. This works for men and women. You can do it yourself, but a professional will always do a better job. The simple details of well-filed nails, clean cuticles and smooth toenails (if you're wearing open-toed shoes) send a signal to bosses, colleagues and clients that you care about the small things as well as the big things.

● **Avoid perspiration stains** If you wear loose-fitting clothes, it will allow air to circulate around your body and perspiration to evaporate. Tight-fitting clothing may cause sweat to become trapped in a film on your skin, which can result in body odour and embarrassing perspiration stains.

● **Wear natural fabrics** Buy clothes made from natural fibres such as cotton. They allow skin to breathe, reducing body odour. Avoid synthetic, man-made fibres, such as nylon or Lycra, which may limit ventilation.

● **Ward off smelly feet** Foot odour is a very common problem. Keep your feet smelling fresh by scrubbing them daily and drying them completely when you get out of the shower. Then insert odour-absorbing insoles into your shoes before putting them on.

● **Use antiperspirant after a shower** Apply antiperspirant when your underarms are a little moist and wet, for example, just after a warm shower or bath. It enables the active ingredients to enter the sweat glands more readily.

● **Avoid sitting in direct sunlight** It heats your body and causes perspiration, especially in warmer weather.

● **Keep your skin dry** Apply a cornflour-based body powder in the morning to help your skin stay drier throughout the day and to reduce odour.

Chlorophyll-rich vegetables have a potent deodorizing effect

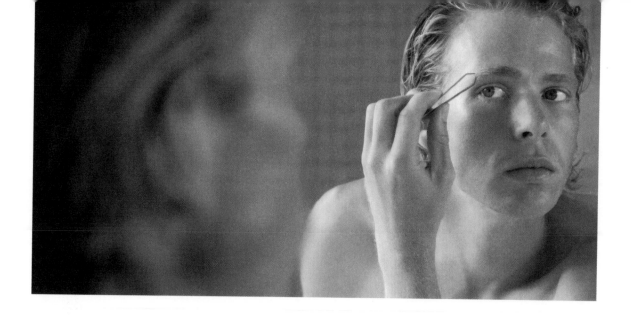

● **Pluck your eyebrows after a shower** Your pores are open just after you've had a shower, enabling the hairs to slide out when you pluck. Avoid brow-shaping when your skin is most sensitive: first thing in the morning, after you've been outside in extremely hot or cold weather, or during your period, when your nerve endings are at their most sensitive.

● **Take up yoga** The stress-management training will help you to control perspiration and body odour better. After heat, stress is probably the top cause of sweating.

● **Prepare some greens for dinner each night** Dark-green leafy vegetables such as spinach, chard, parsley and kale are rich in chlorophyll, which has a potent deodorizing effect on the body.

● **Apply make-up in natural light** Even if this means bringing your make-up and a mirror into the living room. The light from a bulb is often a different shade from that of natural light, and rarely does a bulb-lit room have evenly distributed light. If you must work in a bulb-lit room, be sure to use the correct wattage.

● **Carry a make-up touch-up kit** Take it with you wherever you go. Look for multi-purpose products, such as a lip/cheek/eye cream or a two-ended wand with mascara on one end and eyeliner on the other. Other good kit items include cotton-wool balls soaked in make-up remover, then stored in a film canister, pressed powder, a nail file and lip gloss.

● **Check your face in a hand mirror in front of a window** You'll catch a glimpse of any sun spots or wrinkles you need to cover up or facial hairs you need to pluck, uneven make-up, even long nose hairs. Natural sunlight makes the inspection more revealing.

● **Rub some olive oil on your bikini line** The purpose of this is to keep it soft and free of unsightly red bumps. For best results, apply the olive oil to the area immediately after shaving or waxing.

● **Revive your feet** For instantly fresh feet, spray your soles with chilled cologne, chilled peppermint or rose geranium herbal water. Make your own by adding a couple of drops of the essential oils to a spray bottle of water and storing it in the fridge.

● **Make your eyes appear closer or further apart** To make your eyes appear closer together, tweeze your brows on the outer edges and let them grow in closer towards the nose. To make your eyes appear farther apart, pluck your brows to expand the open space above the nose. In other words, make the brows shorter.

● **Consider laser hair removal** If you are a man with a unibrow, consider laser hair removal to tidy up the area. This procedure can also be used to remove stray nose and ear hairs. Excessive facial hair is generally considered unattractive.

● **Get rid of lumps and bumps** Benzoyl peroxide, an ingredient in many acne creams and face washes, can help to minimize hair bumps. Lotions that contain alpha-hydroxy acids (AHAs) exfoliate your skin and help to cut down on the number of hairs that get trapped under your skin. Apply an AHA lotion morning and night to any skin that you shave regularly. One of these applications should be straight after you've shaved. Be careful, though – AHAs can be irritating, especially if the skin is wet. When you start using an AHA lotion, put it on every other night until you see how well you tolerate it.

● **Choose a conventional razor** It may be faster and simpler to shave with an electric razor, but it's harsher on your skin and can strip away natural oils. Also, an electric razor doesn't shave quite as effectively as a conventional razor.

● **Shave after your shower – or in the shower** Steam and hot water soften the bristles of your beard and open up the pores of your skin, making shaving easier and less painful. Most men can get a terrific shave without any lather or cream by shaving as the last part of a shower. Just 5 minutes of hot, steamy water provides all the moisture and hair softening your beard needs, and the rinse-off and clean-up take just seconds.

● **Prepare your skin** Before your next shave, briskly rub the area with a dry loofah, exfoliating mitt, sponge or flannel. This brushes away dead skin cells that might block hair follicles – a process called exfoliation – and lifts hairs away from their follicles.

● **Shave slowly** Use short strokes and rinse the blade often in hot water. Your skin is not flat, so long strokes increase your chances of cuts or scrapes. Try not to press down with the blade, especially around sensitive areas.

● **Use a shaving brush** Apply your shaving cream with a shaving brush for an extra-lustrous shaving session (whether on your legs or your face). It will create a large quantity of lather, which will make the hairs softer and easier to remove.

● **Shave off some or all of your facial hair** This will give you a more youthful look. If you have a full beard, try a goatee. If you have a goatee, go for the clean-faced look.

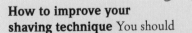

How to improve your shaving technique You should always shave with the 'grain' of your hair growth. When men shave the neck, for instance, they should go down rather than up. When shaving their legs or bikini area, women should follow the same policy. So shave your legs down, not up. This might not give the closest shave, but you won't cut the hair so short that it can burrow under your skin.

● **Trim the other hair on your body**
Many men losing the hair on their heads start to gain it in other places, such as the ears, nose or back. To look clean and contemporary, trim, wax or pluck unwanted hair.

● **Soften bristles and moisten your skin** If you shave with a blade, first ensure that your skin and hairs are wet. Soak in the bath or hold a warm flannel on your face for about 10 minutes before shaving. When skin is wet, the hairs stand up straighter, which makes them easier to shear off. (If you use an electric shaver, the opposite is true: your bristles and skin should be completely dry.)

● **Get a new shaver** If ingrowing hairs keep recurring, changing your shaver might do the trick. If you shave with a blade, switch to an electric shaver. If you use an electric shaver, switch to a blade. Many razors now feature double or even triple blades for an ultra-close shave. But when it comes to preventing ingrowing hairs, an old-fashioned single-bladed razor is often better.

● **Replace aftershaves with witch hazel** Aftershaves contain a large amount of alcohol, which will dry your skin. An effective alternative is witch hazel, which contains just a bit of alcohol and leaves your skin feeling softer and soothed. You can also use it to clean the cut if you nick yourself with the blade.

● **Deal with ingrowing hairs** If a hair has curled back and grown into your skin, you'll probably want to remove it. First, place a flannel soaked in hot water over the area. Leave it on for 5 minutes to soften the hair. Using tweezers, gently pull the tip of the hair away from the skin and remove it.

try it...

Soothing razor rash If you get a rash from shaving, apply a slice of cucumber to the irritated area, or peel a cucumber, whizz it in a blender and apply the purée to the area. Better still, put some avocado in the blender at the same time.
  Aloe vera is one of the best natural ingredients for irritated or burned skin. If you have an aloe plant, cut open the fleshy base of a leaf, squeeze out the clear gel and apply it directly to the skin. Or use a proprietary skin-care product containing the plant extract. Best is 100 per cent pure aloe vera gel. Another alternative is to rub calendula cream onto the affected area.

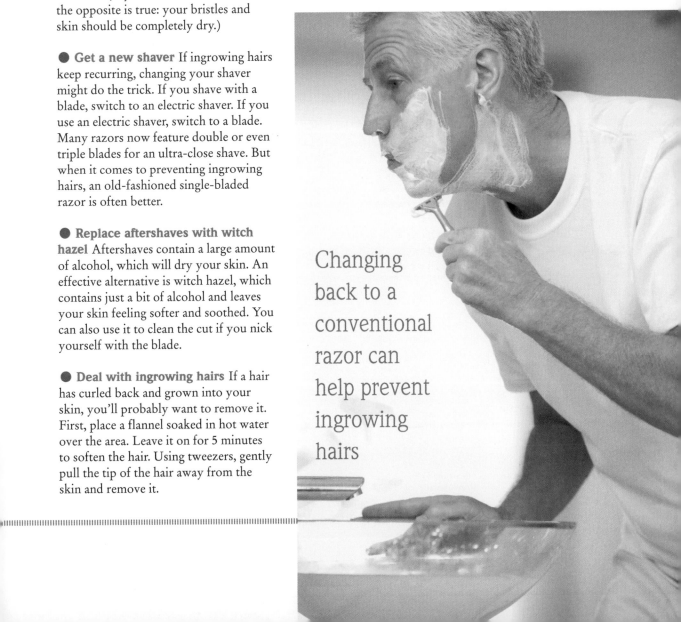

Changing back to a conventional razor can help prevent ingrowing hairs

INDEX

inhalers 103
insect bites and stings 233
insect repellent 233
insomnia 168, 174-175, 218
  medications 176-177
  rebound insomnia 176
insulin 24, 32, 116, 117
  insulin resistance 32, 117
  insulin sensitivity 116, 118
interpersonal therapy 209
intertrigo 231
interval training 41
iron
  sources of 16, 28, 34, 56,
    115, 161, 173
  supplements 56
irritability 82, 187, 206
irritable bowel syndrome
  107, 108, 109, 145
isometric exercises 58, 59, 63
ispaghula husk 108
Italian cuisine 49
  see also pasta; pizzas

J

jasmine 132, 179, 197
jellyfish stings 233
jet lag 177, 201
jogging 123
joint-replacement surgery
  137
jojoba oil 238

K

kale 132
kayaking 70, 71, 90
keratin 243
keyhole surgery 149
kidney beans 11, 21
kind gestures 222
kissing, and calorie burning
  38
kiwi fruit 14, 17, 230
knee circles 57
knee surgery 149

L

lactic acid 234, 235
lactose intolerance 108
lady's mantle 151
laparoscopic surgery 149
laser hair removal 246
laser therapy 150
lateral raise exercise 164
laughter 143, 191, 219, 227
laughter yoga 190
lavender oil 151, 178, 179,
  199, 208, 238
laxatives 20
LDL cholesterol 17, 112,
  113, 121, 125

leapfrog 79
lectucarium 175
legs
  exercises 78-81, 195
  leg lift 81
  leg shake 195
  leg stretch 195
lemon balm 179, 219
lemon drinks 99
lemons 241
lettuces 175
libido 130, 187
life coaches 204-205
lifelong learning 193
lifting heavy objects 79, 138
lime flowers 179
linoleic acid (LA) 42
linseeds 23, 115
lipsticks 237
listeners, good 223
listeria 163, 164
Listerine 238
liver cancer 126, 127
locus of control 190
locust pose (yoga) 215
log chopping 73, 93
loofahs 231
loosening up movements
  194-195
loperamide 107
lunches 24-25, 203
lunge walk 78, 80
lupus 29
lutein 132
lychees 14
lycopene 43, 121, 127
lymph nodes, swollen 97, 99

M

magnesium 17, 32, 134, 173
magnesium citrate 173
make-up
  applying 245
  touch-up kit 245
manganese 29
mangoes 14, 235
manicures 244
martial arts 89
massage 131, 143, 144, 146,
  149, 207, 208, 212-213
  aromatherapy massage 208
  before and after exercise
    212
  foot massage 170
  for headaches 213
  nail massage 243
  scalp massage 171
  self-massage 145, 169,
    212-213
mattresses 181
mayonnaise 35, 45

meal deals 24
meal planning 46
meat 16, 34-35, 113, 177
  fat 34, 35
  processed or cured 21, 51
medications
  administering 162
  caffeine in 175, 176
  salt in 20
  sleep-inducing 176-177
  and snoring 182
  sugar in 19
  see also specific
    medications
meditation 142, 192, 207
  for stress reduction 207
Mediterranean diet 116
melatonin 140, 177
melons 15
memory loss 17, 29
meningitis 157
meningococcal meningitis
  157
menstrual cycle 56
menstrual pain 143, 145
mental stimulation 193, 205
metabolism, boosting 40, 41
migraine 143
milk 17, 32, 35, 140, 177
milk baths 234
mineral water 141
mint
  hair rinse 238
  see also peppermint
mirrors
  eating in front of 38
  exercising in front of 56
MMR vaccine 159
moisturisers 153, 230
moles 97
monosodium benzoate 104
monounsaturated fats 34,
  35, 42
mood swings 217
  see also depression
mood-boosting foods 217
morphine 142
mosquito bites 233
motherhood
  childbirth 154
  new mothers 154-155
  see also babies; children
mould spores 102, 104, 105
mountain pose (yoga) 214
mouth cancer 127
mouthwashes 183, 236
MRSA 148, 150
muesli 22
multi-tasking 198
multiple sclerosis 28, 127
multivitamins and

multiminerals 127, 173,
  216, 231
muscles
  isometric exercises 59, 63
  muscular pain 144
  spasms 138
  strains 146, 147
  tissue 41
music
  exercising to 55, 61, 82
  for depression relief 217
  for stress relief 199
  stroke patients and 124
myalgic encephalopathy
  (ME) 172

N

nail care 242-243
  nail filing 243
  nail polish and removers
    170, 243
nail fungus 242
napping 169, 174, 218
nappy rash 155
nasal congestion 157, 182,
  183, 200
  see also snoring
nature as stress-reliever 193
nausea 128, 129
NEAT (non-exercise activity
  thermogenesis) 118
neck
  exercises 67, 70-71, 143,
    195
  neck brace 183
  neck pillows 180
  neck rolls 68, 70, 143
  neck stretch 195
  neck tilt 195
negative thoughts 218
neroli oil 151
nerve pain 145
nettle tea 183
neurotransmitters 177
nicotine 175
nicotine replacement
  therapy 122
night vision 133
night-eating syndrome 27,
  174
nightclothes 169, 170
nightmares and night terrors
  185
nitrates 120
nitric oxide 130
'no', saying 191, 202, 204
noise decibel levels 134
non-steroidal anti-
  inflammatory drugs
  (NSAIDs) 142
nose blowing 101

PICTURE ACKNOWLEDGMENTS

The following abbreviations are used: t = top, c = centre, b = bottom.
Front cover Getty Images/Imagezoo; 2 ShutterStock, Inc/Kyrylo Grekov; 4 t Getty Images/Fabrice Lerouge, c ShutterStock, Inc/lightpoet, b ShutterStock, Inc/ Yuri Arcurs; 5 t ShutterStock, Inc/Deklofenak, c ShutterStock, Inc/Yuri Arcurs, b Getty Images/Ryan McVay; 6 Getty Images/Rachel Weill; 8 Getty Images/Fabrice Lerouge; 11 iStockphoto.com/Juanmonino; 12 ShutterStock, Inc/wavebreakmedia; 15 ShutterStock, Inc/Paul Maguire; 16 iStockphoto.com/Catherine Yeulet; 18 ShutterStock, Inc/bergamont; 22 ShutterStock, Inc/Africa Studio; 25 ShutterStock, Inc/Dream79; 28 ShutterStock, Inc/Monkey Business Images; 30 ShutterStock, Inc/ stocksolutions; 32 iStockphoto.com/Robyn Mackenzie; 34 ShutterStock, Inc/Irina Solatges; 37 ShutterStock, Inc/Pincasso; 39 iStockphoto.com/largeformat4x5; 40 iStockphoto.com/amete; 42 ShutterStock, Inc/Lisa S.; 44 ShutterStock, Inc/Jag_cz; 47 ShutterStock, Inc/Ariwasabi; 49 ShutterStock, Inc/Santhosh Kumar; 51 ShutterStock, Inc/Jiri Hera; 52 ShutterStock, Inc/lightpoet; 55 ShutterStock, Inc/ Maridav; 56 Getty Images/Tetra Images; 59 ShutterStock, Inc/Yuri Arcurs; 60 ShutterStock, Inc/wavebreakmedia; 61 ShutterStock, Inc/oliveromg; 65 ShutterStock, Inc/Kzenon; 68 Getty Images/Rob Lewine; 71 iStockphoto.com/ ranplett; 72 Reader's Digest/Russell Sadur; 73 Reader's Digest/Russell Sadur; 75 t Reader's Digest/Russell Sadur, b Reader's Digest/Russell Sadur; 76-77 iStockphoto.com/Nirdesha Munasinghe; 79 t Reader's Digest/Russell Sadur, b Reader's Digest/Russell Sadur; 81 ShutterStock, Inc/Robert Kneschke; 82 ShutterStock, Inc/Artem Furman; 85 ShutterStock, Inc/Yuri Arcurs; 86 ShutterStock, Inc/Juriah Mosin; 89 ShutterStock, Inc/Juriah Mosin; 91 ShutterStock, Inc/Margrit Hirsch; 94 ShutterStock, Inc/Yuri Arcurs; 98 Reader's Digest/David Munns; 101 ShutterStock, Inc/Juriah Mosin; 103 iStockphoto.com/Tomo Jesenicnik; 105 iStockphoto.com/ssstep; 106 ShutterStock, Inc/Sergiy Bykhunenko; 109 ShutterStock, Inc/Quanthem; 111 ShutterStock, Inc/Mike Laptev; 113 ShutterStock, Inc/Africa Studio; 115 ShutterStock, Inc/Aleksandr Markin; 118 ShutterStock, Inc/Lars Christensen; 121 ShutterStock, Inc/Mikhail Valeev; 123 ShutterStock, Inc/Mammut Vision; 126 Getty Images/Camille Tokerud; 131 ShutterStock, Inc/prodakszyn; 133 ShutterStock, Inc/Pinkcandy; 136 ShutterStock, Inc/Anneka; 138 ShutterStock, Inc/wavebreakmedia; 141 Reader's Digest/David Munns; 142 ShutterStock, Inc/Yuri Arcurs; 144 ShutterStock, Inc/Alice Day; 148 ShutterStock, Inc/Suzi Nelson; 151 ShutterStock, Inc/photo-oasis; 155 ShutterStock, Inc/Monkey Business Images; 156 Getty Images/Yukmin; 160 Getty Images/RYO/a.collectionRF; 163 ShutterStock, Inc/Goodluz; 166 ShutterStock, Inc/Deklofenak; 169 iStockphoto.com/Nicolas Hansen; 171 Getty Images/Dan Dalton; 172 ShutterStock, Inc/Nitr; 175 ShutterStock, Inc/ Thierry Maffeis; 177 ShutterStock, Inc/karelnoppe; 178 ShutterStock, Inc/Daniel Hughes; 181 iStockphoto.com/Diane Diederich; 182 Getty Images/Keith Goldstein; 184 ShutterStock, Inc/Liv Friis-larsen; 186 ShutterStock, Inc/R. Mackay Photography, LLC; 188 ShutterStock, Inc/Yuri Arcurs; 193 ShutterStock, Inc/Yuri Arcurs; 194 ShutterStock, Inc/Toranico; 197 ShutterStock, Inc/Ron Zmiri; 198 Getty Images/ Cultura/Maiwolf Photography; 200-201 ShutterStock, Inc/lightpoet; 203 ShutterStock, Inc/PeterMooij; 204-205 ShutterStock, Inc/Dudarev Mikhail; 206 ShutterStock, Inc/ Yuri Arcurs; 209 ShutterStock, Inc/Dmitriy Shironosov; 210 ShutterStock, Inc/Dragon Images; 213 ShutterStock, Inc/deepblue-photographer; 214 Getty Images/Thomas Northcut; 216 iStockphoto.com/Chris Fertnig; 219 ShutterStock, Inc/EdBockStock; 220-221 ShutterStock, Inc/Robert Kneschke; 222 iStockphoto.com/londoneye; 224 Getty Images/Ghislain & Marie David de Lossy; 226 ShutterStock, Inc/Yuri Arcurs; 228 Getty Images/Ryan McVay; 231 ShutterStock, Inc/MaxFX; 232 ShutterStock, Inc/ kedrov; 235 ShutterStock, Inc/altafulla; 236 ShutterStock, Inc/Olga Miltsova; 239 ShutterStock, Inc/Piotr Marcinski; 241 ShutterStock, Inc/StefanK; 242 ShutterStock, Inc/Blaz Kure; 245 ShutterStock, Inc/bikeriderlondon; 247 ShutterStock, Inc/Monkey Business Images.

All other images are copyright Reader's Digest. Every effort has been made to find and credit the copyright holders of images in this book. We will be pleased to rectify any errors or omissions in future editions. Email us at gbeditorial@readersdigest.co.uk

1,001 Best Health Hints and Tips Published in 2013 in the United Kingdom by Vivat Direct Limited (t/a Reader's Digest), 157 Edgware Road, London W2 2HR for The Reader's Digest Association, Inc. Based on selected text from Reader's Digest health titles.

1,001 Best Health Hints and Tips is owned and under licence from The Reader's Digest Association, Inc. All rights reserved.
Copyright © 2013 The Reader's Digest Association, Inc.
Copyright © 2013 Reader's Digest Association Far East Limited
Philippines Copyright © 2013 Reader's Digest Association Far East Limited
Copyright © 2013 Reader's Digest (Australia) Pty Limited
Copyright © 2013 Reader's Digest India Pvt Limited
Copyright © 2013 Reader's Digest Asia Pvt Limited

We are committed both to the quality of our products and the service we provide to our customers. We value your comments, so please do contact us on **0871 351 1000** or via our website at **www.readersdigest.co.uk** If you have any comments or suggestions about the content of our books, email us at **gbeditorial@readersdigest.co.uk**

FOR VIVAT DIRECT
Project editor Rachel Warren Chadd
Senior editor Henrietta Heald
Designer Sailesh Patel
Proofreader Barry Gage
Indexer Marie Lorimer

Editorial director Julian Browne
Art director Anne-Marie Bulat
Managing editor Nina Hathway
Picture resource manager Eleanor Ashfield
Pre-press technical manager Dean Russell
Product production manager Claudette Bramble
Production controller Jan Bucil

Colour origination FMG
Printed in China

ISBN: 978-1-78020-170-2
Book Code: 400-636 UP0000-1